NEUROBIOLOGY
OF INCONTINENCE

The Ciba Foundation is an international scientific and educational charity. It was established in 1947 by the Swiss chemical and pharmaceutical company of CIBA Limited—now CIBA-GEIGY Limited. The Foundation operates independently in London under English trust law.

The Ciba Foundation exists to promote international cooperation in biological, medical and chemical research. It organizes about eight international multidisciplinary symposia each year on topics that seem ready for discussion by a small group of research workers. The papers and discussions are published in the Ciba Foundation symposium series. The Foundation also holds many shorter meetings (not published), organized by the Foundation itself or by outside scientific organizations. The staff always welcome suggestions for future meetings.

The Foundation's house at 41 Portland Place, London W1N 4BN, provides facilities for meetings of all kinds. Its Media Resource Service supplies information to journalists on all scientific and technological topics. The library, open five days a week to any graduate in science or medicine, also provides information on scientific meetings throughout the world and answers general enquiries on biomedical and chemical subjects. Scientists from any part of the world may stay in the house during working visits to London.

Ciba Foundation Symposium 151

NEUROBIOLOGY
OF INCONTINENCE

A Wiley-Interscience Publication

1990

JOHN WILEY & SONS

Chichester · New York · Brisbane · Toronto · Singapore

Published in 1990 by John Wiley & Sons Ltd.
Baffins Lane, Chichester
West Sussex PO19 1UD, England

Other Wiley Editorial Offices

John Wiley & Sons, Inc., 605 Third Avenue,
New York, NY 10158-0012, USA

Jacaranda Wiley Ltd, G.P.O. Box 859, Brisbane,
Queensland 4001, Australia

John Wiley & Sons (Canada) Ltd, 22 Worcester Road,
Rexdale, Ontario M9W 1L1, Canada

John Wiley & Sons (SEA) Pte Ltd, 37 Jalan Pemimpin 05-04,
Block B, Union Industrial Building, Singapore 2057

Suggested series entry for library catalogues:
Ciba Foundation Symposia

Ciba Foundation Symposium 151
ix + 336 pages, 52 figures, 18 tables

Library of Congress Cataloging-in-Publication Data
Neurobiology of incontinence.
      p. cm.—(Ciba Foundation symposium : 151)
      Based on a symposium held at the Ciba Foundation, London, Oct.
11–13, 1989.
      Edited by Greg Bock (organizer) and Julie Whelan.
      'A Wiley–Interscience publication.'
      Includes bibliographical references.
      ISBN 0 471 92687 6
      1. Urinary incontinence—Congresses. 2. Fecal incontinence—
Congresses. 3. Urinary organs—Innervation—Congresses.
4. Intestines—Innervation—Congresses.   I. Bock, Gregory.
II. Whelan, Julie.   III. Series.
      [DNLM: 1. Fecal Incontinence—congresses. 2. Neurobiology—
congresses. 3. Urinary Incontinence—congresses. W3 C161F v. 151
/WI 600 N494 1989]
RC921.I5N48   1990
616.8'49—dc20
DNLM/DLC
for Library of Congress   90-12321
                                              CIP

British Library Cataloguing in Publication Data
Neurobiology of incontinence.
  1. Man. Incontinence
  I. Bock, Greg II. Whelan, Julie III. Series
  616.63

  ISBN 0 471 92687 6

Phototypeset by Dobbie Typesetting Limited, Devon.
Printed and bound in Great Britain by Biddles Ltd., Guildford.

Contents

Participants

K.-E. Andersson Department of Clinical Pharmacology, University of Lund, S-221/85 Lund, Sweden

P. Arhan Faculté Necker, Département de Physiologie, Hôpital des Enfants-Malades, 156 rue de Vaugirard, 75730 Paris cédex 15, France

D. C. C. Bartolo Department of Surgery, Bristol Royal Infirmary, Marlborough Street, Bristol BS2 8HW, UK

J. G. Blaivas Department of Urology, College of Physicians and Surgeons, Columbia University, New York, NY 10032, USA

A. Bourcier IFRUG, 2 Square la Fontaine, F-75016 Paris, France

A. F. Brading University Department of Pharmacology, University of Oxford, South Parks Road, Oxford OX1 3QT, UK

G. S. Brindley MRC Neurological Prostheses Unit, Institute of Psychiatry, De Crespigny Park, Denmark Hill, London SE5 8AF, UK

G. Burnstock Department of Anatomy & Developmental Biology, University College London, Gower Street, London WC1E 6BT, UK

J. Christensen Division of Gastroenterology, Department of Internal Medicine, University of Iowa, College of Medicine, Iowa City, IA 52242, USA

W. C. de Groat Departments of Pharmacology & Behavioral Neuroscience, University of Pittsburgh, School of Medicine, 518 Scaife Hall, Pittsburgh, PA 15261, USA

J. O. L. DeLancey Department of Obstetrics & Gynecology, University of Michigan Medical School, 1500 E Medical Center Drive, Ann Arbor, MI 48109-0718, USA

C. J. Fowler   Uro-neurology Unit, The National Hospital for Nervous Diseases, Queen Square, London WC1N 3BG, UK

R. S. Kirby   Department of Urology, St Bartholomew's Hospital, West Smithfield, London EC1A 7BE, UK

H. C. Kuijpers   Department of Surgery, Academic Hospital, POB 9101, 6500 Nijmegen, The Netherlands

C. A. Maggi   Department of Pharmacology, Division of Smooth Muscle, A Menarini Pharmaceutical Research Laboratories, Via Sette Santi 3, I-50131 Florence, Italy

P. H. G. Mahieu   Department of Radiology, Institut Chirurgical de Bruxelles, Université Catholique de Louvain, 59 Square Marie-Louise, B-1040 Brussels, Belgium

C. D. Marsden *(Chairman)*   Department of Clinical Neurology, Institute of Neurology, The National Hospital, Queen Square, London WC1N 3BG, UK

J. Nordling   Department of Urology, H111, Herlev Hospital, DK-2730 Herlev, Denmark

N. W. Read   Sub-Department of Gastrointestinal Physiology & Nutrition, Floor K, Royal Hallamshire Hospital, Glossop Road, Sheffield S10 2JF, UK

M. Saito *(Ciba Foundation Bursar)*   Department of Urology, Nagoya University School of Medicine, 65 Turumae, Showa, Nagoya 466, Japan

S. L. Stanton   Urodynamic Unit, Department of Obstetrics & Gynaecology, St George's Hospital Medical School, Lanesborough Wing, Cranmer Terrace, London SW17 0RE, UK

D. Staskin   Division of Urology, Harvard University School of Medicine, Beth Israel Hospital, 330 Brookline Avenue, Boston, MA 02215, USA

M. Swash   Department of Neurology, The London Hospital, Whitechapel, London E1 1BB, UK

P. J. Tiseo   Department of Anesthesiology, T-018, University of California at San Diego, La Jolla, CA 92093, USA

G. Toson   Glaxo SpA, Research Department, Via Fleming 2, I-37100 Verona, Italy

W. D. Wong   Division of Colon & Rectal Surgery, Box 450, Mayo Building, University of Minnesota Medical School, 420 Delaware Street, SE, Minneapolis, MN 55455, USA

Introduction

C. D. Marsden

Department of Clinical Neurology, Institute of Neurology, The National Hospital, Queen Square, London WC1N 3BG, UK

Clinical neurologists are constantly referred a collection of patients whom I call the 'wandering wounded'—people with various pain syndromes, such as backache, pain in the head or face, or fatigue syndromes, who are searching for an answer to their problem. They eventually end up in the hands of neurologists who are frequently quite incapable of providing an answer. Unexplained incontinence has been a similar problem, but this picture has totally changed as a result of developments that are discussed in great detail in this symposium.

I had one brief excursion into the field that joins the members of this symposium together. This stemmed from Merton and Morton's demonstration (1980) that you can stimulate the human motor cortex electrically through the scalp. Pat Merton and I were wondering about the capacity of the human motor cortex to command muscles in different parts of the body; our particular interest was in the human hand. It came upon us late one evening that it would be interesting to see whether the external anal sphincter was commanded by the human motor cortex, as would be predicted by its capacity to protect one from emergencies. A small experiment with motor-cortical electrical stimulation demonstrated a very powerful cortico–motoneuron connection to the external anal sphincter.

I raise that simply because it illustrates one new technique that has revolutionized this subject, among a range of physiological methods now available for the assessment of both urinary and rectal continence mechanisms. With the advent of those sorts of techniques, many of the 'wandering wounded' who come to neurologists with complaints of incontinence can perhaps be put into categories that we begin to understand. I perceive this as the purpose of this particular symposium.

Against that background let me add that the first part of the symposium is devoted to discussion of the anatomy, physiology and pharmacology of the areas in question. We shall then move to the more clinically orientated aspects of incontinence in the second part of the symposium.

Reference

Merton PA, Morton HB 1980 Stimulation of the cerebral cortex in the intact human subject. Nature (Lond) 285:227

Innervation of bladder and bowel

G. Burnstock

Department of Anatomy and Developmental Biology and Centre for Neuroscience, University College London, Gower Street, London WC1E 6BT, UK

Abstract. The autonomic neuromuscular junction is described and neuro-transmission, co-transmission and neuromodulation are defined, as well as the 'chemical coding' of sympathetic, parasympathetic, sensory-motor and intrinsic neurons in the wall of the bladder and bowel. A detailed description of the patterns of innervation of smooth muscle of the bowel, bladder and urethra and of the urethral and anal sphincters by intramural and extrinsic autonomic nerves is presented, and the functional and pharmacological features of this innervation are summarized. Finally, changes in the pattern of innervation and expression of co-transmitters and receptors in the bladder and bowel that occur during development and old age and following trauma, surgery and disease are discussed.

1990 Neurobiology of Incontinence. Wiley, Chichester (Ciba Foundation Symposium 151) p 2–26

The objective of this article is to provide an introductory overview of current opinions about mechanisms of autonomic neurotransmission, with particular attention to the innervation of the bladder and bowel.

General principles of autonomic neurotransmission

Definition of the autonomic neuromuscular junction

The autonomic neuromuscular junction differs significantly from the skeletal neuromuscular junction (Burnstock 1986a). The terminal regions of autonomic neurons are long and varicose with transmitter being released from only 1–3% of the varicosities during the passage of a single impulse. The varicosities do not form a fixed relationship with the muscle effectors, so that the geometry of a junction is variable and consequently there is no postjunctional specialization. The junctional cleft can vary between 20 nm and 2 µm, and receptors appear to be homogeneous on smooth muscle membranes. This type of junction means that neuromodulation is an important mechanism, as well as neurotransmission. A neuromodulator is any substance that alters the process of neurotransmission. Neuromodulation can occur in two different ways: prejunctional modulation is when occupation of receptors on nerve varicosities

2

leads to changes in the amount of neurotransmitter released, while postjunctional neuromodulation is when a substance acts at a postjunctional site to alter the time course or extent of neurotransmitter action.

Another important feature of the autonomic neuromuscular junction is that, unlike the striated muscle cell, a single smooth muscle cell is not the effector, but rather a bundle of cells in electrical continuity with each other via gap junctions. Thus, some smooth muscle cells in sparsely innervated tissues like the uterus or ureter may not be directly activated by neurotransmitter released from nearby nerve varicosities, but are activated indirectly by activity spreading through the muscle effector bundle from the directly innervated cells.

Multiple transmitters

For about 50 years it was generally assumed that only two neurotransmitters, namely acetylcholine (ACh) and noradrenaline (NA), were employed by the autonomic nervous system. In the early 1960s, however, it became apparent that there were nerves supplying the smooth muscle of the gut and the bladder that were neither adrenergic nor cholinergic, and, by the end of the 1960s, non-adrenergic, non-cholinergic (NANC) nerves were shown to supply many visceral organs and parts of the cardiovascular system (Burnstock 1969). In the early 1970s it was proposed that the purine nucleotide, adenosine 5'-triphosphate (ATP), was the principal transmitter in the NANC inhibitory nerves of the gut and the NANC excitatory nerves supplying the urinary bladder, and these nerves were termed 'purinergic' (Burnstock 1972). There has been much debate about the validity of this hypothesis but it is now widely accepted for those nerves supplying the intestine and bladder, and purinergic nerves have also been shown to supply the rabbit portal vein and the pulmonary resistance vessels (Burnstock 1986b, Inoue & Kannan 1988). 5-Hydroxytryptamine (5-HT) was also claimed as a neurotransmitter in some of the enteric neurons (Gershon 1979). In the mid-1970s it became clear, from detailed electron microscopic studies of nerve profiles in the gastrointestinal tract (Cook & Burnstock 1976) and from the introduction of immunohistochemistry, that other neurotransmitters, particularly neuropeptides, were present in autonomic nerves. Substances currently recorded as neurotransmitters in the autonomic nervous system are shown in Table 1.

Co-transmission

That some nerve cells release more than one transmitter was suggested in 1976 (Burnstock 1976) and it is now widely accepted that most nerves contain two or more neurotransmitters or neuromodulators in variable proportions. For example, the principal transmitters in most sympathetic nerves are NA, ATP and neuropeptide Y (NPY), although at many neuroeffector junctions the main

TABLE 1   Transmitters proposed in the autonomic nervous system

Acetylcholine

Noradrenaline

Adenosine 5'-triphosphate

5-Hydroxytryptamine

γ-Aminobutyric acid

Dopamine

Peptides
  Enkephalin/Endorphin
  Vasoactive intestinal polypeptide/Peptide histidine isoleucine
  Substance P
  Gastrin-releasing peptide/Bombesin
  Somatostatin
  Neurotensin
  Luteinizing hormone-releasing hormone
  Cholecystokinin/Gastrin
  Neuropeptide Y/Pancreatic polypeptide
  Galanin
  Angiotensin
  Adrenocorticotropic hormone
  Calcitonin gene-related peptide

role of NPY is as a postjunctional modulator potentiating the actions of both NA and ATP, while at higher concentrations NPY acts as a prejunctional modulator inhibiting NA and ATP release (see Fig. 1). The principal co-transmitters in parasympathetic nerves appear to be ACh and vasoactive intestinal polypeptide (VIP) (Lundberg 1981, Edwards & Bloom 1982), while in many sensory nerves (or 'sensory-motor nerves', as I believe they should now be termed), substance P, calcitonin gene-related peptide (CGRP) and ATP appear to coexist. Intrinsic nerves in the heart, bladder and airways also contain particular combinations of neurotransmitters.

Chemical coding of autonomic nerves

Currently many studies are being carried out to identify the precise combinations of substances contained in individual or groups of autonomic neurons, their projections and their central connections. This type of analysis has been termed 'chemical coding' and has been developed to the most sophisticated extent in the enteric nervous system (see Furness & Costa 1987). For example, neurons have been identified containing up to five neuropeptides that project to different effectors in the gut (Fig. 2).

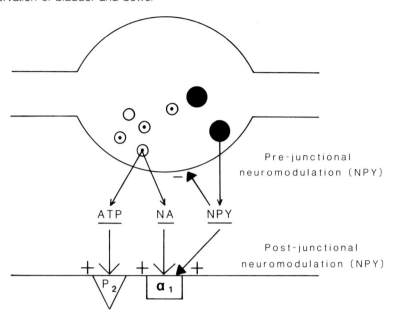

FIG. 1. Schematic representation of different interactions that occur between neuropeptide Y (NPY) and ATP and noradrenaline (NA) released from a single sympathetic nerve varicosity, in the vas deferens and many blood vessels. NA and ATP, probably released from small granular vesicles, act synergistically to contract (+) the smooth muscle via α_1-adrenoceptors and P_2 purinoceptors, respectively. NPY, which is also released from the nerve, has little, if any, direct action on the muscle cell, but exerts potent neuromodulatory actions, both prejunctional inhibition (−) of the release of NA and postjunctional enhancement (+) of the action of NA. (From Burnstock 1987, by permission of the Raven Press.)

Dual control of blood flow

The pioneering work of Furchgott & Zawadzki (1980) has shown that blood vessels are controlled not only by perivascular nerves, but also by endothelial cell factors. Receptors for a variety of substances, including ACh, ATP, substance P, 5-HT and angiotensin II, are located on endothelial cells and when occupied lead to the release of endothelium-derived relaxing factor (EDRF) and consequent vasodilatation. Recent studies in our laboratory have shown that the origin of these substances, for all but the smallest vessels, is subpopulations of endothelial cells which release them during changes in flow (shear stress) or hypoxia, as a pathophysiological mechanism that protects tissues like the brain and heart from hypoxic damage (Burnstock 1988).

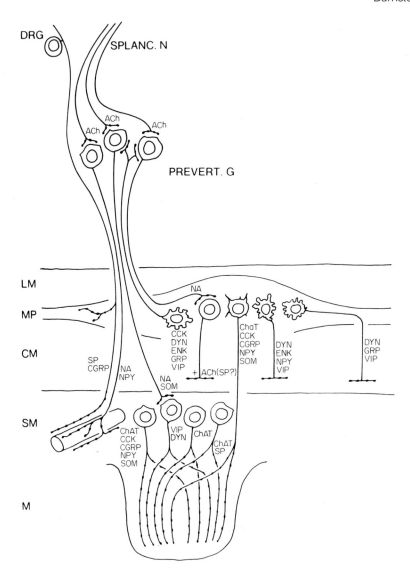

FIG. 2. 'Chemical coding' of neurons in the intestine, showing their projections and, in part, their central connections. DRG, dorsal root ganglion; SPLANC. N, splanchnic nerve; PREVERT. G, prevertebral ganglion; LM, longitudinal muscle; MP, myenteric plexus; CM, circular muscle; SM, submucosa; M, mucosa; ACh, acetylcholine; CCK, cholecystokinin; CGRP, calcitonin gene-related peptide; ChAT, choline acetyltransferase; DYN, dynorphin; ENK, enkephalin; GRP, gastrin-releasing peptide; NA, noradrenaline; NPY, neuropeptide Y; SOM, somatostatin; SP, substance P; VIP, vasoactive intestinal peptide. (From Costa et al 1986, by permission of Elsevier Science Publishers.)

Innervation of the bladder

Bladder body

It has been known since the turn of the century that the responses of the detrusor to pelvic (parasympathetic) nerve stimulation were only partially blocked by atropine (Langley & Anderson 1895). Various explanations were put forward to account for atropine-resistant responses but, by the late 1960s, it was widely accepted that the atropine-resistant response was due to a NANC transmitter (Burnstock 1969, Ambache & Zar 1970, Moss & Burnstock 1985). Evidence was later presented that the identity of the NANC transmitter causing contraction of the detrusor was ATP (Burnstock et al 1972, 1978a, Dean & Downie 1978, Theobald 1982, Kasakov & Burnstock 1983, Levin et al 1986). This evidence included: close mimicry of the response to nerve stimulation and exogenously applied ATP; release of ATP during NANC nerve stimulation which was Ca^{2+} dependent; fluorescence localization of nerves in the bladder positively stained for quinacrine, a compound known to bind very strongly to ATP (Da Prada et al 1978). More recently, the NANC responses have been shown to be blocked by arylazidoaminopropionyl ATP (ANAPP$_3$), an ATP receptor antagonist, and by α,β-methylene-ATP, a stable analogue of ATP that specifically desensitizes P$_2$ purinoceptors. Furthermore, excitatory junction potentials recorded in the smooth muscle of the bladder in response to NANC stimulation are also abolished by α,β-methylene-ATP (Hoyle & Burnstock 1985, Fujii 1988). It has been suggested that ACh and ATP may be co-transmitters in intrinsic parasympathetic neurons in bladder (MacKenzie et al 1982). In recent experiments in our own laboratory, we have demonstrated autoradiographic localization of the P$_{2X}$ purinoceptor in the detrusor muscle of the rat and guinea pig and also in man (Bo & Burnstock 1989, and unpublished observations) (Fig. 3). Although it has been claimed that a NANC component is not present in human bladder (Sibley 1984), others have demonstrated atropine-resistant responses (Hindmarsh et al 1977, Sjögren et al 1982, Cowan & Daniel 1983, Negårdh & Kinn 1983). The current demonstration of ATP receptor binding (X. Bo & G. Burnstock, unpublished observations) and the recent work from Alison Brading's laboratory (Speakman et al 1989) and our own (Hoyle et al 1989) confirm that this component is present and suggest that it is likely to be purinergic, although there seem to be marked regional variations in its distribution; for example, ATP responses and receptors are dense in the trigone region, but very low or perhaps even absent in the tip of the bladder dome. A NANC-mediated slow relaxation has also been described in human detrusor (Klarskov 1987).

In addition to the parasympathetic nerve pathway, there are sympathetic (hypogastric) nerves supplying the bladder which contain NPY as well as NA, and a number of neuropeptides have been localized in nerves in the bladder wall (Gu et al 1984, Crowe & Burnstock 1989). It seems likely that SP and CGRP

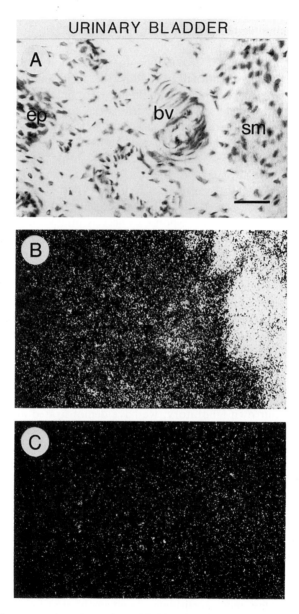

FIG. 3.   (A) shows a section of rat urinary bladder viewed with bright-field optics (stained with 0.5% Toluidine blue). Autoradiograph (B) shows the overall distribution of binding sites of [^{3}H]α,β-methylene-ATP over (A) viewed with dark-field optics. Autoradiograph (C) shows the distribution of non-specific binding sites of [^{3}H]α,β-methylene-ATP over the adjacent section to (A). bv, blood vessel; ep, epithelium; sm, smooth muscle. Calibration bar = 50 μm. (From Bo & Burnstock 1989, by permission of Elsevier Science Publishers.)

are contained in sensory-motor nerves which are abundant (Maggi et al 1988), especially in the trigone region, while VIP and [Leu]enkephalin immunofluorescence may be located in some parasympathetic nerves and/or in projections from intrinsic ganglia (Alm et al 1980, Kawatani et al 1983, Crowe et al 1986a). There are marked species variations in regional innervation and in the transmitters used (Moss & Burnstock 1985, Maggi et al 1987).

Both 5-HT (Holt et al 1985) and γ-aminobutyric acid (GABA) (Kusonoki et al 1984) have been implicated as neuromodulators in the bladder. Prostaglandins produced by ATP released from pelvic nerves also play a part in the contractile responses of the bladder (Burnstock et al 1978b, Andersson et al 1980).

Urethra

Not surprisingly, innervation of the urethra differs substantially from that of the bladder body (Klarskov et al 1983, Slack & Downie 1983, Ito & Kimoto 1985). There is a powerful innervation by adrenergic excitatory nerves, as well as a cholinergic innervation (Ekström & Malmberg 1984). In addition, there are NANC inhibitory nerves and there is some evidence to suggest that VIP and 5-HT, both of which relax the urethra, are NANC transmitter contenders (Hills et al 1984). ATP also relaxes the urethra, but only after it breaks down to adenosine, which then acts on P_1 purinoceptors. Consistent with this finding is the absence of ATP binding in the urethra (Bo & Burnstock 1989).

Intrinsic ganglia

Whereas the presence of intrinsic ganglia in the wall of the bladder has been recognized for some time, only in recent years has it become apparent that these are not simple nicotinic parasympathetic relay stations, but consist of sophisticated local circuitry with the potential to support integrative activities in the bladder and urethra (Crowe et al 1986a, Burnstock et al 1987, Kumamoto & Shinnick-Gallagher 1987, Pittam et al 1987). NPY and somatostatin (SOM) are co-localized in many of the intrinsic neurons (James & Burnstock 1988, 1989). Receptors for ACh (muscarinic as well as nicotinic), VIP, substance P, enkephalin and ATP have been demonstrated on sub-populations of these neurons with electrophysiological and autoradiographic methods (Pittam et al 1987, James & Burnstock 1989). Intramural ganglia have been identified recently in the human urethra (Crowe et al 1988). It is not yet known whether the neuronal circuitry in the wall of the bladder and urethra includes sensory nerves that would allow local reflexes to occur independently of the central nervous system (CNS) (see also de Groat & Kawatani 1985).

Urethral sphincter-striated muscle

The intriguing possibility has been raised that there may be direct interactions between the autonomic nervous system and voluntary system in this sphincter, since both noradrenaline- and VIP-containing nerve fibres have been shown to run in close proximity to both individual and bundles of striated muscle fibres in this sphincter (Crowe et al 1986b, 1989, Lincoln et al 1986). These bundles are varicose and not simply related to blood vessels, but it is not known yet whether they have direct effects on the excitability of the striated muscle membrane or whether they act as modulators of neuromuscular transmission. There appears to be a substantial compensatory increase in the density of noradrenaline-containing fibres after sacral spinal injury in man (Crowe et al 1989).

Innervation of the bowel

Myenteric ganglia

There are two ganglionate plexuses in the wall of the gut, the myenteric plexus lying between the longitudinal and circular muscle coats, and the submucous plexus. Scanning and transmission electron microscopic studies have shown that the organization of these ganglia is closer to that of the CNS than that of sympathetic or parasympathetic ganglia (Paton 1957, Gershon 1979, Wood 1979, Jessen & Burnstock 1982). Glial cells and neurons are in close relationship and their processes form a dense neuropil; neither connective tissue nor blood vessels penetrate into the ganglia. Many neuropeptides, monoamines, purines and amino acids have been identified in subpopulations of neurons within these ganglia (see Fig. 2) (Burnstock 1982, 1986b, Furness & Costa 1987).

Innervation of smooth muscle

The main neural components innervating the bowel smooth muscle are: NANC excitatory nerves utilizing, as co-transmitters, ACh (which produces rapid excitatory junction potentials) and substance P (which produces slow responses); and NANC inhibitory nerves utilizing, probably as co-transmitters, ATP (which produces rapid inhibitory junction potentials) and VIP (which produces slow-onset, sustained relaxations) (see Hoyle & Burnstock 1989). The accumulation of evidence suggests that ATP is the dominant co-transmitter for the NANC inhibitory nerves in the small intestine and colon, while VIP is the dominant transmitter in the stomach. Subtance P excitation of smooth muscle appears to be dominant in the ileum. A diagram proposed by Marcello Costa illustrating the involvement of these nerves in peristalsis is shown in Fig. 4.

ORAL   ANAL

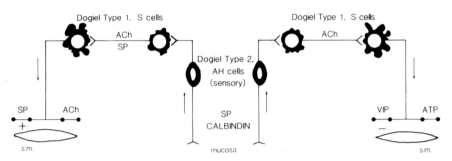

FIG. 4. This model has been put forward by Marcello Costa (Flinders University, Adelaide) to illustrate current views about the neural pathways involved in the peristalsis reflex. Sensory neurons (Dogiel Type 2 cells showing AH-type electrical activity and containing substance P and calbindin) carry impulses generated by stretching of the gut wall to activate, via interneurons (Dogiel Type 1 cells showing S-type electrical activity utilizing ACh), orally directed excitatory motor neurons utilizing ACh and substance P and anally directed NANC inhibitory neurons utilizing ATP and VIP. s.m., smooth muscle. (Figure first presented at the International Congress on Gastroenterology, Digestive Endoscopy and Colo-proctology organized by the Italian Society of Gastroenterology, Rome, 4–10 September 1988.)

It has become apparent (see Thuneberg 1982) that the interstitial cells of Cajal play a role as pacemakers in the activity of smooth muscle and, because these cells are innervated, it is important to take this system into consideration when investigating neuromuscular activity in the gastrointestinal tract.

Sphincters

In general, the sphincters are neurally controlled independently from the non-sphincteric smooth muscle. Stimulation of sympathetic (hypogastric) nerves leads to depolarization and contraction of the circular muscle of the internal anal sphincter, which is blocked by α-adrenoceptor antagonists, whereas stimulation of the parasympathetic nerves supplying this sphincter (second ventral sacral root, VS2) inhibits spontaneous activity resulting in relaxation mediated by NANC nerves in animals and man (Frenckner & Ihre 1976, Bouvier & Gonella 1981). ACh contracts the sphincter in most species. The identity of the NANC transmitter, however, is not clearly resolved (Burleigh 1983, Crema et al 1983, Biancani et al 1985, Goldberg et al 1986, Rattan & Shah 1988), although, since inhibitory junction potentials are evoked in the guinea pig internal sphincter, this would favour a purinergic mechanism in this species; VIP has never been shown to produce rapid hyperpolarizations of this kind, in contrast to ATP (Lim & Muir 1986).

Intrinsic enteric neurons containing a number of neuropeptides, although sparsely distributed in the anal canal, are also likely to project into the internal anal sphincter (Bouvier et al 1986, Krier 1989).

The external anal sphincter is innervated by the perineal inferior haemorrhoidal branches of the pudendal nerves (S2, S3, S4) as well as branching from the coccygeal plexus (S4, S5) (Schuster 1968, Krier 1985). Sensory and sensory-motor fibres containing neuropeptides and possibly ATP are also present in this sphincter as well as the internal anal sphincter (Krier 1989).

The relationship between the neural control of the smooth muscle of the internal anal sphincter and the striated muscle of the external anal sphincter is not resolved (see Krier 1989). Neuronally mediated interactions between motility of internal anal sphincter and bladder, however, have been examined (Bouvier & Grimaud 1984).

Plasticity of autonomic nerves

An important recent development has been to examine the changes in expression of co-transmitters and receptors in ageing and after surgery or trauma (see Burnstock 1990). Some examples follow.

Plasticity of nerves in the bladder

Long-term sympathectomy.   Substantial increases in CGRP-immunofluorescent nerves were seen in rat bladder six or 20 weeks after sympathectomy by chronic exposure to guanethidine. The possibility that sympathetic nerve growth factor is involved in the mechanism of hyperinnervation by CGRP-containing sensory nerves has been raised (Aberdeen et al 1990).

Spinal injury.   Relatively little attention has been paid to the autonomic innervation of the bladder and urethra after spinal cord injury, but some interesting examples of changes in expression of transmitters and receptors in the nerves that remain are beginning to be recognized. For example, adrenergic nerves appear to be increased in relation to the striated muscle of the external urethral sphincter of patients with sacral, but not cervical or thoracic, spinal lesions (Crowe et al 1989). In contrast, dense VIP-immunoreactive, but not noradrenaline-containing nerves, were found in the urethral smooth muscle in patients with thoracic lesions (Crowe et al 1988).

Diabetes.   Taking into account the hypertrophy and distension of bladders from eight-week streptozotocin-treated diabetic rats, there was an increase in the activity of choline acetyltransferase and acetylcholinesterase and in dopamine levels, probably indicating an increase in activity of both sympathetic and parasympathetic nerves (Lincoln et al 1984).

Plasticity of enteric nerves

Hirschsprung's and Crohn's diseases. It has been known for some years now that in the absence of enteric ganglia in the colon of man in Hirschsprung's disease, there is a striking hyperinnervation of the musculature by both adrenergic and cholinergic nerves (Gannon et al 1969). It is interesting that recent studies show that, in contrast to these extrinsic nerves, projections of the intrinsic enteric neurons containing peptides and purines do not appear to enter the aganglionic bowel (Hamada et al 1987). In contrast, in Crohn's disease there appears to be a compensatory increase in VIP in the diseased intestine (Bishop et al 1980).

Diabetes. Faecal incontinence associated with diabetes mellitus may be due to neuropathy (Schiller et al 1982). The streptozotocin-treated rat has been used as a model for diabetes mellitus; for example, there is good correlation between the loss of the VIPergic innervation of penile erectile tissue in rats and in impotent diabetic man (Crowe et al 1983). Increases in VIPergic innervation of the small and large intestine have been reported (Belai et al 1985), but there are concomitant decreases in CGRP-immunoreactive nerves (Belai et al 1987). Despite the increase in VIP levels in enteric nerves of diabetic rats there is no release of VIP from these nerves, although this can be reversed by acute application of insulin (Burnstock et al 1988).

Laxatives. Long-term use of purgative laxatives formulated from anthraquinone derivatives such as sennosides A and B, as in cascara and senna pods, causes neuropathy of the enteric plexuses of the large intestine. Smooth muscle atrophy accompanies loss of intrinsic innervation, myenteric nerve terminal damage and submucosal nerve terminal damage, leading to the condition known as cathartic colon. The typical lesions of cathartic colon implicate loss of absorptive and secretory function as well as loss of motor function. Although anthraquinone-derived laxatives can result in general neuropathy, the adrenergic neurons appear to be less susceptible than either cholinergic or peptidergic and purinergic neurons (Reimann et al 1980). Also, neurons that selectively take up quinacrine (an acridine dye related to anthraquinone, which binds to high concentrations of ATP) are damaged early (Smith 1968). The relationship between anthraquinone and NANC neurons is consistent with the observation that Reactive Blue 2, which is a sulphonic acid anthraquinone derivative, antagonizes purinergic inhibitory neuromuscular transmission and exogenous ATP in the large intestine of the rat and guinea pig and in the rat duodenum (Manzini et al 1986).

Comment

In view of the growing number of examples of autonomic nerve plasticity in adult animals and man it is suggested that neuropathologists need to pay attention to compensatory increases in expression of transmitters, as well as seeking evidence for degrees of damage or loss of nerves; and that when new strategies for drug development are being considered, the age and pathological history of the patient should be taken into account. An exciting question to ask during the next phase of research is: 'what are the molecular mechanisms that control the expression of co-transmitters and receptors in ageing and disease?'

References

Aberdeen J, Corr L, Milner P, Lincoln J, Burnstock G 1990 Marked increases in calcitonin gene-related peptide-containing nerves in the developing rat following long-term sympathectomy with guanethidine. Neuroscience 35:175–184

Alm P, Alumets J, Håkanson R, Owman Ch, Sjöberg N-O, Sundler F, Walles B 1980 Origin and distribution of VIP (vasoactive intestinal polypeptide)-nerves in the genito-urinary tract. Cell Tissue Res 205:337–347

Ambache N, Zar MA 1970 Non-cholinergic transmission by post-ganglionic motor neurones in the mammalian bladder. J Physiol (Lond) 210:761–783

Andersson K-E, Husted S, Sjögren C 1980 Contribution of prostaglandins to the adenosine triphosphate-induced contraction of rabbit urinary bladder. Br J Pharmacol 70:443–452

Belai A, Lincoln J, Milner P, Crowe R, Loesch A, Burnstock G 1985 Enteric nerves in diabetic rats: increase in vasoactive intestinal polypeptide, but not substance P. Gastroenterology 89:967–976

Belai A, Lincoln J, Burnstock G 1987 Lack of release of vasoactive intestinal polypeptide and calcitonin gene-related peptide during electrical stimulation of enteric nerves in streptozotocin-diabetic rats. Gastroenterology 93:1034–1040

Biancani P, Walsh J, Behar J 1985 Vasoactive intestinal peptide: a neuro-transmitter for relaxation of the rabbit internal anal sphincter. Gastroenterology 89:867–874

Bishop AE, Polak JM, Bryant MG, Bloom SR, Hamilton S 1980 Abnormalities of vasoactive intestinal polypeptide containing nerves in Crohn's disease. Gastroenterology 79:853–860

Bo X, Burnstock G 1989 [^{3}H]-α,β-Methylene ATP, a radioligand labelling P$_2$-purinoceptors. J Auton Nerv Syst 28:85–88

Bouvier M, Gonella J 1981 Nervous control of the internal anal sphincter of the cat. J Physiol (Lond) 310:457–469

Bouvier M, Grimaud JC 1984 Neuronally mediated interactions between urinary bladder and internal anal sphincter motility in the cat. J Physiol (Lond) 346:461–469

Bouvier M, Kirschner G, Gonella J 1986 Actions of morphine and enkephalins on the internal anal sphincter of the cat: relevance for the physiological role of opiates. J Auton Nerv Syst 16:219–232

Burleigh DE 1983 Non-cholinergic, non-adrenergic inhibitory neurons in human internal anal sphincter muscle. J Pharm Pharmacol 35:258–260

Burnstock G 1969 Evolution of the autonomic innervation of visceral and cardiovascular systems in vertebrates. Pharmacol Rev 21:247–324

Burnstock G 1972 Purinergic nerves. Pharmacol Rev 24:509–581

Burnstock G 1976 Do some nerve cells release more than one transmitter? Neuroscience 1:239–248

Burnstock G 1982 Cytochemical studies in the enteric nervous system. In: Chan-Palay V, Palay SL (eds) Cytochemical methods in neuroanatomy. Alan R Liss, New York, p 129–149

Burnstock G 1986a Autonomic neuromuscular junctions: current developments and future directions. (The Anatomical Society Review Lecture.) J Anat 146:1–30

Burnstock G 1986b The changing face of autonomic neurotransmission. (The First von Euler Lecture in Physiology.) Acta Physiol Scand 126:67–91

Burnstock G 1987 Mechanisms of interaction of peptide and nonpeptide vascular neurotransmitter systems. J Cardiovasc Pharmacol 10, suppl 12:S74–S81

Burnstock G 1988 Regulation of local blood flow by neurohumoral substances released from perivascular nerves and endothelial cells. Acta Physiol Scand 133, suppl 571:53–59

Burnstock G 1990 Changes in expression of autonomic nerves in aging and disease. J Auton Nerv Syst, suppl, in press

Burnstock G, Dumsday BH, Smythe A 1972 Atropine-resistant excitation of the urinary bladder: the possibility of transmission via nerves releasing a purine nucleotide. Br J Pharmacol 44:451–461

Burnstock G, Cocks T, Crowe R, Kasakov L 1978a Purinergic innervation of the guinea-pig urinary bladder. Br J Pharmacol 63:125–138

Burnstock G, Cocks T, Kasakov L, Wong H 1978b Direct evidence for ATP release from non-adrenergic, non-cholinergic ('purinergic') nerves in the guinea-pig taenia coli and bladder. Eur J Pharmacol 49:145–149

Burnstock G, Allen TGJ, Hassall CJS, Pittam BS 1987 Properties of intramural neurones cultured from the heart and bladder. Exp Brain Res series 16:323–328

Burnstock G, Mirsky R, Belai A 1988 Reversal of nerve damage in streptozotocin-diabetic rats by acute application of insulin in vitro. Clin Sci 75:629–635

Cook RD, Burnstock G 1976 The ultrastructure of Auerbach's plexus in the guinea-pig. I. Neuronal elements. J Neurocytol 5:171–194

Costa M, Furness JB, Gibbins IL 1986 Chemical coding of enteric neurons. In: Hökfelt T et al (eds) Coexistence of neuronal messengers: a new principle in chemical transmission. Elsevier, Amsterdam (Progress in Brain Research vol 68) p 217–239

Cowan WD, Daniel EE 1983 Human female bladder and its noncholinergic contractile function. Can J Physiol Pharmacol 61:1236–1246

Crema A, Frigo GM, Lecchini S, Manzo L, Onori L, Tonini M 1983 Purine receptors in the guinea-pig internal anal sphincter. Br J Pharmacol 78:599–603

Crowe R, Burnstock G 1989 A histochemical and immunohistochemical study of the autonomic innervation of the lower urinary tract of the female pig. Is the pig a good model for the human bladder and urethra? J Urol 141:414–422

Crowe R, Lincoln J, Blacklay PF, Pryor JP, Lumley JSP, Burnstock G 1983 Vasoactive intestinal polypeptide-like immunoreactive nerves in diabetic penis: a comparison between streptozotocin-treated rats and man. Diabetes 32:1075–1077

Crowe R, Haven AJ, Burnstock G 1986a Intramural neurones of the guinea-pig urinary bladder: histochemical localization of putative neurotransmitters in cultures and newborn animals. J Auton Nerv Syst 15:319–339

Crowe R, Light K, Chilton CP, Burnstock G 1986b Vasoactive intestinal polypeptide-, somatostatin- and substance P-immunoreactive nerves in the smooth and striated muscle of the intrinsic external urethral sphincter of patients with spinal cord injury. J Urol 136:487–491

Crowe R, Burnstock G, Light JK 1988 Intramural ganglia in the human urethra. J Urol 140:183–187

Crowe R, Burnstock G, Light JK 1989 Adrenergic innervation of the striated muscle of the intrinsic external urethral sphincter from patients with lower motor spinal cord lesion. J Urol 141:47–49

Da Prada M, Richards JG, Lorez HP 1978 Blood platelets and biogenic mono-amines: biochemical, pharmacological and morphological studies. In: de Gaetano G, Garattini S (eds) Platelets: a multidisciplinary approach. Raven Press, New York, p 331–353

Dean DM, Downie JW 1978 Contribution of adrenergic and 'purinergic' neurotransmission to contraction in rabbit detrusor. J Pharmacol Exp Ther 207:431–445

de Groat WC, Kawatani M 1985 Neural control of the urinary bladder: possible relationship between peptidergic inhibitory mechanisms and detrusor instability. Neurourol Urodynam 4:285–300

Edwards AV, Bloom SR 1982 Recent physiological studies of the alimentary autonomic innervation. Scand J Gastroenterol 17, suppl 71:77–89

Ekström J, Malmberg L 1984 On a cholinergic motor innervation of the rat urethra. Acta Physiol Scand 120:237–242

Frenckner B, Ihre T 1976 Influence of autonomic nerves on the internal anal sphincter in man. Gut 17:306–312

Fujii K 1988 Evidence for adenosine triphosphate as an excitatory transmitter in guinea-pig, rabbit and pig urinary bladder. J Physiol (Lond) 404:39–52

Furchgott RF, Zawadzki JV 1980 The obligatory role of endothelial cells in the relaxation of arterial smooth muscle by acetylcholine. Nature (Lond) 288:373–376

Furness JB, Costa M 1987 The enteric nervous system. Churchill Livingstone, Edinburgh

Gannon BJ, Burnstock G, Noblett H, Campbell G 1969 Histochemical diagnosis of Hirschsprung's disease. Lancet 1:894–895

Gershon MD 1979 Non-adrenergic, non-cholinergic autonomic neurotransmission mechanisms. In: Burnstock G et al (eds) Neurosciences research program bulletin. MIT Press, Cambridge, Massachusetts, vol 17:414–424

Goldberg M, Hanani M, Nissan S 1986 Effects of serotonin on the internal anal sphincter: in vivo manometric study in rats. Gut 27:49–54

Gu J, Blank MA, Huang WM et al 1984 Peptide-containing nerves in human urinary bladder. Urology 24:353–357

Hamada Y, Bishop AE, Federici G, Rivosecchi M, Talbot IC, Polak JM 1987 Increased neuropeptide Y-immunoreactive innervation of aganglionic bowel in Hirschsprung's disease. Virchows Arch A 411:369–377

Hills J, Meldrum L, Klarskov P, Burnstock G 1984 A novel non-adrenergic, non-cholinergic nerve-mediated relaxation of the pig bladder neck: an examination of possible neurotransmitter candidates. Eur J Pharmacol 99:287–293

Hindmarsh JR, Idowu OA, Yeates WK, Zar MA 1977 Pharmacology of electrically evoked contractions of human bladder. Br J Pharmacol 61:115P

Holt SE, Cooper M, Wyllie JH 1985 Evidence for purinergic transmission in mouse bladder and for modulation of responses to electrical stimulation by 5-hydroxytryptamine. Eur J Pharmacol 116:105–111

Hoyle CHV, Burnstock G 1985 Atropine-resistant excitatory junction potentials in rabbit bladder are blocked by α,β-methylene ATP. Eur J Pharmacol 114:239–240

Hoyle CHV, Burnstock G 1989 Neuromuscular transmission in the gastrointestinal tract. In: Wood JD (ed) Motility and circulation. American Physiological Society, Bethesda, Maryland (Handbook of physiology, section 6: The gastrointestinal tract, vol I) p 435–464

Hoyle CHV, Chapple C, Burnstock G 1989 Isolated human bladder: evidence for an adenine dinucleotide acting on P_{2X}-purinoceptors and for purinergic transmission. Eur J Pharmacol 174:115–118

Inoue T, Kannan MS 1988 Nonadrenergic and noncholinergic excitatory neurotransmission in rat intrapulmonary artery. Am J Physiol 254:H1142–H1148

Ito Y, Kimoto Y 1985 The neural and non-neural mechanisms involved in urethral activity in rabbits. J Physiol (Lond) 367:57–72

James S, Burnstock G 1988 Neuropeptide Y-like immunoreactivity in intramural ganglia of the newborn guinea pig urinary bladder. Regul Pept 23:237–245

James S, Burnstock G 1989 Localization of muscarinic receptors on somatostatin-like immunoreactive neurones of the newborn guinea pig urinary bladder in culture. Neurosci Lett 106:13–18

Jessen KR, Burnstock G 1982 The enteric nervous system in tissue culture, a new mammalian model for the study of complex nervous networks. In: Kalsner S (ed) Trends in autonomic pharmacology. Urban & Schwarzenberg, Baltimore, vol II:95–115

Kasakov L, Burnstock G 1983 The use of the slowly degradable analog, α,β-methylene ATP, to produce desensitisation of the P_2-purinoceptor: effect on non-adrenergic, non-cholinergic responses of the guinea-pig urinary bladder. Eur J Pharmacol 86:291–294

Kawatani M, Lowe IP, Booth AM, Backes MG, Erdman SL, de Groat WC 1983 The presence of leucine-enkephalin in the sacral preganglionic pathway to the urinary bladder of the cat. Neurosci Lett 39:143–148

Klarskov P 1987 Non-cholinergic, non-adrenergic nerve-mediated relaxation of pig and human detrusor muscle in vitro. Br J Urol 59:414–419

Klarskov P, Gerstenberg T, Ramirez D, Hald T 1983 Non-cholinergic, non-adrenergic nerve mediated relaxation of trigone, bladder neck and urethral smooth muscle in vitro. J Urol 129:848–850

Krier J 1985 Discharge patterns of pudendal efferent fibres innervating the external anal sphincter of the cat. J Physiol (Lond) 368:471–480

Krier J 1989 Motor function of anorectum and pelvic floor musculature. In: Schultz SG et al (eds) Motility and circulation. American Physiological Society, Bethesda, Maryland (Handbook of physiology, section 6: The gastrointestinal system, vol I) part 2:1025–1053

Kumamoto E, Shinnick-Gallagher P 1987 Postganglionic stimulation activates synaptic potentials in cat bladder parasympathetic neurons. Brain Res 435:403–407

Kusunoki M, Taniyama K, Tanaka C 1984 Neuronal GABA release and GABA inhibition of ACh release in guinea pig urinary bladder. Am J Physiol 246:R502–R509

Langley JN, Anderson HK 1895 The innervation of the pelvic and adjoining viscera. IV. The internal generative organs. J Physiol (Lond) 19:122–130

Levin RM, Ruggieri MR, Wein AJ 1986 Functional effects of the purinergic innervation of the rabbit urinary bladder. J Pharmacol Exp Ther 236:452–457

Lim SP, Muir TC 1986 Neuroeffector transmission in the guinea-pig internal anal sphincter: an electrical and mechanical study. Eur J Pharmacol 128:17–24

Lincoln J, Crockett M, Haven AJ, Burnstock G 1984 Rat bladder in the early stages of streptozotocin-induced diabetes: adrenergic and cholinergic innervation. Diabetologia 26:81–87

Lincoln J, Crowe R, Bokor J, Light JK, Chilton CP, Burnstock G 1986 Adrenergic and cholinergic innervation of the smooth and striated muscle components of the urethra from patients with spinal cord injury. J Urol 135:402–408

Lundberg JM 1981 Evidence for coexistence of vasoactive intestinal polypeptide (VIP) and acetylcholine in neurons of cat exocrine glands. Morphological, biochemical and functional studies. Acta Physiol Scand, suppl 496:1–57

MacKenzie I, Burnstock G, Dolly JO 1982 The effects of purified botulinum neurotoxin type A on cholinergic, adrenergic and non-adrenergic, atropine-resistant autonomic neuromuscular transmission. Neuroscience 7:997–1006

Maggi CA, Giuliani S, Santicioli P, Abelli L, Geppetti P, Somma V, Renzi D, Meli A 1987 Species-related variations in the effects of capsaicin on urinary bladder functions:

relation to bladder content of substance P-like immunoreactivity. Naunyn-Schmiedeberg's Arch Pharmacol 336:546-555

Maggi A, Santicioli P, Patacchini R et al 1988 Regional differences in the motor response to capsaicin in the guinea-pig urinary bladder: relative role of pre- and postjunctional factors related to neuropeptide-containing sensory nerves. Neuroscience 27:675-688

Manzini S, Hoyle CHV, Burnstock G 1986 An electrophysiological analysis of the effect of reactive blue 2, a putative P_2-purinoceptor antagonist, on inhibitory junctional potentials of rat caecum. Eur J Pharmacol 127:197-204

Moss HE, Burnstock G 1985 A comparative study of electrical field stimulation of the guinea-pig, ferret and marmoset bladder. Eur J Pharmacol 114:311-316

Nergårdh A, Kinn A-C 1983 Neurotransmission in activation of the contractile response in the human urinary bladder. Scand J Urol Nephrol 17:153-157

Paton WDM 1957 The action of morphine and related substances on contraction and on acetylcholine output of coaxially stimulated guinea-pig ileum. Br J Pharmacol 12:119-127

Pittam BS, Burnstock G, Purves RD 1987 Urinary bladder intramural neurones: an electrophysiological study utilizing a tissue culture preparation. Brain Res 403:267-278

Rattan S, Shah R 1988 Influence of purinoceptors' agonists and antagonists on opossum internal anal sphincter. Am J Physiol 255:G389-G394

Reimann JF, Schmidt H, Zimmermann W 1980 The fine structure of colonic submucosal nerves in patients with chronic laxative abuse. Scand J Gastroenterol 15:761-768

Schiller LR, Santa Ana CA, Schmulen AC, Hendler RS, Harford WV, Fordtran MD 1982 Pathogenesis of fecal incontinence in diabetes mellitus. N Engl J Med 307:1666-1671

Schuster MM 1968 Motor action of rectum and anal sphincters in continence and defecation. In: Code CF (ed) Motility. American Physiological Society, Washington DC (Handbook of physiology, section 6: Alimentary canal, vol IV) p 2121-2146

Sibley GNA 1984 A comparison of spontaneous and nerve-mediated activity in bladder muscle from man, pig and rabbit. J Physiol (Lond) 354:431-443

Sjögren C, Andersson K-E, Husted S, Mattiasson A, Moller-Madsen B 1982 Atropine resistance of transmurally stimulated isolated human bladder muscle. J Urol 128:1368-1371

Slack BE, Downie JW 1983 Pharmacological analysis of the responses of the feline urethra to autonomic nerve stimulation. J Auton Nerv Syst 8:141-160

Smith BG 1968 Effect of irritant purgatives on the myenteric plexus in man and in the mouse. Gut 9:139-143

Speakman MJ, Walmsley D, Brading AF 1989 An in vitro pharmacological study of the human trigone—a site of non-adrenergic, non-cholinergic neurotransmission. Br J Urol 61:304-309

Theobald RJ Jr 1982 Arylazido aminopropionyl ATP (ANAPP₃) antagonism of cat urinary bladder contractions. J Auton Pharmacol 3:175-179

Thuneberg L 1982 Interstitial cells of Cajal: intestinal pacemaker? Adv Anat Embryol Cell Biol 71:1-130

Wood JD 1979 Neurophysiology of the enteric nervous system. In: Brooks CMcC, Koizumi K, Sato A (eds) Integrative functions of the autonomic nervous system. University of Tokyo Press, Tokyo; Elsevier, Amsterdam, p 177-193

DISCUSSION

Brindley: On the question of non-cholinergic, non-adrenergic nerves to the human bladder, there seems to be a straightforward, almost directly clinical answer, namely that large doses of anticholinergic drugs paralyse the human detrusor completely. Over 30 years ago, Cullumbine and others (1955) gave 5 mg of atropine to soldiers, in connection with protection against nerve gas, and found that they could not urinate. My colleagues have tested the effects of atropine in baboons, cats and New World monkeys (Craggs et al 1986). Complete unresponsiveness of the bladder to sacral root stimulation is produced in baboons, but not in the New World monkeys, and in the cats there is only a very small blocking effect. So the non-cholinergic mechanisms are very powerful in cats, weak in New World monkeys, and virtually absent in baboons. We could find no bladder pressure response to sacral anterior root stimulation in one human patient under atropine. There are now many patients with sacral anterior root stimulator implants and several with hypogastric plexus stimulators, so the opportunity now exists for discovering whether anticholinergic drugs block the human bladder completely. The right drug to use may be glycopyrrolate, which is shorter-acting than atropine, as well as not crossing the blood–brain barrier. If we find that large doses of this drug abolish the responses of the detrusor to sacral anterior root stimulation, and excitatory responses (if there are any) to hypogastric stimulation, what do the purinergic receptors do?

Burnstock: The muscarinic and ATP effects potentiate each other, so there is synergism between the two neurotransmitters. I am not surprised that you reduce excitability with a muscarinic antagonist, but with an ATP antagonist you might also considerably reduce activity. I think acetylcholine and ATP have different excitatory roles in the bladder: ATP produces rapid short-lasting contractions, whereas acetylcholine produces a longer-lasting maintained contraction.

Brindley: The brief effects are the ones most strikingly knocked out by atropine, however.

Burnstock: The literature on human bladder is ambiguous. Some people say, as you do, that there is no non- adrenergic, non-cholinergic (NANC) component in the human bladder. I would be surprised if this were so, because although one expects species differences, one does not often find something which is present in all other mammals to be totally absent in man. Also, in some pathological states the NANC component has been claimed to *emerge* in the human bladder. Then one must consider the difference between male and female bladder (Ed Daniel has claimed a strong NANC component in the female bladder), and also differences in the regional distribution of NANC nerves. Most pharmacological studies of human bladder have been carried out on the dome, which is free of a NANC component, unlike the trigone region (as Alison Brading has found). We plan to do a careful localization of both muscarinic and purinergic receptors in the human bladder to map the regional variations.

Brading: In our experiments on human bladder we find very clear evidence (unpublished), as you do, for the presence of purinergic receptors, but no evidence for any nerve-mediated purinergic response (Sibley 1984). This seems difficult to understand. I am particularly interested in where the ATP comes from. Certainly in the lower mammals, where one sees a marked purinergic response on stimulating the intrinsic nerves, I have always assumed that the ATP is coming from the same nerve terminals as the acetylcholine is. Therefore in the human bladder, if you have acetylcholine coming from nerves, and ATP receptors there, why are we not getting any purinergic response? In some of the lower areas of the bladder, such as the trigone, we do find purinergic responses to nerve stimulation, but not in the dome.

Burnstock: When we looked at six samples of human bladder, in four we had clear evidence for purinergic responses, but in two we did not. To repeat myself, we need to know more about the regional distribution of purinergic nerves and receptors.

Blaivas: I am interested in the question of distinguishing transmitters that perform different functions. When we look at the actions of purinergic agonists in the rabbit and the rat whole bladder model, there is a rapid increase in detrusor pressure which occurs much earlier, but is less sustained than that due to cholinergic agonists. There is a cholinergic response which empties the bladder more slowly, but more effectively. Yet the concept of co-transmission to me implies that two transmitters are working together to perform a single function. We are working on the hypothesis that ATP, at least in the rabbit and rat, is useful in starting the micturition process— in particular, in opening the urethra. If you simply measure tension and force in muscle strips, it doesn't have a direction and doesn't enable you to look at function. In a whole bladder and urethra model you can see whether ATP is necessary to start the contractions and open the urethra, and then whether the cholinergic influence comes in to empty the bladder.

Burnstock: That is an interesting point. If I might draw an analogy with noradrenaline and ATP as co-transmitters in sympathetic nerves to blood vessels, during homeostatic conditions, such as gentle exercise, there are long trains of impulse discharge in sympathetic nerves, which favours the noradrenaline component. However, in stress, there are brief bursts of impulses in sympathetic nerves, and that favours the ATP component, since it works through a different receptor mechanism involving voltage-dependent calcium channels. The same might be true in the bladder; if acetylcholine and ATP coexist in the same neurons in the bladder, they may turn out to play different roles, if we can establish the physiological circumstances which favour one or the other.

Blaivas: We need to look at serial sections, from the urethra up to the neck of the bladder, because there is probably little purinergic activity at the dome, but it may play a major role in the trigone and in the urethra.

Christensen: Since the bladder and rectum have similar embryological origins, I have always thought that their innervation must be much the same. I have looked at the rectum quite carefully and it's not homogeneous in terms of the anatomy of the nerve density. We see a steep decline in the density of ganglia, and of ganglion cells, from the sigmoid colon to the anal canal, a 10-fold reduction. Is there a gradient in the density of innervation in the intrinsic nerves of the bladder? And in the rectum, virtually all the ganglion cells are of Dogiel Type 1, with lamellar dendrites. Is this also true of the urinary bladder—or do we know anything about that?

Burnstock: We know a bit about it. The intrinsic neurons in the bladder are very few in comparison with those in the gut. There is a very sophisticated intrinsic innervation in the gut and we know that if you cut the extrinsic nerves, peristaltic and other intrinsic reflexes can occur, so even intrinsic sensory neurons are present. In the bladder, the intrinsic neurons are far fewer and much less well defined in functional terms. Interneurons are present in the ganglia and there are many different receptors present on the neurons. Therefore, these are not simple, parasympathetic nicotinic relay stations; rather they are capable of coordinating and integrating neural activity, although clearly less sophisticated than in the gut.

Christensen: The rectum is very unsophisticated too, neuroanatomically, because there are only about 100–200 ganglion cells per cm^2 of surface area. Is it the same order in the bladder?

Burnstock: It depends on species. In the rat there are no neurons actually in the wall of the bladder; they are mostly on the outside. In the guinea pig and in man we have seen groups of ganglia within the wall. The ganglia are small, containing only 5–20 neurons. We have never carried out a quantitative study of the whole bladder. While the total is unlikely to be large, it may be enough to be effective functionally, because of the long varicose branching terminals of these neurons.

Andersson: On the question of atropine resistance in the human bladder, it is clear that there are differences between the detrusor muscle, the trigone, and the bladder neck and proximal urethra. At present there is little evidence for atropine resistance in the normal human detrusor muscle (Andersson 1986). I don't think anybody denies that there is an atropine-resistant component in the trigone or in the bladder neck and proximal urethra.

It is also important to stress that there is a good correlation between the lack of atropine resistance in the normal human bladder *in vivo* and *in vitro*. I also think there might be changes within the detrusor muscle, in connection with, for example, outflow obstruction, that could alter the innervation. Normally, peptidergic innervation is centred in the lower third of the bladder, but this might change during outflow obstruction.

There are clinical correlates to the occurrence of hyperactivity of the bladder and sensitivity to atropine. Dr Blaivas and his coworkers (Blaivas et al 1980) did some interesting trials in which they titrated the dose of propantheline in patients with bladder hyperactivity and found that most patients responded well to this anticholinergic drug; so in many cases hyperactivity of the bladder is mediated through muscarinic cholinergic receptors. This is an important way of seeing whether the hyperactive bladder contraction is mediated entirely through one transmitter, or if more than one is involved.

Swash: I want to turn to the sensory side of things, because sensation is very important in the context of this symposium. It has intrigued me for some time how we sense bladder or rectal fullness. We know something about the importance of the afferent mechanisms in peristalis. You used the word 'sensory' deliberately vaguely, Professor Burnstock, when you spoke about 'sensory-motor' neurons. Which aspects of these cells are sensory? Are they, or are some of them, just sensory, or do some have motor functions as well? If so, which of their neurotransmitters and co-modulators are important in determining sensory function? CGRP is obviously important in the myenteric plexus in the gut; is it relevant here too?

Burnstock: Substance P, calcitonin gene-related peptide and ATP are the established transmitters in sensory nerves, but other peptides have also been described in some sensory nerves. I think there are also sensory endings of the more traditional type in the bladder, containing many small mitochondria. The proportion of these two types is not yet clear. The first type I have called 'sensory-motor' nerves because they contain substances that are extremely potent when released, and likely to have an efferent role during 'axon reflex' activity. This doesn't exclude their being sensory too.

Maggi: In connection with that, is there any evidence that at least some of the intrinsic neurons of the bladder might be sensory neurons, or at least neurons projecting to prevertebral ganglia, in such a way as to provide some information for the activation of reflexes?

Burnstock: This is a fascinating question, but we do not know yet. I am interested to know whether there is any evidence that after cutting the extrinsic nerves to the bladder you can still get reflex activity in the bladder. If you do, you would have to say that there probably are sensory neurons. The same is true in the heart: one talks about 'intercoronary reflexes' when the extrinsic nerves are cut, but the evidence is unclear. The same goes for the lung.

Brindley: It's clear that there is not much reflex activity left in a complete cauda equina lesion, but I would like to know whether there are slight traces. David Thomas of Sheffield might be able to give an answer, because he has the biggest experience of doing cystometry in patients with cauda equina lesions.

de Groat: A number of studies have been done on afferent pathways to the cat bladder. As I shall discuss in my paper (p 27), there are two kinds of afferents, small myelinated Aδ fibres and unmyelinated C fibres. Jänig & Morrison (1986) made the interesting observation that the myelinated fibres which are activated by distension of the bladder are fired by low levels of bladder pressure and increase their activity as the pressure in the bladder increases, so they grade almost linearly the tension in the bladder wall. These afferents are probably involved in signalling that the bladder is filling, and are involved in triggering reflexes; on the other hand, the large majority (95%) of the unmyelinated C fibres are silent and cannot be activated under normal conditions, even by extreme distension of the bladder (Häbler et al 1988). These afferents are referred to as 'sleeping' or 'silent' C fibres. They have been identified at other sites in the body, in particular the joints. These afferents are turned on by inflammation or irritation of the bladder, just as they are in the joints.

The next question is whether the bladder has local reflexes like the gut. My view is that the bladder is quite different from the gut. It is dependent upon the CNS for control, whereas the gut has a myenteric plexus and thus has considerable intrinsic control.

However, there are local responses which appear sometimes in the bladder in pathological conditions. In cats, we have damaged the sacral efferent outflow, which is essentially equivalent to a cauda equina lesion (de Groat & Kawatani 1989). Under these conditions we can demonstrate that afferents which arise from dorsal root ganglion cells generate reflexes locally through the parasympathetic ganglia, back to the bladder. These are not obvious in normal cats but are apparent after nerve injury. This experimental pathological condition would be similar to a patient with a myelomeningocele or a cauda equina lesion.

So I would agree with Geoff Burnstock that the conditions of the preparation, or the condition of the patient, will influence to some extent the organization of the neural pathways. The interesting point is that the local reflexes in the bladder are triggered by the unmyelinated, not the myelinated afferents; thus this is another example of pathology unmasking reflexes to the bladder. I would also agree with Geoff that in certain conditions, such as hyperactive bladder or urinary incontinence, local reflexes and abnormal central reflexes may contribute to the symptoms.

Marsden: In the normal subject, there appears to be relatively little local control of the bladder.

de Groat: If the human is like the cat and the rat.

Marsden: Which takes us back to Giles Brindley's question.

Brindley: It is clear from cystometry that there is very little local reflex activity but it is not clear to me whether it is 'very little', or zero.

Blaivas: Dr de Groat mentioned that tension or pressure stimulates the Aδ fibres. Morrison refers to 'pressure' and shows a graded stimulation response due to increasing pressure, but I don't know how that could be achieved in the whole bladder model. Is the implication that when you fill the bladder, it elicits afferent impulses, and the greater the pressure, the greater the impulse? Normally, when you fill the bladder, in an animal, you don't get a graded pressure response; you get very little rise in pressure at all. Are you talking about tension in the wall of the bladder, or pressure? A cystometrogram in an animal shows a flat response, but Morrison showed a very nice gradation of responses. Is he doing something to make the pressure go up, artificially?

de Groat: Yes! Dr Morrison connected the bladder to a fluid reservoir which could be raised to various levels above the bladder; if the reservoir were 20 cm above the bladder, there would be a pressure of 20 cm of water in the bladder.

Blaivas: That isn't necessarily true; that only happens when the flow stops.

de Groat: I presume he did the experiments under constant pressure conditions. I agree that this is not what happens in a normal person whose bladder is filling naturally.

Staskin: This discussion illustrates a problem that we shall face throughout the symposium: we shall be trying to extrapolate from experimental models to clinical situations. Observations at the various levels of experimentation—the molecular level, smooth muscle behaviour in the muscle bath, behaviour of the whole organ during *in vitro* or *in vivo* experiments, clinical obervations during urodynamic evaluation—are not comparable, because of differences in the models as well as artifacts of the testing situations. Non-physiological responses are commonly elicited by the nature of the stimulus, for instance pharmacological dosages in the muscle bath which cannot be tolerated clinically. It has become quite obvious to those interested in urodynamics that the urodynamic situation may not reproduce the clinical symptoms. In this instance, if one wants to create increased pressure within the bladder, over-distension provides increased pressure which would not be observed clinically. In addition, cystometry measures intravesical pressure, but it does not reflect wall tension, which is determined by the radius of the sphere, or, in this case, bladder volume.

A question which interests me is whether the stimuli for uninhibited bladder contractions, which are a major cause of clinically observed incontinence, are myogenic and originate locally within the bladder musculature, or are neurogenic and reflect a change in the reflex neural pathways.

Maggi: Some people believe that a part of detrusor instability, which by definition occurs without any overt sign of accompanying neurological disease, has a myogenic origin; for example, there is a change in the bladder muscle. Professor Burnstock mentioned the existence of 'pacemaker' cells in the gut, the Cajal cells. Is there any morphological or functional evidence for pacemaker cells in the bladder muscle, in the normal or diseased state?

Brading: We certainly believe that a lot of bladder instability is myogenic. In all our experimental animal models and in humans that we have examined, we find clear denervation of the detrusor associated with bladder instability. Professor T. Tomita from Japan was working in my laboratory recently, looking at the spread of electrical impulses between bladder smooth muscle cells, in the guinea pig. In normal bladder, the electrical spread turned out to be far less than in almost any other smooth muscle (Brading et al 1989). This suggests that although the individual smooth muscle cells may be connected together in bundles, the impulses from one small area of the bladder don't spread. However, we have evidence that in bladder instability there is probably an increased spread of electrical impulses from cell to cell. In mini-pigs with detrusor instability, we can cut the sacral roots and still get the unstable contractions continuing perfectly. This doesn't mean that there isn't any local reflex activity. Evidence for some reflex control of unstable contractions is that in obstructed pigs, during bladder filling, the contractions are small at first and get bigger as you increase the fill, but in transected bladders with no sacral root input the unstable contractions increase less with filling, which suggests that there may be some reflex inhibition of the early contractions during filling with intact sacral roots (Sethia 1988).

Stanton: It has been suggested that there might be a pacemaker centre in the intramural ureter, associated with vesico-ureteral reflux. I don't know how relevant that is, or whether it has been confirmed.

I have two questions for Geoff Burnstock. I was interested in the concept of sexual difference in noradrenergic response. I wonder whether this is because of the large numbers of noradrenergic receptors in the prostatic capsule, in the male, or whether this sex difference is mediated by oestrogen/progesterone receptors in the female. As a second, more functional question: do you really feel that it will be feasible to treat sphincter incompetence with purinergic substances, bearing in mind their toxicity?

Burnstock: On the first question, I mainly discussed changes in *transmitter* expression, but *receptor* expression is even more important in terms of the development of new drugs. Receptor expression is sometimes secondary to changes in nerve innervation, but sometimes independent of it. Hormones can certainly change receptor expression, and there are increasing numbers of examples of large differences in the behaviour of tissues in the male and female. In atherosclerosis, there are differences in responses of the same vessels from males and females. Furthermore, if you grow vascular smooth muscle in tissue culture from males and females, they behave differently in terms of proliferation, probably because of differences in hormone exposure. So I expect to find big differences between the behaviour of male and female bladders. We need to know more about the control of receptor expression in males and females, and also in pathological situations.

On the second question, the development of purinergic drugs is in its infancy. Many companies are becoming interested in purines, although this has so far been concentrated on the adenosine P_1 purinoceptor. Suramin [sym-bis(*m*-aminobenzoyl-*m*-amino-*p*-methyl benzoyl-1-naphthylamino-4,6,8-trisulphonate) carbamide] has recently been recognized as a competitive antagonist of the ATP P_2 purinoceptor and it is very effective in the bladder. Unlike the selective 'desensitizer' of the P_2 purinoceptor, α,β-methylene-ATP, analogues of Suramin could be developed for therapeutic purposes, but we are not at that stage yet.

As a reply to Dr Brading's comments, finally, there is now a fluorescent antibody to gap-junction protein available. Using a confocal microscope, the whole pattern of gap-junction distribution in a big piece of smooth muscle from the bladder could be determined. It would be very interesting to consider making a comparative analysis of this kind on normal and hyperactive bladder.

References

Andersson K-E 1986 Clinical relevance of some findings in neuro-anatomy and neurophysiology of the lower urinary tract. Clin Sci 70 (Suppl 14):21s–32s

Blaivas JG, Labib KB, Michalik J, Zayed AAH 1980 Cystometric response to propantheline in detrusor hyperreflexia: therapeutic implications. J Urol 124:259–262

Brading AF, Parekh AB, Tomita T 1989 Tissue impedance of smooth muscles isolated from guinea pig. J Physiol (Lond) 417:63P

Craggs MD, Rushton DN, Stephenson JD 1986 A putative non-cholinergic mechanism in urinary bladders of new but not old world primates. J Urol 136:1348–1350

Cullumbine H, McKee WHE, Creasey NH 1955 Effects of atropine sulphate upon healthy male subjects. Q J Exp Physiol 40:309–319

de Groat WC, Kawatani M 1989 Reorganization of sympathetic preganglionic connections in bladder ganglia following sacral parasympathetic denervation. J Physiol (Lond) 409:431–449

Häbler H-J, Jänig W, Koltzenburg M 1988 A novel type of unmyelinated chemosensitive nociceptor in the acutely inflamed urinary bladder. Agents Actions 25:219–221

Jänig W, Morrison JFB 1986 Functional properties of spinal visceral afferents supplying abdominal and pelvic organs, with special emphasis on visual nociception. In: Cervero F, Morrison JFB (eds) Visceral sensation. Elsevier Science Publishers, Amsterdam (Progress in Brain Research vol 67) p 87–114

Sibley GNA 1984 A comparison of spontaneous and nerve-mediated activity in bladder muscle from man, pig and rabbit. J Physiol (Lond) 354:431– 443

Sethia KK 1988 The pathophysiology of detrusor instability. DM thesis, Oxford University

Central neural control
of the lower urinary tract

William C. de Groat

Departments of Pharmacology and Behavioral Neuroscience, Center for Neuroscience, University of Pittsburgh, Pittsburgh, PA 15261, USA

Abstract. The lower urinary tract has two main functions, the storage and periodic elimination of urine, which are regulated by a complex neural control system in the brain and spinal cord. This neural system exhibits switch-like patterns of activity that are generated by visceral reflex circuits, some of which are under voluntary control. Experimental studies in animals indicate that the micturition reflex is mediated by a spinobulbospinal pathway passing through a coordination centre (the pontine micturition centre) located in the rostral brainstem. This reflex pathway is, in turn, modulated by higher centres in the cerebral cortex which are presumably involved in the voluntary control of micturition. Several neurotransmitters (including GABA, opioid peptides and glutamic acid) appear to have a role in the central pathways controlling micturition. Since pharmacological manipulation of putative inhibitory transmitter mechanisms increases bladder activity and decreases bladder capacity it is possible that similar changes induced by pathological conditions may underlie bladder dysfunctions occurring in patients with neurogenic urinary incontinence. Further study of these neurotransmitter systems may yield new therapeutic approaches for the treatment of hyperactive bladder disorders.

1990 Neurobiology of Incontinence. Wiley, Chichester (Ciba Foundation Symposium 151) p 27–56

The excretory function of the lower urinary tract is completely dependent on neural mechanisms that reside in the brain and lumbosacral spinal cord. This dependence on central nervous control distinguishes the urinary tract from many other visceral structures, such as the heart and gastrointestinal tract, that maintain a certain level of function even after elimination of extrinsic neural input.

The lower urinary tract is also unusual in its pattern of activity and in the complexity of its neural regulation. For example, it exhibits only two modes of operation, namely the storage and elimination of urine. Thus, many of the neural circuits controlling micturition exhibit switch-like or phasic patterns of activity (Fig. 1), in contrast to the tonic patterns occurring in autonomic pathways to the cardiovascular organs. In addition, the storage and release of urine are clearly under voluntary control, unlike many other visceral functions which are purely involuntary. Micturition is therefore dependent on learned behaviour which emerges during maturation of the nervous system as well as on primitive reflexes which are present in the neonate. The storage and release of urine also require the integration of autonomic and somatic efferent mechanisms within the spinal cord. This is necessary to coordinate the activity

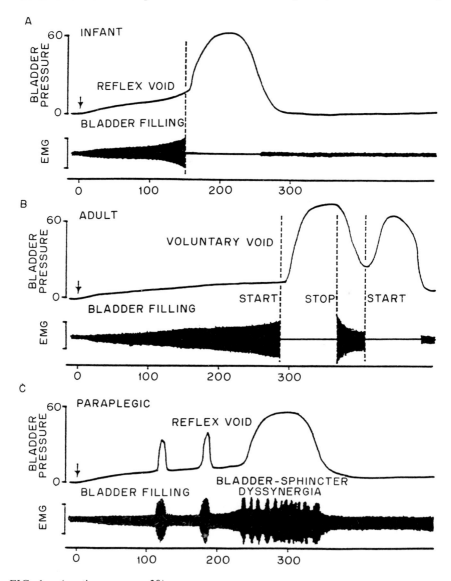

FIG. 1.   *(caption on page 29)*

of pelvic visceral structures with that of the perineal and extra-urethral striated muscles.

The dependence of lower urinary tract functions on complex central networks which extend from the cerebral cortex to the sacral spinal cord renders these functions very susceptible to a considerable number of neurological disorders. Indeed, changes in the activity of the lower urinary tract are often the first signs of such disorders. Thus, neurological mechanisms are an important consideration in the diagnosis and treatment of urinary tract dysfunctions, such

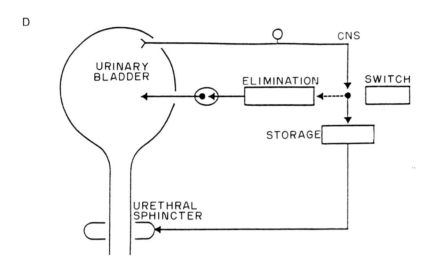

FIG. 1.   Combined cystometrograms and sphincter electromyograms (EMG) comparing reflex voiding responses in an infant (A) and in a paraplegic patient (C) with a voluntary voiding response in an adult (B). The abscissa in all records represents bladder volume in millilitres and the ordinates represent bladder pressure in cm H_2O and electrical activity of the EMG recording. On the left side of each trace the arrows indicate the start of a slow infusion of fluid into the bladder (bladder filling). Vertical dashed lines indicate the start of sphincter relaxation which precedes by a few seconds the bladder contraction in A and B. In part B note that a voluntary cessation of voiding (stop) is associated with an initial increase in sphincter EMG followed by a reciprocal relaxation of the bladder. A resumption of voiding is again associated with sphincter relaxation and a delayed increase in bladder pressure. On the other hand, in the paraplegic patient (C) the reciprocal relationship between bladder and sphincter is abolished. During bladder filling, transient uninhibited bladder contractions occur in association with sphincter activity. Further filling leads to more prolonged and simultaneous contractions of the bladder and sphincter (bladder–sphincter dyssynergia). Loss of the reciprocal relationship between bladder and sphincter in paraplegic patients interferes with bladder emptying. (Parts A–C from de Groat & Steers, 1990, with permission.) (D) Diagram indicating the switch-like function of the micturition reflex pathway. During urine storage low level of afferent activity activates efferent input to the urethral sphincter. During urine elimination a high level of afferent activity activates efferent input to the bladder.

as incontinence. This paper will review anatomical and physiological studies in animals that have provided insights into the reflex pathways and transmitters involved in the neural control of micturition.

Anatomy and innervation of the lower urinary tract

The storage and periodic elimination of urine are dependent upon the activity of two functional units in the lower urinary tract: (1) a reservoir (the urinary bladder) and (2) an outlet consisting of bladder neck, urethra and striated muscles of the urethral sphincter. These structures are in turn controlled by three sets of peripheral nerves: sacral parasympathetic (pelvic nerves), thoracolumbar sympathetic (hypogastric nerves and sympathetic chain) and sacral somatic nerves (pudendal nerves) (Fig. 2) (Kuru 1965, de Groat & Kawatani 1985, Torrens & Morrison 1987, Wein & Barrett 1988).

The sacral parasympathetic outflow provides the major excitatory input to the urinary bladder. This input is mediated by cholinergic as well as non-cholinergic (purinergic) transmitters. Thoracolumbar sympathetic pathways elicit a variety of responses in the lower urinary tract including: (1) inhibition of detrusor smooth muscle, (2) excitation of the bladder base and urethra, and (3) modulation of cholinergic transmission in bladder parasympathetic ganglia (Fig. 3). These effects promote the storage of urine and facilitate urinary continence. The efferent innervation of the peri-urethral and external urethral striated muscles is carried by axons in the pudendal nerve from somatic motoneurons in the lumbosacral spinal cord. The sphincter moto-neurons in the cord have a close morphological and functional relationship with the autonomic neurons in the same segments of the cord (Thor et al 1989).

Afferent axons innervating the urinary tract are present in the three sets of nerves (de Groat 1986, Jänig & Morrison 1986). The most important afferents for initiating micturition are those passing in the pelvic nerve to the sacral spinal cord (Kuru 1965). These afferents are small myelinated (Aδ) and unmyelinated (C) fibres which convey impulses from tension receptors in the bladder wall to neurons in laminae I, V, VII and X of the spinal cord (Figs. 4 & 5) (Morgan et al 1981). Aδ bladder afferents in the cat respond in a graded manner to passive distension as well as active contraction of the bladder (Jänig & Morrison 1986) and exhibit pressure thresholds in the range of 5–15 mmHg, which are similar to those pressures at which humans report the first sensation of bladder filling. These fibres also code for noxious stimuli in the bladder. On the other hand, C fibre bladder afferents have very high thresholds and commonly do not respond to even high levels of intravesical pressure (Habler et al 1988). However, activity in these afferents is unmasked or enhanced by chemical irritation of the bladder mucosa. These findings indicate that C fibre afferents in the cat have specialized functions, such as the signalling of inflammatory or noxious events in the lower urinary tract.

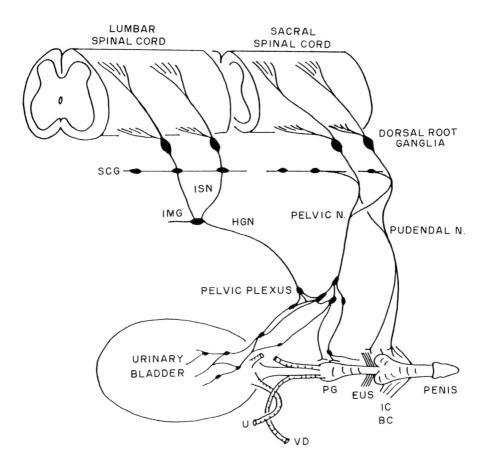

FIG. 2. Diagram showing the sympathetic, parasympathetic, and somatic innervation of the urogenital tract of the male cat. Sympathetic preganglionic pathways emerge from the lumbar spinal cord and pass to the sympathetic chain ganglia (SCG) and then via the inferior splanchnic nerves (ISN) to the inferior mesenteric ganglia (IMG). Preganglionic and postganglionic sympathetic axons then travel in the hypogastric nerve (HGN) to the pelvic plexus and the urogenital organs. Parasympathetic preganglionic axons which originate in the sacral spinal cord pass in the pelvic nerve to ganglion cells in the pelvic plexus and to distal ganglia in the organs. Sacral somatic pathways are contained in the pudendal nerve, which provides an innervation to the penis, the ischiocavernosus (IC), bulbocavernosus (BC), and external urethral sphincter (EUS) muscles. The pudendal and pelvic nerves also receive postganglionic axons from the caudal sympathetic chain ganglia. These three sets of nerves contain afferent axons from the lumbosacral dorsal root ganglia. U, ureter; PG, prostate gland; VD, vas deferens. (From de Groat & Steers 1988, with permission.)

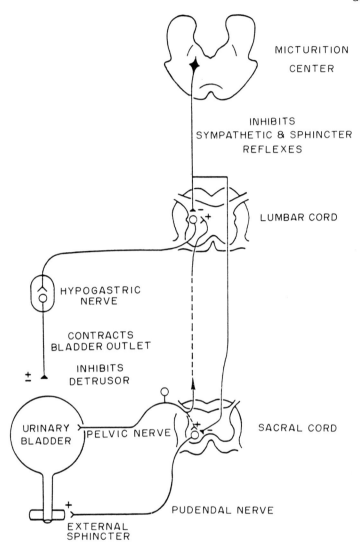

MICTURITION
CENTER

INHIBITS
SYMPATHETIC & SPHINCTER
REFLEXES

LUMBAR CORD

HYPOGASTRIC
NERVE

CONTRACTS
BLADDER OUTLET

INHIBITS
DETRUSOR

URINARY
BLADDER

PELVIC NERVE

SACRAL CORD

PUDENDAL NERVE

EXTERNAL
SPHINCTER

FIG. 3. Diagram showing detrusor–sphincter reflexes. During the storage of urine, distension of the bladder produces low level vesical afferent firing, which in turn stimulates (1) the sympathetic outflow to the bladder outlet (base and urethra) and (2) pudendal outflow to the external urethral sphincter. These responses occur by spinal reflex pathways and represent 'guarding reflexes', which promote continence. Sympathetic firing also inhibits detrusor muscle and transmission in bladder ganglia. At the initiation of micturition, intense vesical afferent activity activates the brainstem micturition centre, which inhibits the spinal guarding reflexes. (From de Groat & Booth 1984, with permission.)

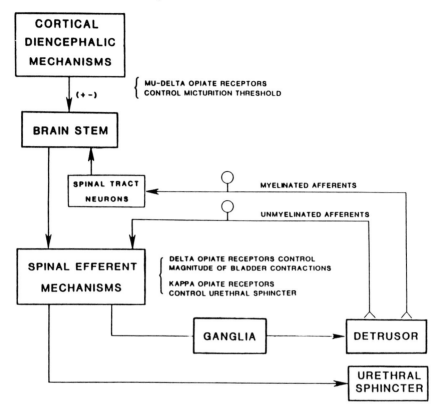

FIG. 4. Diagram of the central reflex pathways and enkephalinergic mechanisms which regulate micturition in the cat. In animals with an intact neuraxis, micturition is initiated by a supraspinal reflex pathway passing through a centre in the brainstem. The pathway is triggered by small myelinated afferents (Aδ) connected to tension receptors in the bladder wall. In chronic spinal animals, connections between the brainstem and the sacral spinal cord are interrupted and micturition is initially blocked. However, in chronic spinal animals a spinal reflex mechanism emerges which is triggered by unmyelinated (C fibre) vesical afferents. The C fibre reflex pathway is usually weak or undetectable in animals with an intact nervous system. Pharmacological studies have shown that in the brain μ or δ opiate receptors control micturition threshold and bladder capacity, whereas in the spinal cord δ opiate receptors control the magnitude of bladder contractions, κ opiate receptors mediate a depression of the pudendal motor outflow to the external urethral sphincter. (From de Groat & Kawatani 1985, with permission.)

Reflex mechanisms controlling the lower urinary tract

The central pathways controlling lower urinary tract function are organized as simple on–off switching circuits (Fig. 1D) that maintain a reciprocal relationship between the urinary bladder and urethral outlet. The principal reflex components of these switching circuits are listed in Table 1 and illustrated in Fig. 1.

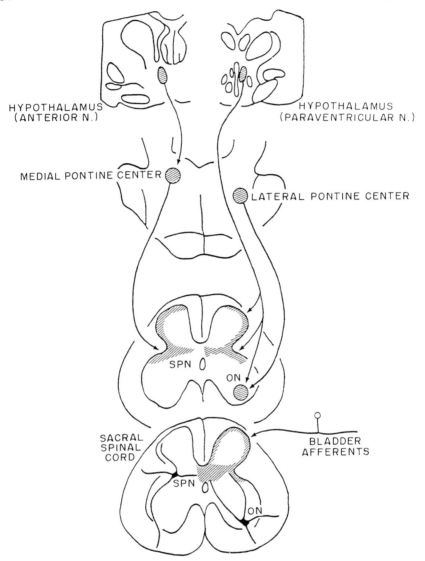

FIG. 5.   Neural connections between the brain and the sacral spinal cord that may be involved in the regulation of the lower urinary tract in the cat. Lower section of spinal cord shows the location and morphology of: (1) a preganglionic neuron in the sacral parasympathetic nucleus (SPN), (2) a sphincter motoneuron in Onuf's nucleus (ON) and (3) the sites of central termination of afferent projections from the urinary bladder. (Based on the studies of Nadelhaft et al 1980, Morgan et al 1981 and Thor et al 1989.) Upper section of spinal cord shows the sites of termination of descending pathways arising in the pontine micturition centre (medial), the pontine sphincter or urine storage centre (lateral) and the paraventricular nuclei of the hypothalamus. Section through the pons shows projection from anterior hypothalamic nuclei to the pontine micturition centre. (Based on studies of Holstege 1987 and Holstege et al 1986.) (From de Groat & Steers 1990, with permission.)

TABLE 1 Reflexes to the lower urinary tract

Afferent pathway	Efferent pathway	Central pathway
Urine storage		
Low level vesical afferent activity (pelvic nerve)	1. External sphincter contraction (somatic nerves) 2. Internal sphincter contraction (sympathetic nerves) 3. Detrusor inhibition (sympathetic nerves) 4. Ganglionic inhibition (sympathetic nerves) 5. Sacral parasympathetic outflow inactive	Spinal reflexes
Micturition		
High level vesical activity (pelvic nerve)	1. Inhibition of external sphincter activity 2. Inhibition of sympathetic outflow 3. Activation of parasympathetic outflow	Spinobulbospinal reflexes

From de Groat & Booth 1984.

Intravesical pressure measurements during bladder filling in both man and animals reveal that bladder pressure is maintained at a low and relatively constant level (5–10 cmH$_2$O) when bladder volume is below the threshold for inducing voiding (Fig. 1A, B). A low intravesical pressure during urine storage is essential to allow urine flow from the kidney through the ureters at a low pressure head. The accommodation of the bladder to increasing volumes of urine is primarily a passive phenomenon dependent upon the intrinsic properties of the vesical smooth muscle and quiescence of the parasympathetic efferent pathway (de Groat et al 1982, Torrens & Morrison 1987, Wein & Barrett 1988). In addition, in some species urine storage is also facilitated by sympathetic reflexes which mediate an inhibition of bladder activity, closure of the bladder neck and contraction of the proximal urethra (Table 1, Fig. 3). Although the importance of these sympathetic reflexes in man is still uncertain, their contribution to urine storage in animals is generally accepted. During bladder filling the activity of the sphincter electromyogram (EMG) also increases, reflecting an increase in efferent firing in the pudendal nerve and an increase in outlet resistance which contributes to the maintenance of urinary continence. The somatic and sympathetic reflexes that occur during urine storage are initiated by a low level of afferent activity conveyed in the pelvic nerve to the sacral spinal cord from tension receptors in the bladder wall (Table 1, Fig. 3).

The storage phase of the urinary bladder can be switched to the voiding phase either involuntarily (reflexly) or voluntarily (Fig. 1). The former is readily demonstrated in the human infant or in the anaesthetized animal when the volume of urine exceeds the micturition threshold. At this point, increased afferent firing from tension receptors in the bladder reverses the pattern of efferent outflow, producing firing in the sacral parasympathetic pathways and inhibition of sympathetic and somatic pathways. The expulsion phase consists of an initial relaxation of the urethral sphincter (Fig. 1A) followed in a few seconds by a contraction of the bladder, an increase in bladder pressure and flow of urine. Secondary reflexes elicited by the passage of urine through the urethra reinforce the bladder contraction and facilitate bladder emptying (Kuru 1965, Wein & Barrett 1988).

These reflexes require the integrative action of neuronal populations at various levels of the neuraxis (Figs. 3–5). Certain reflexes, for example, those mediating the excitatory outflow to the sphincters and the sympathetic inhibitory outflow to the bladder, are organized at the spinal level (Fig. 3), whereas the parasympathetic outflow to the detrusor has a more complicated central organization involving spinal and spinobulbospinal pathways (Fig. 4).

Electrophysiological and neuroanatomical studies in animals indicate that the spinobulbospinal parasympathetic pathway passes through a centre in the rostral brainstem (the pontine micturition centre) which is located in the region of the locus ceruleus or locus ceruleus alpha in the cat and in the lateral dorsal tegmental nucleus in the rat (de Groat 1975, Torrens & Morrison 1987). This centre, in conjunction with neuronal circuitry in adjacent areas of the brain (e.g., the locus subceruleus, lateral parabrachial nucleus), appears to play a major role in coordinating the neuronal mechanisms underlying both urine storage and release. Thus, destruction of the pontine micturition centre or interruption of the neuraxis below the pons causes the immediate elimination of the micturition reflex and the slow development of involuntary, uncoordinated, spinal voiding mechanisms (Fig. 1C) which mediate automatic voiding in the paraplegic patient.

The central pathways which are likely to mediate the spinobulbospinal micturition reflex have been demonstrated with axonal tracing techniques. For example, it has been shown that the dorsal pontine tegmentum receives inputs from neurons located in lateral laminae I, V and VII of the sacral spinal cord. Neurons in these areas of the spinal cord receive dense projections from bladder afferent pathways (Fig. 5) and respond to distension or contraction of the bladder (de Groat et al 1981). It is assumed that these neurons represent the spinal ascending limb of the micturition reflex pathway.

Descending projections from the pontine micturition centre to the spinal cord have also been identified in the cat and rat (Loewy et al 1979, Holstege et al 1986) (Fig. 5). In the cat, neurons in the dorsolateral pons send direct projections to the sacral parasympathetic nucleus and to lamina I on the lateral edge of the sacral dorsal horn, an area that contains dendritic projections from the sacral preganglionic neurons and afferent inputs from the bladder (Nadelhaft et al 1980, Morgan et al 1981, de Groat et al 1986). Thus, the sites of termination of descending projections from the pontine micturition centre are optimally located to regulate reflex mechanisms at the spinal level. A second area located somewhat more laterally in the pons sends projections to the sphincter motor nucleus in the sacral spinal cord (Holstege et al 1986) (Fig. 5). Electrical stimulation of this dorsolateral area elicits sphincter contractions and inhibits bladder activity, whereas stimulation of the more medial pontine micturition centre produces the opposite effects: inhibition of sphincter activity and excitation of the bladder.

Neurophysiological data are consistent with the concept of a spinobulbospinal micturition reflex pathway. In both cat and rats stimulation of bladder afferents activates neurons in the pons at latencies of 30–40 ms, whereas electrical stimulation in the pons excites sacral preganglionic neurons at latencies of 45–60 ms (de Groat 1975). The sum of latencies for the spinobulbar and bulbospinal components of the reflex pathway approximate the latency (65–100 ms) for the entire reflex.

Single-unit recordings in the pontine micturition centre of the cat and rat have identified several populations of cells exhibiting firing correlated with bladder activity. One group of cells fires just prior to and during reflex contractions of the bladder, whereas another group is inhibited during bladder contractions. The all-or-none-pattern of activity of these units, coupled with pharmacological data (see below), provides support for the view that this region of the pons contains the neuronal switching circuit responsible for controlling the storage–voiding cycle of the lower urinary tract.

On the other hand, there is also evidence that a switching or gating circuit is present in the spinal cord (de Groat & Ryall 1969, de Groat 1975, McMahon & Morrison 1982). For example, in chronic spinal animals, reflex mechanisms within the lumbosacral spinal cord are capable of duplicating many of the functions performed by the reflex pathways in the intact animal. In addition, the firing of sacral preganglionic neurons elicited by bladder distension in chronic spinal cats after recovery from spinal shock is similar to that occurring in intact cats (de Groat & Ryall 1969, de Groat et al 1982).

However, despite these similarities, electrophysiological studies in rats and cats have shown that the reflex pathways in intact and chronic animals are markedly different. In both species the central delay for the micturition reflex in chronic spinal animals is considerably shorter (< 5 ms in rats; 15–40 ms in cats) than in intact animals (60–75 ms). In addition, in chronic spinal cats the afferent limb of the micturition reflex consists of unmyelinated (C fibre) afferents, whereas in intact cats it consists of myelinated (Aδ) afferents (Fig. 4) (see de Groat et al 1981, 1986 for reviews). Thus, there seems to be a considerable reorganization of reflex connections in the spinal cord after the interruption of descending pathways from the brain. C fibre afferent-evoked reflexes, which are weak and occur in only 50% of cats with an intact neuraxis, are facilitated, whereas Aδ afferent reflexes are completely eliminated in chronic spinal animals.

These data indicate that two distinct central pathways (supraspinal and spinal) utilizing different peripheral afferent limbs (A and C fibre) can mediate bladder reflexes (Fig. 4). The supraspinal pathway seems to have the major role in the initiation of bladder contractions in animals with an intact neuraxis. Although the function of the spinal reflex pathway in normal animals is uncertain, this pathway is essential for the development of automatic micturition in paraplegic animals. It is not known whether the spinal switching circuit which mediates automatic micturition is functional in normal animals or whether this circuit becomes functional as a consequence of synaptic reorganization after spinal cord damage (Thor et al 1986) or other pathological disorders such as urethral obstruction (Steers & de Groat 1988).

The organization of suprapontine pathways controlling micturition is less well defined, despite the fact that there is a large body of literature dealing with the responses of the lower urinary tract to lesions or electrical stimulation of the brain (Torrens & Morrison 1987, Wein & Barrett 1988). In brief, it appears that the voluntary control of micturition in humans is dependent upon (1) connections between the frontal cortex and the septal and the preoptic regions of the hypothalamus, and (2) connections between the paracentral lobule and the brainstem and spinal cord. Lesions to these areas of cortex resulting from tumours, aneurysms or cerebrovascular disease appear to remove inhibitory control over the anterior hypothalamic area which normally provides an excitatory input to micturition centres in the brainstem.

Electrical stimulation of anterior and lateral hypothalamic regions induces bladder contractions and voiding, whereas stimulation of posterior and medial hypothalamic areas inhibits bladder activity (Torrens & Morrison 1987). According to results obtained in cats, the inhibitory and excitatory effects of hypothalamic stimulation are believed to be mediated, respectively, by activation of sympathetic inhibitory pathways and activation of parasympathetic excitatory pathways to the bladder (Torrens & Morrison 1987).

Axonal tracing studies in cats have shown that the anterior hypothalamic area sends direct projections through the medial forebrain bundle to the pontine micturition centre (Fig. 5) (Holstege 1987). On the other hand, medial and posterior hypothalamic areas, including the paraventricular nucleus, send direct projections to the sacral parasympathetic nucleus, to the sphincter motor nucleus (Onuf's nucleus), and to certain sites of bladder afferent termination (laminae I and X) in the sacral spinal cord (Holstege 1987). Thus the modulatory effects of hypothalamic centres on the reflex pathways to the lower urinary tract are probably mediated by direct inputs to both pontine and sacral micturition centres.

Neurotransmitters in micturition reflex pathways

The sacral parasympathetic reflex pathway to the urinary bladder is essentially a positive feedback circuit. In the absence of inhibitory modulation this circuit would trigger voiding at very low bladder volumes and therefore not allow adequate urine storage, a situation that does occur with injuries or diseases of the central nervous system (Torrens & Morrison 1987, Wein & Barrett 1988). Thus, it is clear that the reflex must be under tonic inhibitory control. There has been considerable interest in defining the properties of and in particular the neurotransmitters involved in the putative inhibitory mechanisms.

Enkephalins

Immunocytochemical and pharmacological experiments have focused attention on the role of enkephalinergic inhibitory mechanisms in the regulation of micturition. Enkephalinergic varicosities are very prominent in the region of the sacral parasympathetic nucleus and the external urethral sphincter motor nucleus (Onuf's nucleus) in the sacral spinal cord as well as in the region of the pontine micturition centre of various species (de Groat et al 1983, 1986). Administration of exogenous enkephalins or opiate drugs to the brain by intracerebroventricular injection, microinjection into the pontine micturition centre, or intrathecal injection to sacral spinal cord in the cat and rat depresses micturition and sphincter reflexes (de Groat & Kawatani 1985, de Groat et al 1986,

Maggi & Meli 1986). Three types of opiate receptors mediate these depressant effects, μ and δ and κ. In the cat spinal cord δ opiate receptors are primarily responsible for inhibition of the micturition reflex, whereas both μ and δ opiate receptors mediate inhibition in the cat brain (Fig. 4) or the rat and human spinal cord. Sphincter reflexes are resistant to the actions of μ and δ opiate agonists administered to the spinal cord, but are inhibited by the intrathecal administration of κ receptor agonists.

A role of endogenous opioids in the control of micturition has been suggested by the effects of the opioid antagonist naloxone (de Groat et al 1983, 1986, Maggi & Meli 1986). The administration of naloxone systemically, intrathecally, intracerebroventricularly or by microinjection into the pontine micturition centre facilitates the micturition reflex. In low doses, naloxone reduces the bladder volume necessary to evoke micturition. Naloxone also increases the frequency and magnitude of low amplitude pressure waves on the tonus limb of the cystometrogram in chloralose-anaesthetized cats. These pressure waves are similar to the uninhibited contractions seen in patients with hyperactive bladder reflexes. The injection of small doses of naloxone into the pontine micturition centre of decerebrate cats also lowers the micturition threshold. In high doses, the drug produces sustained contractions of the bladder and firing on bladder postganglionic nerves. The effect is noted in anaesthetized animals with an intact neuraxis or in decerebrate unanaesthetized animals, but not in acute spinal animals where the spinobulbospinal micturition reflex pathway is interrupted.

However, in chronic paraplegic cats and rats which exhibit automatic micturition, naloxone administered systemically or injected intrathecally induces rhythmic bladder contractions, as well as spontaneous urination, and facilitates somato–bladder reflexes (Thor et al 1986, de Groat et al 1986). These data indicate that the spinal pathways mediating micturition in paraplegic cats are also under a tonic enkephalinergic inhibitory control. This is in contrast to normal animals, where intrathecal naloxone does not change bladder capacity. Thus, bladder capacity in normal animals appears to be controlled by enkephalinergic mechanisms in the brain, whereas in paraplegic animals this function shifts to the spinal cord.

Naloxone also affects bladder function in man (de Groat & Kawatani 1985). In normal patients, a significant rise in intravesical pressure (i.e. decreased bladder compliance) has been noted during cystometry after naloxone administration. Naloxone also increases instability during cystometry in patients with incomplete suprasacral spinal cord lesions, reducing by approximately one-third the bladder volume necessary to induce micturition. These data suggest that endogenous enkephalinergic mechanisms in the brain and spinal cord have an important role in regulating the storage and release of urine (Fig. 6).

γ-Aminobutyric acid (GABA)

Injections of GABA agonists intracerebroventricularly, into the pontine micturition centre or intrathecally inhibit the micturition reflex. Bicuculline, a GABA$_A$ receptor antagonist, administered into the pontine micturition centre in decerebrate unanaesthetized cats, blocks the inhibitory effects of GABA agonists and also decreases the bladder volume threshold for the induction of micturition (Roppolo et al 1986). The latter result indicates that GABAergic inhibitory mechanisms in the pons are involved in regulating bladder capacity (Fig. 6).

GABA also inhibits bladder reflex pathways when applied to the sacral spinal cord. Baclofen, a GABA$_B$ receptor agonist which mimics the inhibitory effect of GABA, has been used clinically via intrathecal administration in patients with hyperactive bladders to suppress bladder activity and to promote urine storage.

Other putative transmitters

The role of other transmitters in reflex pathways to the lower urinary tract is less clear. For example, exogenous glutamic acid and dopamine injected into the pontine micturition centre facilitate bladder reflexes, whereas injections of cholinergic muscarinic receptor agonists inhibit the reflexes (Fig. 6). Further studies are necessary to determine whether endogenously released substances can duplicate these effects. Preliminary experiments focusing on this question have

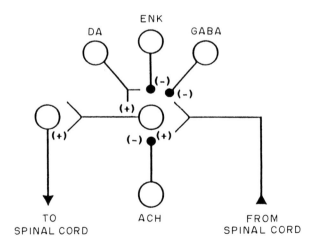

FIG. 6. Diagram showing the variety of neurotransmitters that may regulate transmission in the pontine micturition centre. DA, dopamine; ENK, enkephalins; GABA, γ-aminobutyric acid; ACH, acetylcholine; +, excitatory; −, inhibitory.

revealed that in cats and rats the systemic administration of MK-801, a substance that blocks NMDA (N-methyl-D-aspartate) channels, increases bladder capacity and inhibits reflex bladder contractions (Roppolo & de Groat 1989). These data implicate glutamic acid as an excitatory transmitter at some point in the micturition reflex pathway, although the specific site is uncertain.

5-Hydroxytryptamine (serotonin) may also have a transmitter role in central pathways to the lower urinary tract, because the lumbosacral sympathetic and parasympathetic autonomic centres receive a dense serotonergic input from the raphe nuclei in the caudal brain stem. In addition, the systemic administration of the serotonin precursor, 5-hydroxytryptophan, inhibits the parasympathetic micturition reflex and facilitates the vesicosympathetic urine storage reflex (de Groat et al 1979). Since electrical stimulation of the serotonergic neurons in raphe nuclei also inhibits bladder activity (Torrens & Morrison 1987), it is possible that bulbospinal serotonergic pathways are involved in modulating the micturition reflex pathway.

Conclusions

During the past decade there has been a considerable advance in our understanding of the neural mechanisms underlying micturition. Electrophysiological studies in animals have provided detailed information about the organization of the central reflex pathways which coordinate the activities of the bladder and urethral sphincters. In addition, pharmacological experiments have identified various substances that may function as neurotransmitters in these reflex pathways. It is anticipated that this information will lead to more effective diagnosis and treatment of neurogenic bladder dysfunction.

Acknowledgements

Supported by grant AM-31788 from the National Institutes of Health, grant BNS-08348 from the National Science Foundation, and a Clinical Research Center grant (MH-30915).

References

de Groat WC 1975 Nervous control of the urinary bladder of the cat. Brain Res 87:201–211
de Groat WC 1986 Spinal cord projections of visceral afferent neurones. In: Cervero F, Morrison JFB (eds) Visceral sensation. Elsevier Science Publishers, Amsterdam. (Progress in Brain Research vol 67) p 165–188
de Groat WC, Booth AM 1984 Autonomic systems to the urinary bladder and sexual organs. In: Dyck PJ et al (eds) Peripheral neuropathy, vol 1, 2nd edn. W. B. Saunders, Philadelphia, p 285–299
de Groat WC, Kawatani M 1985 Neural control of the urinary bladder: possible relationship between peptidergic inhibitory mechanisms and detrusor instability. Neurourol Urodyn 4:285–300

de Groat WC, Ryall RW 1969 Reflexes to sacral preganglionic parasympathetic neurones concerned with micturition in the cat. J Physiol (Lond) 200:87–108

de Groat WC, Steers WD 1988 Neural control of the urinary bladder and sexual organs: experimental studies in animals. In: Bannister R (ed) Autonomic failure, 2nd edn. Oxford University Press, Oxford, p 196–222

de Groat WC, Steers WD 1990 Autonomic regulation of the urinary bladder and sexual organs. In: Loewy A, Spyer KM (eds) The autonomic nervous system: central regulation of autonomic functions. Oxford University Press, Oxford, in press

de Groat WC, Booth AM, Krier J, Milne RJ, Morgan C, Nadelhaft I 1979 Neural control of the urinary bladder and large intestine. In: Brooks CM et al (eds) Integrative functions of the autonomic nervous system. University of Tokyo Press, Tokyo, p 50–67

de Groat WC, Nadelhaft I, Milne RJ, Booth AM, Morgan C, Thor K 1981 Organization of the sacral parasympathetic reflex pathways to the urinary bladder and large intestine. J Auton Nerv Syst 3:135–160

de Groat WC, Booth AM, Milne RJ, Roppolo JR 1982 Parasympathetic preganglionic neurons in the sacral spinal cord. J Auton Nerv Syst 5:23–43

de Groat WC, Kawatani M, Hisamitsu T et al 1983 The role of neuropeptides in the sacral autonomic reflex pathways of the cat. J Auton Nerv Syst 7:339–350

de Groat WC, Kawatani M, Hisamitsu T et al 1986 Neural control of micturition: the role of neuropeptides. J Auton Nerv Syst, Suppl p 369–387

Habler H-J, Jänig W, Koltzenburg M 1988 A novel type of unmyelinated chemosensitive nociceptor in the acutely inflamed urinary bladder. Agents Actions 25:219–221

Holstege G 1987 Some anatomical observations on the projections from the hypothalamus to brainstem and spinal cord: an HRP and autoradiographic tracing study in the cat. J Comp Neurol 260:98–126

Holstege G, Griffiths D, De Wall H, Dalm E 1986 Anatomical and physiological observations on supraspinal control of bladder and urethral sphincter muscles in the cat. J Comp Neurol 250:449–461

Jänig W, Morrison JFB 1986 Functional properties of spinal visceral afferents supplying abdominal and pelvic organs with special emphasis on visceral nociception. In: Cervero F, Morrison JFB (eds) Visceral sensation. Elsevier Science Publishers, Amsterdam (Progress in Brain Research vol 67) p 87–114

Kuru M 1965 Nervous control of micturition. Physiol Rev 45:425–494

Loewy AD, Saper CB, Baker RP 1979 Descending projections from the pontine micturition center. Brain Res 172:533–538

Maggi CA, Meli A 1986 The role of neuropeptides in the regulation of the micturition reflex. J Auton Pharmacol 6:133–162

McMahon SB, Morrison JFB 1982 Spinal neurones with long projections activated from the abdominal viscera of the cat. J Physiol (Lond) 332:265–281

Morgan C, Nadelhaft I, de Groat WC 1981 The distribution of visceral primary afferents from the pelvic nerve within Lissauer's tract and the spinal gray matter and its relationship to the sacral parasympathetic nucleus. J Comp Neurol 201:415–440

Nadelhaft I, Morgan C, de Groat WC 1980 Localization of the sacral autonomic nucleus in the spinal cord of the cat by the horseradish peroxidase technique. J Comp Neurol 193:265–281

Roppolo JR, de Groat WC 1989 The effects of MK-801 on the micturition reflex in the cat. Soc Neurosci Abstr 15:630

Roppolo JR, Mallory BS, Ragoowansi A, de Groat WC 1986 Modulation of bladder function in the cat by application of pharmacological agents to the pontine micturition center. Soc Neurosci Abstr 12:644

Steers WD, de Groat WC 1988 Effect of bladder outlet obstruction on micturition reflex pathways in the rat. J Urol 140:864–871

Thor K, Kawatani M, de Groat WC 1986 Plasticity in the reflex pathways to the lower
    urinary tract of the cat during postnatal development and following spinal cord injury.
    In: Golberger M et al (eds) Development and plasticity of the mammalian spinal cord.
    Fidia Research Series, vol III. Fidia Press, Padova, Italy, p 65–81
Thor K, Morgan C, Nadelhaft I, Houston M, de Groat WC 1989 Organization of afferent
    and efferent pathways in the pudendal nerve of the cat. J Comp Neurol 288:263–279
Torrens M, Morrison JFB 1987 The physiology of the lower urinary tract. Springer-
    Verlag, Berlin
Wein AJ, Barrett DM 1988 Voiding function and dysfunction: a logical and practical
    approach. Year Book Medical Publishers, Chicago

DISCUSSION

Read: I am interested in the extent to which there is a parallelism between what
Professor de Groat described in the bladder and what is observed in the anorectal
region. To be specific, I wonder whether the paradoxical contraction of the
external anal sphincter, which is described in some patients with severe constipation, is a parallel phenomenon to bladder detrusor–sphincter dyssynergia—in
other words, a dyssynergia between the rectum and the anal sphincter.

Professor de Groat, to what extent is the control of the bladder and rectal
function, and defaecation, integrated? Some people say it's not possible to
micturate and defaecate simultaneously. I think it probably is, but do you see
any integration of function between the two organs?

de Groat: The idea that normal humans do not micturate and defaecate
simultaneously goes back to the early part of this century. However, Denny-
Brown & Robertson (1933, 1935) reported that after spinal injury, simultaneous
micturition and defaecation could occur, the implication being that differential
activation of the two excretory systems was dependent on an intact nervous
system, whereas in a paraplegic patient with a damaged spinal cord the two
systems could be turned on simultaneously.

In cats the reflexes operate reciprocally: if both the rectum and the bladder
are distended and maintained under constant volume conditions they exhibit
reciprocal patterns of activity. John Morrison (McMahon & Morrison 1982)
described this phenomenon in the cat and we have seen it as well. Furthermore,
distension of the bladder inhibits defaecation reflexes, and distension of the
colon or rectum inhibits micturition reflexes. So they are reciprocally organized.

This reciprocal inhibition occurs not only with the organ response, but also
with interneuronal pathways in the spinal cord. Neurons activated by rectal
distension are inhibited by bladder distension. Interestingly, vaginal stimulation
seems to mimic rectal stimulation in terms of interneuronal firing; for example,
many interneurons in the cord that receive excitatory input from the colon and
rectum also receive an excitatory input from the vagina and an inhibitory input
from the bladder.

There is also controversy about whether the anal and urethral sphincters are activated simultaneously. This seems to occur under normal conditions, but there are situations where the anal sphincter can be activated separately from the urethral sphincter.

Blaivas: It is our clinical experience that in certain pathological states the sphincters can be activated separately. Most neurologically normal people, when asked, can contract both. The problem is that it is difficult to ask someone to contract one sphincter and relax the other. One usually says 'if you are in the middle of urinating or in the middle of a bowel movement, try to stop'; and clinically they always contract the whole pelvic floor, so I don't think that in a normal person there is the separation.

Brindley: In relation to simultaneous defaecation and micturition, the obvious thing is to ask people whether they can or cannot do this. I can; I think many other people can, but some can't. Why can some people not do it? I relate this to another question. If you ask people: 'can you accelerate micturition by straining?' some people say 'yes, if I strain during micturition, the flow increases'; others say that if they strain during micturition the flow stops. It could be that those who can't defaecate and micturate at the same time are those in whom straining (which is usual in defaecation but unusual in micturition) activates the pelvic floor and they cannot then micturate.

Fowler: I would like to ask Professor de Groat more about the voluntary reflex of micturition in neurologically normal patients. Is it not right to equate voluntary control with connections down the corticospinal pathways, and in fact the only part of the lower urinary tract that has this connection is the urethral sphincter? And is it not generally agreed that the first act of voluntary micturition is inhibition of the urethral sphincter; that is, electrical silence in this sphincter is the first process in the micturition reflex? Would you therefore agree that this is the most likely mechanism whereby voluntary micturition is achieved; and, if so, it's a very interesting neurological example of a mechanism that is achieved by a voluntary inhibition down the corticospinal pathway, rather than an activation?

de Groat: I agree with virtually all these comments. It seems that relaxation of the pelvic floor and the sphincter is the first act of voluntary micturition. Apparently it's the first part of reflex micturition as well. This raises the possibility that voluntary control of the bladder (an organ composed of visceral smooth muscle) is mediated through a complicated indirect pathway from the brain to striated muscle, and then via afferent feedback from the muscle into the spinal cord, to influence the visceral reflex pathway. This scheme does not require the cerebral cortex to control directly visceral reflex mechanisms.

In early experiments by Lapides and co-workers, patients were paralysed with a neuromuscular blocking agent, curare; the patients were then asked to urinate, and could do so voluntarily. They could also voluntarily stop urination (Lapides & Diokno 1976).

Blaivas: It took longer, however.

de Groat: Yes. That implies that the mechanism described by Dr Fowler is probably important, and probably the first event; but these experiments by Lapides suggest that there may also be a cerebral voluntary control of the visceral pathways but that this control may be slower.

Fowler: Surely in the curarized patients one simply did not see the effect in the periphery, because neuromuscular transmission was blocked? This doesn't mean that an inhibitory drive on the anterior horn cells didn't initiate the whole reflex arc. Admittedly, you didn't see the end results, but I don't think that's compelling evidence against there being such a mechanism.

de Groat: That is true. However, you are now suggesting something very unusual, that motoneurons in the spinal cord communicate with the autonomic pathways. I don't know of any evidence for such connections.

Marsden: There is an alternative, namely that the corticomotoneuron pathway to the external sphincter, which has extensive collaterals, will have collaterals onto the pontine micturition centre.

de Groat: I agree. This would be another central mechanism for the voluntary control of visceral reflex pathways.

Fowler: Does urethral sphincter relaxation always precede detrusor contraction?

Nordling: You have to be cautious about the interpretation of the timing because the target organs are different. You measure the EMG instantaneously, whereas the measurement of bladder function is a measurement of bladder *pressure*, and it takes time for the smooth muscles to contract enough to build up the pressure inside the bladder; this happens within several seconds, but nervous activity might go on simultaneously. You have to measure activity in the nerves, to clarify whether it is going on at the same time.

Brindley: Professor de Groat said that the afferents from the bladder travel in the sacral roots. It is important from the clinical point of view to know whether this is exactly true, or only roughly true. This question will surely be answered before long, because in patients with spinal injuries, if one wants to block the micturition reflex and also block reflex low compliance of the bladder, a remedy that has been used very successfully is to cut the sacral posterior roots at the level of the conus medullaris. The posterior roots can be cut here without risk of damaging the anterior roots. It is not so easy to know how far up you are going in the operation, but you can be sure of cutting S5 up to S2 posterior, and not damaging L5. An unknown amount of the S1 posterior root will be cut, but this is unimportant.

In 10 of the 11 patients whom I know to have had this procedure, it has abolished all reflex bladder activity. It greatly improved compliance in both of the two patients in whom this was previously bad. In the one patient in whom the procedure did not wholly succeed, the operation was well done; so evidently the information from the bladder that is responsible for the persisting reflex activity in this one patient is not entirely carried in sacral posterior roots. One possibility is that it is local reflex activity, not a spinal reflex at all. A second possibility is the activity comes via anterior rather than posterior roots. The third possibility is that it comes in higher up, by lumbar or even thoracic roots, perhaps with the sympathetics. But for most patients it seems that what you say is right: all or nearly all bladder reflex afferents enter the cord by sacral posterior roots.

de Groat: There is some evidence in animals that afferents project through the ventral roots to the spinal cord. However, many afferent axons in the ventral roots loop back and enter the spinal cord via the dorsal roots. The large majority of these afferents are unmyelinated.

Another issue regarding the surgical approach to blocking afferent pathways is whether this is too extreme and whether it could be replaced by a more limited destruction of a specific afferent system, such as the unmyelinated afferents. This might be sufficient to reduce the bladder symptoms but not completely block the micturition reflex or interfere with other kinds of afferent projections (like those to the sexual organs) that are carried in the sacral roots. The chemical destruction of a specific axonal population, for example the fibres which mediate certain types of bladder reflexes, may be much better than a surgical destruction of the entire population.

Bourcier: When we are treating female or male patients by physiotherapy, we are surprised to find that whereas men can control their pelvic floor activity properly and stop the urine stream, women have a real problem in controlling this inner musculature. The question is why there is this difference between men and women in the awareness of the uro-genital area.

When we use electrostimulation of the pelvic floor by the vaginal or anal route, the EMG activities recorded are not the same: the increase in activity can be in either the urethral sphincter or anal sphincter. Sometimes we have no effect on the urethral sphincter but a normal activity in the puborectalis. So, stimulation of the same pudendal nerve leads to different responses of the pelvic floor muscle. What does it mean?

de Groat: Regarding the first question, it may be simply that women have a smaller sphincter muscle mass and thus a less effective closure of the bladder outlet than men.

Regarding the differential effects of electrical stimulation on various muscle groups, it may be that there are different electrical thresholds or different distributions of efferent axons within the nerves being stimulated. It is possible that during normal reflex responses, all these muscles are activated simultaneously, but under the artificial conditions of electrical stimulation it may be possible to selectively activate specific subpopulations, particularly at low intensities of electrical stimulation.

Stanton: The earlier question of whether a person can activate one or other sphincter may have a sexually conditioned cause. Men, who stand to void, have no trouble in contracting the anal sphincter and inhibiting the urethral sphincter, whereas when sitting, for either male or female this is much less easy to do, and I suspect most women cannot differentiate between the two.

On Alain Bourcier's statement, it is certainly a clinical observation that women have much greater difficulty contracting the anal sphincter or pelvic floor than men. Perhaps they don't do it adequately, either because of denervation following childbirth or because they don't understand the instruction. Clinically when I ask women to squeeze the examining finger in an anal examination, 50% will do this, 45% will *open* the anal sphincter; the remaining 5% actually squeeze the examining finger on the other hand. I suspect there is also a 'teleological' difference, if that's the right term, that men have been conditioned; because of the increase in urethral resistance they have to work very hard to expel urine, and they develop good sphincter mechanisms because they do interrupt their stream during the act of voiding. Whereas a woman can void by one of three mechanisms. She can just relax the pelvic floor and gravity does the rest, and in the 'developed' countries there is no need ever to contract the urethral sphincter mechanism. In countries where there is simply a hole in the floor, the woman has to aim the urine stream accurately to avoid soiling her feet. The anecdotal evidence is that incontinence is much less common in such people than in women in developed countries, because they are using the sphincter mechanism from childhood, and therefore when it comes to childbirth they are able to overcome much better the damage to the pelvic floor. There is no good epidemiological evidence for this, only anecdotal evidence, unfortunately.

Bourcier: When we we are dealing with nulliparous women complaining of stress incontinence or the pelvic floor relaxation syndrome, the response to the order to 'squeeze on the examining fingers' could be wrong. In this group, the subject, instead of squeezing, pushes down; we have called this false manoeuvre the 'inverted perineal command'. When we ask the patient to push, she produces the same downward pressure with a strong contraction of the abdominal wall. This type of patient cannot correct the control very easily, even after several sessions of biofeedback. When the physician advises her to do exercises at home, she could worsen the problem. In studying the voluntary control of the other striated muscles, we have not found this type of reversed command. In men, this perturbation is very rare.

de Groat: In addition to sex differences, the sphincter muscles, and the motoneurons that innervate them, are also unusual in terms of their anatomy, physiology and pathology. Sphincter motoneurons, in contrast to motoneurons innervating limb muscles, have a dendritic morphology very similar to that of sacral autonomic preganglionic neurons, to which they are linked functionally. These motoneurons send their dendrites rostrocaudally along the spinal cord within the nucleus and also send bundles of transverse dendrites to three areas of the cord. The dendritic bundles may be important in coordinating the activity of the entire population of sphincter motoneurons.

Finally, the pathology is different. In amyotrophic lateral sclerosis, most of the motor neurons in the body that innervate the limbs are destroyed, yet the sphincter motor neurons survive. On the other hand, in Shy–Drager's syndrome, a disorder of the autonomic system, the motoneurons survive but the autonomic cells, along with the sphincter motor neurons, degenerate. So these motoneurons of the sphincter muscles are a special group which in part are like autonomic neurons and in part like traditional motoneurons.

Maggi: I am very interested in the bladder–bladder spinal reflex (i.e. the short-loop reflex). You mentioned that in spinally transected cats the spinal reflex emerges some weeks after sectioning the cord. You also say that in rats this reflex can be observed after placing a ligature at the urethral level. From this, one could argue that the spinal reflex is not normally present and requires some time to develop, perhaps as a result of some neuronal plasticity in the cord.

An alternative explanation is that the reflex exists normally but is inhibited by supraspinal descending pathways. If we apply a painful stimulus in rats at the level of the perineal skin, or at the level of the proximal colon by distension of a balloon, and the bladder is empty, we can record a small bladder contraction in acute spinal rats which is sensitive to hexamethonium; so vesico-excitatory responses are present in acute spinal rats. Do you think this bladder-to-bladder short-loop reflex could be present normally, being inhibited by supraspinal centres, or that it requires time to develop?

de Groat: About 50% of our normal cats have shown this C fibre afferent evoked spinal reflex. However, it is weak in normal animals, but is markedly enhanced several weeks after spinal injury.

The spinal reflex is also detectable in about 30% of anaesthetized intact rats but is small and irregular. It emerges after spinal transection or after partial obstruction of the urethral outlet. The reflex could be under bulbospinal inhibitory control, but the fact that it is not enhanced immediately after spinal cord transection suggests that the inhibition is not prominent. Our view is that the spinal reflex in normal animals is mediated by weak synaptic connections whch are strengthened in certain pathological conditions.

We have also shown that after urethral obstruction there is an expansion of the afferent projections from the bladder to the spinal cord and an increase in the size of the bladder afferent neurons. So there is morphological plasticity, which coincides with the physiological plasticity.

We have seen the opposite change in the diabetic rat. The bladder is hypoactive, the spinal reflex is never observed, and there is a reduction in the number of afferent projections from the bladder to the spinal cord. Thus there appears to be a correlation between the level of bladder activity and the prominence of the spinal short-loop reflex.

We are interested in this reflex because it may have a role in certain pathological conditions. It may function to modulate the supraspinal pathway, which is the principal mechanism for initiating voiding.

Blaivas: I would like to consider the all-or-none concept of the induction of the micturition reflex. This clearly exists in the normal state. In pathological states we see many different things that make bladder contraction wax and wane. That is to say, if a person with a stroke, for example, initiates a detrusor contraction, he or she has the same kind of smooth tracing that one sees in a classic micturition reflex. But in patients with a variety of other conditions there is a tremendous variation in detrusor pressure and flow rate without an apparent contraction of the sphincter. This suggests that many things regulate the detrusor contraction once it starts—other reflexes that might make the contraction fade prematurely, or wax and wane. You showed different kinds of activity in the pontine micturition centre. Do you have any feeling for what kind of reflexes operate during micturition?

de Groat: This is an important issue and something that should be explored. I think there probably are conditions where the reflexes will wax and wane in animals, just as they do in humans, and where there can be premature bladder contractions during the filling phase (termed uninhibited contractions in humans).

For example, the administration of naloxone, an opioid antagonist, to a cat elicits uninhibited waves on the filling curve, just as one sees in patients with hyperactive bladders. We believe that inhibitory mechanisms in the brain and spinal cord contribute to the all-or-none property of the pathway. When these inhibitory mechanisms are deficient, the system begins to generate graded responses, at which point patients will begin to exhibit symptoms, such as frequency and urgency. There are also situations where the micturition reflex pathway becomes weaker and disorganized. We see this during long experiments in the cat. At the beginning of an experiment, with the animal in good condition, the sacral preganglionic neurons appears to be strongly coordinated and exhibit similar patterns of activity, but as the experiment progresses and the animal's condition deteriorates and reflexes weaken, the neurons begin to lose their synchrony. When synchrony is lost, you have the condition you just described. Thus a very effective pathway—one that's strongly activated in an all-or-none fashion—will show good synchrony of neural activity, maintained bladder contractions and good urine flow. But in conditions where the reflex is deficient, neuronal coordination is reduced and voiding is less efficient.

Blaivas: Does that manifest itself as a change in the pressure curve?

de Groat: Yes; you would see a low amplitude pressure curve that would be more prolonged than usual. The best condition is short duration, rapid emptying. The worst condition is very slow emptying. This is a sign of pathology. The system works well when it is tightly coupled. Gap junctions, which Geoff Burnstock talked about in smooth muscle, probably have a role in coordinating the activity of neural populations. Gap junctions have been identified in motor nuclei in the spinal cord, and notably in the phrenic motor nucleus, which controls one muscle, the diaphragm, that functions in an all-or-none manner to produce either inspiration or expiration. These motor neurons are linked together. It is likely that similar connections occur with bladder preganglionic neurons and sphincter motoneurons. The lack of coordination can lead to dysfunction.

Marsden: I have a general question about species differences. I am reminded in this discussion about fictive locomotion—the capacity of the cat and rat to be driven to walk if you stimulate locomotor areas in the brainstem. This has been very difficult to demonstrate in the monkey. All the work that you described, Professor de Groat, inevitably has been carried out in cat and rat so far. How much of it has been replicated in a higher primate species?

Second, you demonstrated clearly that the unmyelinated local spinal reflex is weak in the 'intact' animal; it can only be unearthed by spinal transection. Are you not facing the same problem in your decerebrate animal, or in the anaesthetized animal, which is effectively equal to the decerebrate one, of unearthing the strength of the pontine controlling system but hiding the strength of the cortical controlling system?

de Groat: To take the last point first, certainly the decerebrate unanaesthetized animal is not normal, and the anaesthetized but intact animal is also not normal. However, we have obtained similar results in the two preparations. We presume that the basic reflex pathway in the acute decerebrate animal is similar to that in the intact animal; although decerebration may have eliminated certain modulatory mechanisms it does not appear to change the basic pathway. You will hear later from Paul Tiseo, who is using unanaesthetized rats with catheters in the bladder. He finds certain patterns of bladder activity which are similar to those in the decerebrate unanaesthetized rat and the urethane-anaesthetized rat. If these three preparations produce comparable results in the rat, it seems reasonable to assume that a similar situation exists in the cat.

On the question of species differences, the monkey has been difficult to study because in our experience the anaesthetized monkey doesn't generate micturition responses. However, we can say that the neuroanatomy of the monkey looks very similar to that of the cat in regard to the sphincter motor neurons, the afferent pathways from the bladder, and the preganglionic neurons in the spinal cord. I presume that some, if not all, of the responses that we have described in rats, dogs and cats apply to humans as well.

However, there are species differences. In rat and dog there appears to be a bladder–sphincter dyssynergia in the normal animal. That is, when the bladder contracts there is electrical activity of the external urethral sphincter. This activity doesn't seem to interfere with urination. Simultaneous contraction of the bladder and sphincter is never seen in humans, except in pathological conditions, and is rare in cats.

What is the purpose of having a sphincter contraction at the same time as a bladder contraction, in rat and dog? Perhaps one purpose is to generate isometric contractions of the bladder, and therefore during urine flow there are periodic stops in the flow; this may allow very effective and complete emptying. This may be more important in four-legged animals where gravity contributes very little to the voiding mechanism. At any rate, the rat appears to have bladder–sphincter dyssynergia, yet it empties its bladder very effectively. So not everything seen in animals will be found in humans.

Christensen: Dogs, and also cats, use urination for another function than simply to eliminate urine; they mark their hunting territories in this way, and this suggests that they must have a requirement for a special function that primates presumably lack.

As a gastroenterologist, I would like to know how much of what you told us about the pontine micturition centre can be applied to the concept of a central defaecation centre. Is it the same centre, or is it a different one?

de Groat: Jack Krier and I examined reflex control of the distal bowel in cat, and found it to be quite different from the control of the bladder (de Groat & Krier 1976, 1978). The defaecation reflex, at least in the cat, is organized entirely in the lumbosacral spinal cord and is triggered by C fibre afferents. After acute spinal cord transection the reflex pathway remains functional. There is brain control over this pathway, but it is apparently much less important than the spinal cord mechanisms. The defaecation reflex is also dependent in part on peripheral mechanisms, in the myenteric plexus, and on local ganglionic reflexes. The sympathetic pathways to the bowel are also more independent of central control than the sympathetic pathways to the bladder. Thus in paraplegic patients bowel problems are less severe than bladder problems.

In summary, urination is a centrally mediated event that depends on the brain and spinal cord, whereas defaecation has more prominent peripheral control mechanisms.

Swash: A fundamental problem remains about the relationship between the autonomic and somatic nervous systems. I have to say that if I were designing the system, I wouldn't design it the way you described it! It seems a clumsy way of setting the system up, with the detrusor muscle being governed from the top end in the brainstem, and the Onuf nucleus being the switch-off mechanism at the bottom end, albeit triggered from the top by a fast-conducting pathway. It seems difficult to conceive of a control system in which there is not some sort of communication at a distal level, say between the Onuf nucleus and the autonomic system in the sacral cord, because if there is to be adequate control of the Onuf nucleus there must be some input from the distal part of the system to modulate it. We know that the muscle fibres of the external urethral and anal sphincters are in continuous contraction; that activity must be modulated and controlled in some way.

de Groat: What is the basis for that continuous contraction of the sphincter muscles? My reading of the literature, and our studies, indicate that continuous contraction is mediated by reflexes that are triggered by afferents from the bladder and the bowel, and maybe even from the sphincter muscle itself. When the dorsal roots are cut, the activity of these sphincter muscles disappears, so it's generated within the spinal cord. The activity remains in paraplegic animals, so the communication that you describe *is* occurring at the spinal level.

Swash: It is lost in tabes dorsalis as well, and there are a few muscle spindles in the external anal and external urethral sphincter muscles, so there is a distal sensory input from these muscles.

de Groat: So it's designed as you would like it to be?

Swash: It is and it isn't! There must be communication somewhere between the autonomic nervous system and the external sphincter muscle, at a spinal level, to make it work properly. We must also put into the equation the function of the internal sphincter muscles, the innervation of which is obscure at present. They are probably not directly innervated, except by the mechanisms that Geoff Burnstock discussed earlier, namely the close relationship of beaded terminal nerve fibres with the syncytium of smooth muscle cells.

de Groat: In the cat, the internal sphincter (i.e., the bladder neck and proximal urethra) receives a prominent input from the sympathetic hypogastric pathway. This pathway is activated by a spinal reflex mechanism when the bladder is slowly filled. The reflex consists of bladder afferents which pass in the pelvic nerve to the sacral spinal cord, and there interact with propriospinal neurons which carry information to the lumbar cord, and then activate sympathetic efferent pathways passing back to the bladder (see Fig. 3, p 32). This is a local sacral–lumbar reflex which provides negative feedback to the bladder, producing inhibition of bladder smooth muscle, inhibition in bladder ganglia (adrenergic inhibition of cholinergic transmission), and finally activation of the outlet. So there are three components to this reflex, and all three promote urine storage. The reflex pathway is turned off by the brainstem during micturition. The pontine micturition centre in the brainstem also turns off the striated sphincter pathway, and turns on the parasympathetic pathway. It is very nicely organized, just as you might have put it together! In the 'spinal' patient or animal, this sympathetic pathway cannot be turned off, so it continues to promote the storage of urine as the bladder fills. This can account for some of the bladder problems in paraplegic patients.

Marsden: Is that design adequate to meet your purposes, Dr Swash?

Swash: Not really! I still think there has to be a distal connection. Two other points interest me about this. One is detrusor–sphincter dyssynergia, and the other, perhaps, the analogy in the anal system where there is paradoxical contraction of the anal sphincter muscle. In most of those patients, despite the recognized associations with CNS disease, there is no obvious clinical disorder. If there is no discernible lesion in the central nervous system, for example in the spinal cord, there must be one somewhere else, perhaps in the sacral autonomic or peripheral somatic nervous systems.

Blaivas: Didn't Elbadawi show junctions between autonomic and somatic nerve fibres very near the urethra?

de Groat: Geoff Burnstock has pictures of that.

Swash: That's the second point I was going to make. There is a copious innervation of the intramural striated muscle fibres, which are even more extraordinary than the ordinary urethral and anal voluntary sphincter muscles. There must be some synergy there between the autonomic and somatic nervous systems.

de Groat: In Geoff Burnstock's studies, that innervation is most prominent in patients with some pathology.

Burnstock: Yes, in patients with sacral spinal injury.

de Groat: It is clear that peripheral nerves can talk to one another. We have seen this in experiments where we were electrically stimulating bladder strips from rats. In these conditions, the acetylcholine system can modulate noradrenaline release, and, conversely, noradrenaline modulates acetylcholine release. The adrenergic and cholinergic fibres lie close together and presumably interact. We also showed that sympathetic adrenergic input to bladder ganglia can inhibit cholinergic transmission, so at the ganglionic level there is interaction between inhibitory and excitatory pathways (de Groat & Booth 1980). In addition, in the spinal cord, there are mechanisms that coordinate the sympathetic and parasympathetic systems. Thus there are multiple sites of interaction in the reflex pathways. The transmitters presumably interact at the smooth muscle, and at the respective nerve terminals; they interact within the ganglia of the bladder; and they can interact within the central nervous system. It makes sense to coordinate these systems at all levels.

Marsden: Where is the actual termination of the bulbospinal pathway? Is it onto interneurons?

de Groat: This still has to be resolved. As I discussed (p 37), Holstege injected tracer substances into the pontine micturition centre and showed that the tracer was distributed in the general area of the autonomic nucleus. The question remains whether there are direct bulbospinal monosynaptic connections with preganglionic neurons, or whether there are interneurons in the autonomic area which then project to the preganglionic cells. I have indirect, pharmacological evidence to suggest that it's not a direct monosynaptic connection, but an interneuronal pathway (de Groat 1976).

Marsden: The same would be true for the afferents coming into the spinal cord. Once you have input into the spinal interneuronal pool, you have every opportunity for interconnection at any level of any system.

de Groat: We have been using the c-*fos* oncogene to analyse connections within the spinal cord made by afferent pathways from the urinary bladder. Recently it was shown in other laboratories that activation of somatic afferents by painful stimuli turns on the c-*fos* oncogene and increases the levels of c-*fos* proteins in second-order neurons in the spinal cord. There remains the question of whether that occurs only at the first synapse, or also at second- and third-order synapses along the pathway. At any rate, we have shown that in the rat, bladder pain increases the levels of c-*fos* protein in some sacral preganglionic neurons. This suggests that some of these neurons may receive direct monosynaptic inputs from the bladder nociceptive afferents. Such a pathway could mediate the short latency spinal reflex, in the rat.

Swash: This neural system may not be unique. Clinical pathological observations, for example in progressive autonomic failure, show that the abductor muscle of the larynx is selectively denervated. These patients have a peculiar snoring breathing pattern during sleep, because the laryngeal folds are passively opposed. The vagus nerve therefore is another system in which there are autonomic and special visceral and somatic efferents, in functional relationship to each other. The cricopharyngeal muscle at the oral end of the gut is in continuous activity as well. There is also an interesting interaction between the voluntary striated and smooth involuntary muscles in the oesophagus. During swallowing the upper striated part of the oesophagus discharges an oral–anal wave of contraction, that is smoothly taken up by the lower unstriated part of the oesophagus to transport the bolus by peristalsis into the stomach.

de Groat: I believe that the movement of solid material into and out of the gut requires similar mechanisms. It requires somato-visceral integration at the proximal end and viscero-somatic integration at the distal end. We can learn a lot about the integration and coordination of visceral and somatic systems by studying swallowing, defaecation or urination.

Brindley: The coordination of sphincter relaxation with bladder contraction depends, of course, on the central nervous system. On the question of whether any of it can be done by the spinal cord in man, the evidence is strongly against. If you look at the pattern of reflex micturition in tetraplegics in whom the whole lumbosacral cord and most of the thoracic cord are intact, the common situation is true active detrusor–sphincter dyssynergia; when the bladder contracts, the pelvic floor *actively* contracts. In the minority of such patients, the pelvic floor has tone, which is unchanged during micturition. But I have never seen, or heard of, a tetraplegic patient showing relaxation of the pelvic floor during bladder contraction.

Christensen: Thank you for mentioning the oesophagus, Dr Swash! I would make one point and ask one question. The striated muscle of the oesophagus contains a large number of VIP-staining fibres which surround muscle cells. These are not spindles, but they look as if they are innervating striated muscle cells, much as you have described in the urethra.

My question concerns the size of the motor unit in the urethral striated muscle. In the oesophagus the motor units are very small, less than 10 muscle cells per nerve fibre. Do we know anything about the size of motor units in urethral striated muscle?

Burnstock: They are surely small too?

Fowler: Yes.

Burnstock: This is a very interesting close parallel, then. Someone should put a microelectrode into these striated fibres and examine the actions of VIP in both preparations.

Swash: It would be easy in the oesophagus.

Burnstock: Professor de Groat, I am intrigued that there is a reflex that emerges in pathological situations. What does this mean in evolutionary terms? What advantage in terms of survival could this have?

de Groat: It's a reserve! Why indeed should we have an entire population of afferent fibres that are inactive except under pathological conditions? It's intriguing that the afferent pathway for the spinal micturition reflex in cats is the same as the 'silent' afferent group—that is, the silent C fibres. What would be the function of C fibre evoked reflexes? Let's consider a situation where the bladder is infected or irritated. The spinal pathway can be activated when there is a need to empty the bladder completely, and perhaps to make it hyperactive over a period of time when there is need to eliminate irritating substances. The spinal reflex could also help to reduce the urine volume under conditions where there is partial obstruction, and where the bladder has to contract more forcefully to pass urine by that obstruction. Thus an auxiliary 'motor' comes into play to turn on the bladder and to make it contract more strongly. There is redundancy in the nervous system, which may be held in abeyance for special situations when a stronger response is needed.

Blaivas: It's not a 'stronger' response. What is happening is that the sphincter is contracting and the pressure is going up. It's the same bladder, contracting the same way, against a different resistance.

References

de Groat WC 1976 Mechanisms underlying recurrent inhibition in the sacral parasympathetic outflow to the urinary bladder. J Physiol (Lond) 257:503–513

de Groat WC, Booth AM 1980 Inhibition and facilitation in parasympathetic ganglia. Fed Proc 39:2990–2996

de Groat WC, Krier J 1976 An electrophysiological study of the sacral parasympathetic pathway to the colon of the cat. J Physiol (Lond) 260:425–445

de Groat WC, Krier J 1978 The sacral parasympathetic reflex pathway regulating colon motility and defaecation in the cat. J Physiol (Lond) 276:481–500

Denny-Brown D, Robertson EG 1933 On the physiology of micturition. Brain 56:149–190

Denny-Brown D, Robertson EG 1935 An investigation of the nervous control of defaecation. Brain 58:256–310

Lapides J, Diokno AC 1976 Urine transport, storage and micturition. In: Lapides J (ed) Fundamentals of urology. Saunders, Philadelphia, p 190–220

McMahon SB, Morrison JFB 1982 Factors that determine the excitability of parasympathetic reflexes to the bladder. J Physiol (Lond) 332:35–43

Functional anatomy of the female lower urinary tract and pelvic floor

John O. L. DeLancey

Division of Gynecology, Department of Obstetrics and Gynecology, University of Michigan Medical School, 1500 E. Medical Center Drive, Ann Arbor, Michigan 48109-0718, USA

Abstract. Stress continence depends upon three factors: proximal urethral support, vesical neck closure, and urethral contractility. The position of the vesical neck is not static but mobile and under voluntary control. Its support depends upon connections of the urethrovaginal endopelvic fascia to the medial aspect of the levator ani. In addition, these fasciae are attached to the arcus tendineus fasciae pelvis which supports the urethra during levator relaxation, and probably during stress. Levator contraction supports the proximal urethra and also pulls the vesical neck anteriorly against a band of endopelvic fascia which is suspended between the arcus tendinei, compressing it closed. Relaxation of the muscles allows the vesical neck to descend, and facilitates its opening. The connective tissue and smooth muscle of the trigonal ring encircles the vesical neck's lumen, and may contribute to closure of this area. The striated urogenital sphincter muscle can contract to assist in maintaining continence in *continent* women whose vesical neck is not competent. It has a circular sphincteric portion from 20 to 60% of urethral length. From 60 to 80% it has a considerable bulk of muscle which forms an arch at the perineal membrane that would compress the urethra from above.

1990 Neurobiology of Incontinence. Wiley, Chichester (Ciba Foundation Symposium 151) p 57–76

'In our endeavour to understand reality we are somewhat like a man trying to understand the mechanism of a closed watch. He sees the face and the moving hands, even hears its ticking, but he has no way of opening the case. If he is ingenious he may form some picture of a mechanism which could be responsible for all the things he observes, but he may never be quite sure his picture is the only one which could explain his observations. He will never be able to compare his picture with the real mechanism.' (Einstein & Infield 1938.)

With this metaphor, Einstein has beautifully captured the problem of learning how something works, and this paradigm can be applied to the problem of studying the urinary continence mechanism. Our indirect observations of function (analogous to the clock's hand motion and ticking) include pressure measurements, electromyography, and radiographic observation. As our technological ability to study these parameters has increased during the last two decades, many observations have come to light which do not agree with the mechanical structure of the continence mechanism previously thought to be responsible for urinary control.

Unlike Einstein's poor horologist, who is denied the chance to examine the inner workings of his watch, we have the opportunity to inspect the mechanism which we wish to study and can directly compare its mechanics with our functional findings. It is the purpose of this chapter to examine the structure of the urinary continence mechanism in the female as it relates to clinical and physiological observations.

The phenomenon of stress urinary incontinence

Stress urinary incontinence is a common problem in women, although it is rare in men. It occurs when a defective 'sphincteric mechanism' is unable to withstand the rise in intravesical pressure which occurs when increases in intra-abdominal pressure compress the bladder. In continent women, increases in abdominal pressure would overwhelm the normal resting pressure within the urethra, were it not for a concomitant rise in intra-urethral pressure (Enhorning 1961). The normal urethral pressure rise during a cough maintains a positive pressure gradient during this event and prevents urine loss. This rise in urethral pressure is lost during a cough in patients with stress incontinence (Hilton & Stanton 1983, Bump et al 1988) because of poor urethral support. The structural hypothesis proposed to explain this observation contends that the proximal urethra and vesical neck are normally within the abdomen, above some theoretical floor, where they would be compressed by intra-abdominal pressure to the same extent as the bladder. In this paradigm, stress incontinence would occur if the urethra fell below this 'floor', and lay outside the region where it could be compressed shut by abdominal pressure.

Many theories have been proposed to explain the mechanical alterations associated with stress incontinence. They are usually based on the idea that there is a ligamentous connection between the urethra and pubic bones (pubo-urethral ligament) which would hold the urethra above a 'floor' where it can be influenced by increases in intra-abdominal pressure. Damage to these ligaments allowing the vesical neck to drop below the floor would cause stress incontinence. Although this is an attractive hypothesis, it does not fit the available clinical facts. Specifically, it does not explain neurophysiological observations that stress incontinence is associated with denervation of the urethral sphincter and pelvic floor (Snooks et al 1985, Smith et al 1989a,b) and that there is not a good relationship between the position or the urethra and the problem of stress incontinence (Fantl et al 1986). The following morphological description examines the relationship between pelvic floor structure and clinical observations of continence.

Anatomical materials

Table 1 summarizes the anatomical material upon which these findings are based. A diversity of observational methods has consciously been used to avoid artifacts in any one technique. In addition, care has been used to avoid spatial distortions involved in embalming and dissection, by emphasizing serial-section study on specimens fixed by immersion.

Structure and function of the continence mechanism

Vesical neck support and continence

Clinical observations (Fig. 1).   The support of the vesical neck is dynamic rather than static, as was previously thought. The vesical neck descends when the urine stream begins and is elevated at the end of micturition, a motion which has been ascribed to the levator ani muscles (Muellner 1951). In addition, the vesical neck and proximal urethra lie some 2–3 cm above the lower border of the pubic symphysis (Noll & Hutch 1969)—above the level of the attachment of the pubo-urethral ligaments. These observations indicate that structures in addition to the pubo-urethral ligaments must be involved in vesical neck support.

Anatomy.   In considering the support of the vesical neck it is important to recognize that the urethra and anterior vaginal wall are not two separate adjacent structures like the gall bladder and transverse colon, but are structures embedded

TABLE 1   Anatomical materials

Serial histological sections[a]
Eight individuals, 0–37 years
Serial whole pelvis sections
Four individuals, 14–33 years
Fixed cadaver dissections
15 individuals, 45–86 years
Unembalmed cadaver dissections
49 individuals, 0–79 years
Clinical radiographic studies
48 individuals, 26–78 years

[a]Available to the author from Dr Thomas Oelrich, who prepared these sections for his study of the striated urogenital sphincter muscle in the female (Oelrich 1983). Sections contained at least urethra, vesical neck, vagina, levator ani, pubic bones, endopelvic connective tissue; and, at most, the whole pelvis.

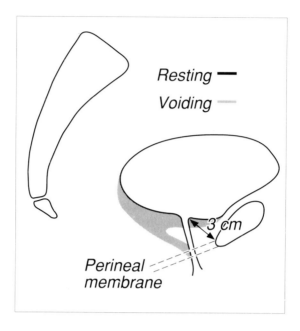

FIG. 1. Topography and mobility of the normal proximal urethra and vesical neck, based upon resting and voiding in normal women. (Reprinted from DeLancey 1990 with permission of J. B. Lippincott Co.)

in a single malleable mass, similar to adjacent nuclei in the brain. They are bound within the endopelvic connective tissue which unites them. Therefore, the support of the urethra and vesical neck depends upon the support of the endopelvic fascia and anterior vaginal wall. It is these tissues, along with their lateral attachments, that we shall refer to functionally as the 'urethral supports'.

Three structures are involved in the normal support of the proximal urethra and vesical neck (DeLancey 1989, Richardson et al 1981), namely the arcus tendineus fasciae pelvis (white line), the levator ani, and the endopelvic fascia and anterior vaginal wall.

The arcus tendineus fasciae pelvis is a band of dense regular connective tissue which is suspended between the pubis and ischial spine (Fig. 2). Its point of origin lies 1 cm above the inferior border of the pubis, and 1 cm from the midline. Near the pubis, it lies on the inner surface of the medial levator ani (pubococcygeus-puborectalis portion) while posteriorly it lies over the obturator internus muscle. In this dorsal region it fuses with the origin of the iliococcygeus muscle (the arcus tendineus *levatoris ani*). Portions of the smooth muscle and inert connective tissue which make up the endopelvic connective tissue attach the anterior vaginal wall and urethra to the white line in its anterior half. This connection is densest at the urethrovesical junction and would limit the amount of downward excursion which can take place in these tissues, and would to some extent explain static support of the upper urethra and vesical neck. These fascial attachments of the urethral supports, however, form only a part of vesical neck support.

As previously mentioned, the medial portions of the levator ani muscles pass lateral to the arcus tendineus fasciae pelvis. Just caudal to the arcus, and above the level of the perineal membrane (= urogenital diaphragm), the endopelvic fascia surrounding the wall of the vagina attaches to the margin of the levator ani which borders the urogenital hiatus (pubovaginalis portion of the levator ani) opposite the upper half of the urethra and forms the muscular attachment of the urethral supports (DeLancey 1988) (Figs. 3 and 4). The medial portion of the levator ani muscles has been shown to have a substantial quantity of Type I striated muscle (Gosling et al 1981). This specialization permits the constant tone which has been observed in the levators (Parks et al 1962) and would reinforce the concept that they can be important to vesical neck support even when the muscle is not wilfully contracted. There is no attachment of the levators to the urethra in the female, and it is because of the intimate union of the urethra, endopelvic connective tissue and vaginal wall that the connection of these latter two structures to the levators allows the activity of this muscle to assist in the control of vesical neck position.

Functional correlates.   Several observations about patients with stress urinary incontinence can provide physiological ideas against which our anatomical observations can be tested. Although most would agree intuitively that *support* of the vesical neck is important to stress incontinence, when one looks at the data on the relationship between vesical neck *position* (as determined by urethral axis or radiography) and continence, there is not a direct relationship between position and sphincteric function (Fantl et al 1981, 1986). This is exemplified by patients who have significant cysto-urethrocele where the urethra is outside of the introitus, but are frequently continent. This implies that it is not the actual *position* of the urethra relative to some fixed floor which is important.

The importance of vesical neck support but not of position can be explained by looking at the anatomical relationship between the urethra and its surrounding tissues. Rather than the urethra piercing some floor, above which it is influenced by abdominal pressure and below which it is not, it is itself a part of the pelvic floor. Its function is determined not only by its own contractility but also by the impact of structures which surround it.

As the pressure in the abdomen rises, it forces the pelvic viscera downward. It may be that it is the impact of the urethra against the urethral supports which favours its closure, rather than that any specific position is important. These issues deserve further consideration in our study of the way in which this mechanism works. The relative support of the urethra and bladder is important. If the bladder is poorly supported, as is true with a large cystocele, then it is

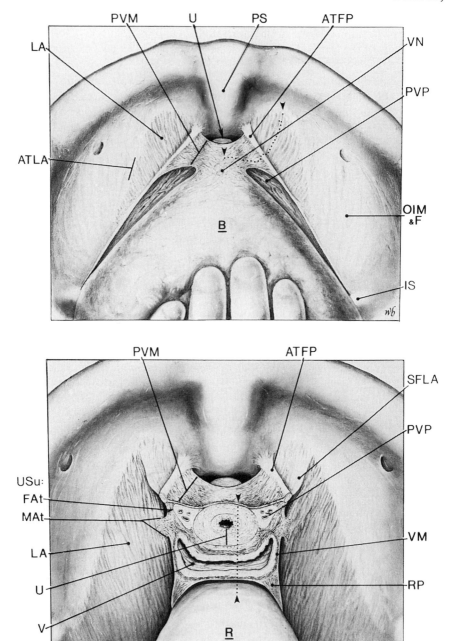

FIGS. 2 & 3 *(captions opposite)*

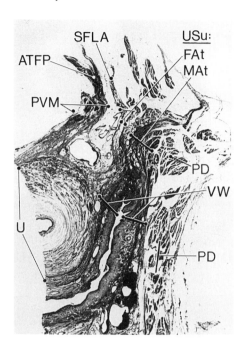

FIG. 4. Cross-section of the urethra (U), vaginal wall (VW), and levator ani muscles (LA) from the right half of the pelvis taken just below the vesical neck at approximately the same level as shown in Fig. 3. The pubovesical muscles (PVM) can be seen anterior to the urethra and the periurethral vascular plexus (PVP), and attach to the arcus tendineus fasciae pelvis (ATFP). Urethral supports (USu) run underneath (dorsal to) the urethra and vessels. Some of its fibres (MAt) attach to the muscle of the levator ani (LA) while others (FAt) are derived from the vaginal wall (VW) and vaginal surface of the urethra (U) and attach to the superior fascia of the levator ani (SFLA). (Reprinted from DeLancey 1989 with permission of Alan R. Liss.)

FIG. 2. Space of Retzius (drawn from cadaver dissection). Pubovesical muscle (PVM) can be seen going from vesical neck (VN) to arcus tendineus fasciae pelvis (ATFP) and running over the paraurethral vascular plexus (PVP). ATLA, arcus tendineus levator ani; B, bladder; IS, ischial spine; LA, levator ani muscles; OIM&F, obturator internus muscle and fascia; PS, pubic symphysis; and U, urethra. Dotted lines indicate plane of section of Figs. 3 and 4. (Reprinted from DeLancey 1989 with permission of Alan R. Liss.)

FIG. 3. Cross-section of the urethra (U), vagina (V), arcus tendineus fasciae pelvis (ATFP), and superior fascia of levator ani (SFLA) just below the vesical neck (drawn from cadaver dissection). Pubovesical muscles (PVM) lie anterior to urethra and anterior and superior to para-urethral vascular plexus (PVP). The urethral supports (USu) ('the pubo-urethral ligaments') attach the vagina and vaginal surface of the urethra to the levator ani muscles (MAt, muscular attachment) and to the superior fascia of the levator ani (FAt, fascial attachment). Additional abbreviations: R, rectum; RP, rectal pillar; and VM, vaginal wall muscularis. (Reprinted from DeLancey 1989 with permission of Alan R. Liss.)

difficult for increases in abdominal pressure to raise intravesical pressure because the bladder simply expands below the introitus. Therefore the urethra in this situation need only be supported somewhat better than the bladder, explaining continence when the urethra is poorly supported, but better supported than the bladder.

Vesical neck mobility and voiding

Clinical observations.   Because support of the urethra is so important, one would at first expect that strong fibrous tissues would fix it immovably in place, yet the structural arrangement described above contains a connection to the levator ani. This muscular attachment is responsible for the vesical neck motion associated with the initiation of micturition (Muellner 1951). The importance of this mobility is supported by the clinical fact that fixing the urethra immovably in place, as is done during some urethral suspension operations, can sometimes be associated with voiding difficulty, while reattaching the supportive tissues to their normal lateral attachments is not (Richardson et al 1981).

Anatomy.   Some further structural features of this region also favour this concept. The point of flexion between the upper mobile urethra and the lower fixed portion of the urethra has been referred to as the knee of the urethra (Westby et al 1982) and occurs at 56% of urethral length. This is the area where it becomes fixed to the pubic bones by the perineal membrane, with the attachment to the levator ani muscles lying just cephalad to this point (DeLancey 1986).

Within the space of Retzius there exist bilateral bands of connective tissue which attach the vesical neck to the two arcus tendinei anteriorly and may influence vesical neck closure. They are the structures anatomists refer to as the pubovesical ligaments (pubovesical muscles, Figs. 3 & 4) and are separated from the urethral supports by a small plexus of vessels (DeLancey 1989). Olsen et al (1980) refers to them as the anterior suspensory mechanism of the vesical neck and feels that they restrain anterior displacement of the vesical neck and favour its closure when the urethra is in its normal high retropubic position. The positions of these tissues and the mobility of the vesical neck raise the question of whether the location of the vesical neck relative to this restraining band has a role in the closure of the vesical neck in its normal high position, and in the facilitation of voiding when it falls back away from the pubic bones.

Sphincteric function

So far, I have presented the anatomy of this region as if control of vesical neck position was the only factor important to stress continence. Although support of the lower urinary tract is undoubtedly important to urinary continence during stress, it is not the only important factor when pressure in the abdomen rises. Two observations help to reveal what these other factors are. First, in patients whose vesical neck is open at rest, or closes poorly, stress incontinence can occur despite normal support (McGuire 1981). Second, patients having excision of the distal urethra during radical vulvectomy can develop stress incontinence postoperatively despite a lack of change in urethral support or resting sphincteric function (Reid et al 1990). These observations demonstrate the importance of the sphincteric function of the lower urinary tract itself, both the internal and external sphincteric mechanisms.

Topography (Fig. 5).   Anatomically, the spatial relationships of the lower urinary tract sphincteric mechanism can be understood by dividing the urethral lumen into five equal parts, each being 20% of the urethral *luminal* length (DeLancey 1986). The first fifth of the urethral lumen is actually surrounded by the vesical neck and not the urethral wall and constitutes the internal sphincter. This is the region which is inadequate in Type III stress incontinence (see below). The distal 20% of the urethra is simply a fibrous nozzle, and is

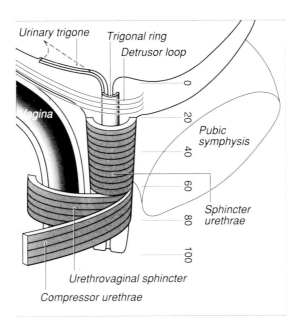

FIG. 5.   Diagrammatic representation showing the component parts of the internal and external sphincteric mechanisms and their locations. The sphincter urethrae, urethrovaginal sphincter and compressor urethrae are all parts of the striated urogenital sphincter muscle. (Reprinted from DeLancey 1990 with permission of J. B. Lippincott Co.)

devoid of sphincteric function. The area from 20 to 80% of urethral length comprises the external sphincter. It contains the striated urogenital sphincter muscle, a scant amount of circular smooth muscle, considerable longitudinal smooth muscle, and the other elements of the urethral wall (blood vessels, mucosa, and connective tissue).

Internal sphincter.   Observation of an open vesical neck in patients with stress incontinence was made by Howard Kelly in his original description of this condition. Documentation of the clinical importance of this condition as differentiated from stress incontinence caused by poor urethral support was made by McGuire (1981), and the condition was termed Type III stress incontinence. In these individuals the proximal centimetre of the urethra has poor intrinsic closure. This can occur because of either defective innervation to the region, or surgical trauma.

Lying in this region are two tissues which surround the proximal centimetre of the urethra. These are the detrusor loop and the trigonal ring. The former is a localized loop of detrusor muscle which forms a U-shaped loop open posteriorly and courses anterior to the vesical neck. A localized innervation of the base of the bladder may allow this to function in a different way from the muscle of the dome (Elbadawi 1988). In addition, the trigonal ring is also found in this region (Huisman 1983). Woodburne (1968) has further reported a high concentration of elastin here which may contribute to closure. Finally, as discussed previously, mechanical factors may favour compression of-the vesical neck here.

External sphincter.   Although continence at the level of the vesical neck is ideal, only 50% of women proved to be continent always maintain continence at this level (Versi et al 1986). In the other 50% of individuals, urine sometimes enters the urethra during a cough. In these women, the sphincteric mechanism below this level is the difference between continence and incontinence. Previously this mechanism was felt to be unimportant because *dorsal* incision during Spence diverticulectomy of the distal urethra did not cause incontinence. Excision of the distal urethra, during radical vulvectomy, however, has been found to be highly associated with incontinence (Reid et al 1990).

Understanding the difference to continence between incising the ventral urethral wall and excising the urethra illustrates the importance of the recent contribution of Oelrich (1983), which corrected significant errors in the description of the striated urogenital sphincter muscle in the female. In the distal portion of the urethra, the sphincter is formed by two arch-shaped bands of muscle, the compressor urethrae and the urethrovaginal sphincter. Incision of the dorsal urethra would not affect these muscles, but excision of the distal urethra would.

TABLE 2 Hypotheses concerning function of elements of the urinary continence mechanism

Structure	Hypothesized function
Levator ani	Tonic contraction maintains high position of vesical neck and may contract during cough to support vesical neck. Relaxes to change position of vesical neck relative to pubovesical muscles to facilitate micturition
Endopelvic connection to arcus tendineus	Assists levators in support and limits the downward excursion of the vesical neck when the levators are relaxed, or overcome during cough
Pubovesical muscles	May facilitate vesical neck opening by pulling on vesical neck when levators relax and may contribute to closure when they are contracted
Internal sphincteric mechanism	Maintains vesical neck closure at rest and is necessary in addition to normal support for continence during cough
Extrinsic sphincteric mechanism	Resting tone contributes to resting urethral pressure, and contraction prevents incontinence when marginally compensated proximal mechanism leaks

Summary

The urinary continence mechanism (Table 2) is a logical one which involves the interplay of the urethral supports and the internal and external sphincteric mechanisms. The pelvic floor musculature has an important role in the urinary continence mechanism. An appreciation of the relationship between structure and clinical function should help us to interpret the role of damage to the pelvic floor muscles and connective tissue in the development of stress urinary incontinence. Further, knowledge of the role of normal proximal urethral mobility in voiding may permit us to minimize the voiding dysfunction which sometimes accompanies urethral suspension operations which fix the urethra immovably in place.

Acknowledgements

The author would like to thank Dr Thomas Oelrich for the use of his histological materials, Mr Arthur Rathburn for assistance with specimen preparation, and the Department of Anatomy, University of Michigan Medical School, for the use of their dissection facilities.

References

Bump RC, Copeland WE, Hurt WG, Fantl AJ 1988 Dynamic urethral pressure/profilometry pressure transmission ratio determinations in stress-incontinent and stress-continent subjects. Am J Obstet Gynecol 159:749–755

DeLancey JOL 1986 Correlative study of paraurethral anatomy. Obstet Gynecol 68:91–97

DeLancey JOL 1988 Structural aspects of the extrinsic continence mechanism. Obstet Gynecol 72:296–301

DeLancey JOL 1989 Pubovesical ligament: a separate structure from the urethral supports (pubo-urethral ligaments). Neurourol Urodynam 8:53–61

DeLancey JOL 1990 Anatomy and physiology of urinary continence. Clin Obstet Gynecol, in press

Einstein A, Infield L 1938 The evolution of physics. Simon & Schuster, New York

Elbadawi A 1988 Neuromuscular mechanisms of micturition. In: Yalla SV et al (eds) Neurourology and urodynamics. Macmillan, New York, p 3–35

Enhorning G 1961 Simultaneous recording of the intravesical and intra-urethral pressures. Acta Obstet Gynecol Obstet Suppl 276:1–68

Fantl JA, Hurt WG, Beachley MC, Bosch HA, Konerding KF, Smith PJ 1981 Bead-chain cystourethrogram: an evaluation. Obstet Gynecol 58:237–240.

Fantl JA, Hurt WG, Bump RC, Dunn LJ, Choi SC 1986 Urethral axis and sphincteric function. Am J Obstet Gynecol 155:554–558

Gosling JA, Dixon JS, Critchley HOD, Thompson SA 1981 A comparative study of the human external sphincter and periurethral levator ani muscles. Br J Urol 53:35–41

Hilton P, Stanton SL 1983 Urethral pressure measurement by microtransducer: the results in symptom-free women and in those with genuine stress urinary incontinence. Br J Obstet Gynaecol 90:919–933

Huisman AB 1983 Aspects on the anatomy of the female urethra with special relation to urinary continence. Contrib Gynecol Obstet 10:1–31

McGuire EJ 1981 Urodynamic findings in patients after failure of stress incontinence operations. Prog Clin Biol Res 78:351–360

Muellner SR 1951 Physiology of micturition. J Urol 65:805–810

Noll LE, Hutch JA 1969 The SCIPP line—an aid in interpreting the voiding lateral cystourethrogram. Obstet Gynecol 33:680–689

Oelrich TM 1983 The striated urogenital sphincter muscle in the female. Anat Rec 205:223–232

Olsen KP, Walter S, Hald T 1980 Anterior bladder suspension defects in the female: radiological classification with urodynamic evaluation. Anatomically corrective operations. Acta Obstet Gynecol Scand 59:535–542

Parks AG, Porter NH, Melzak J 1962 Experimental study of the reflex mechanism controlling muscles of the pelvic floor. Dis Colon Rectum 5:407–414

Reid GC, DeLancey JOL, Hopkins MP, Roberts JA, Morley GW 1990 Urinary incontinence following radical vulvectomy. Obstet Gynecol, in press

Richardson AC, Edmonds PB, Williams NL 1981 Treatment of stress urinary incontinence due to paravaginal fascial defect. Obstet Gynecol 57:357–362

Smith ARB, Hosker GL, Warrell DW 1989a The role of partial denervation of the pelvic floor in the aetiology of genitourinary prolapse and stress incontinence of urine. A neurophysiological study. Br J Obstet Gynaecol 96:24–28

Smith ARB, Hosker GL, Warrell DW 1989b The role of pudendal nerve damage in the aetiology of genuine stress incontinence in women. Br J Obstet Gynaecol 96:29–32

Snooks SJ, Badenoch DF, Tiptaft RC, Swash M 1985 Perineal nerve damage in genuine stress urinary incontinence. Br J Urol 57:422–426

Versi E, Cardozo LD, Studd JWW, Brincat M, O'Dowd TM, Cooper DJ 1986 Internal urinary sphincter in maintenance of female continence. Br Med J 292:166–167

Westby M, Asmussen M, Ulmsten U 1982 Location of maximum intraurethral pressure related to urogenital diaphragm in the female subject as studied by simultaneous urethrocystometry and voiding urethrocystography. Am J Obstet Gynecol 144:408–412

Woodburne RT 1968 Anatomy of the bladder and bladder outlet. J Urol 100:474–487

DISCUSSION

Bartolo: I am interested in the question of whether the pressure acting on the urethra has any sphincteric action. Sid Phillips some years ago proposed a similar hypothesis on rectal continence, suggesting that a flutter valve might be responsible for anorectal continence (Phillips & Edwards 1965). Then Sir Alan Parks developed his hypothesis that continence was related to the anorectal angle and a flap valve mechanism. Nick Read and I have worked quite independently, looking at these theories, and Duthie (1971) has also criticized Phillips' hypothesis, showing that anatomically the anal sphincter was below the pelvic floor, so there was no way in which intra-abdominal pressure could act on that sphincter. Therefore a sphincteric mechanism rather than a flutter valve must be involved.

We (Bartolo et al 1986) looked at the anorectal angle, because Parks had said that anorectal continence is not so much sphincteric, but related to the fact that the anterior rectal wall was driven down into the anal canal. We filled the rectum with liquid barium sulphate and simultaneously measured rectal pressure and anal sphincter pressure, with EMGs from external sphincter and the puborectalis muscle; we asked patients to do a Valsalva manoeuvre, blowing up the sphygmomanometer. We imaged the rectum on a screen radiologically. We never saw evidence of a flap valve, and we always found that sphincter pressure exceeded rectal pressure. So we had no evidence for the concept of a valve, whether a flutter valve or a flap valve. We would agree entirely with your hypothesis.

DeLancey: It's an interesting point to decide whether to look for the *one* thing that determines continence, or the many things. My guess is that several factors each play some role. As in most areas of the body, there is a redundancy in design. You can for example, remove one lung, and the other can provide for relatively normal function. In sorting out causation, therefore, it is difficult to select only one part of a system for study without the others. The empirical observation is that intraurethral pressure goes up during a cough, more than we can account for simply by contraction of the pelvic floor musculature. The thought is that it is the support of the urethra which somehow allows this to occur. How this occurs is unknown. I suppose that you are saying that the angulation isn't the only thing that determines continence, but it's the relative pressure between the two parts of the bowel. But, as I understand it, one of the primary findings in patients with anal incontinence is the loss of the anorectal angulation?

Bartolo: Yes, but I think that's an epiphenomenon, if you like. We find that people with the worst incontinence (usually incontinence seen in rectal prolapse) have a very obtuse anorectal angle. But we can successfully correct the prolapse surgically and make that angle even more obtuse. We find the same with idiopathic incontinence or neurogenic incontinence, where we operate, but success does not correlate with improvement in the anorectal angle.

Bourcier: Is there any anatomical or physiological relation between the compressor urethrae and the paraurethral sphincter? Is it the same muscle?

DeLancey: The terminology of the area is just as confused as that of all the other areas of the pelvis! There is only one body of striated muscle in the area which is inherent within the urethra. It has two components, but it is one muscular group; the components are the urethral sphincter and the compressor urethrae/urethrovaginal sphincter. The second striated muscle that could influence the urethra is the levator ani, through its connections with the tissue around the urethra. It does not lie within the urethra.

Bourcier: As there is a direct connection between the vagina and the puborectalis muscle, why do we not start the treatment of vaginal prolapse by increasing the tone and power of this muscle by direct stimulation, instead of surgery?

DeLancey: A number of things would be necessary for that treatment to work. One is that the connections to the puborectalis muscle must still be present. In some women, during vaginal birth, when you pull on the forceps, you feel something tear, and it could be one of a number of things, including a connection to that muscle. So you would have to depend upon that connection being intact, in order to improve support through exercise. The second is that you would have to depend upon the person being able to exercise that muscle, so the innervation would need to be intact. If those two things were true, I suspect you could influence that one portion of the sphincteric mechanism. At present we don't know how important that part is, but certainly improving the strength of those muscles would improve that component of the continence mechanism.

Blaivas: I have a number of clinical observations for you to comment on. Firstly, the structures that you so nicely demonstrate are very flimsy in the living person. You can very easily dissect these tissues off. The only strong structure I ever notice between the urethra and the side wall of the pelvis is the arcus tendineus, which is very obvious; all the tissue between seems to me very flimsy.

Secondly, anyone who works with electromyography in patients can document that a woman can very quickly voluntarily contract whatever muscles make urethral diameter smaller. They do that so fast that it is unlikely to be other than a normal, fast-twitch striated muscle.

Thirdly, on the concept about the bladder neck descending during voiding, my feeling is that the bladder neck does not descend. Rather, it simply widens and assumes a funnel shape. As it gets wider, the posterior position gives the appearance of descent.

The fourth point is on the concept of the distal urethral segment having the highest pressure transmission. That may be artifact, because it is the only part of the urethra that is fixed to the undersurface of the pubis, and that's the fulcrum point around which movement occurs, and I think it is the place where the catheter is most likely to bend during a cough and perhaps cause an artifactual rise in pressure.

The last point relates to the effects of anaesthesia on urethral sphincter function. Under spinal or epidural anaesthesia, increased intra-abdominal pressure almost always results in urinary loss. If manual suprapubic pressure is exerted with a full bladder, the resulting urinary stream seems to be related entirely to how much pressure is exerted. The greater the pressure, the more forceful the stream. This is true even in patients who have severe prostatic obstruction. This suggests that there is an essential neuromuscular mechanism which normally keeps the urethral sphincter closed and that this mechanism is blocked by spinal or epidural anaesthesia.

DeLancey: I agree fully that what you dissect in front of the urethra—that is, between urethra and the pubic bones—is flimsy, and has nothing to do with urethral support. The intriguing point is that the urethra itself can be removed relatively easily, down to the area of the urogenital diaphragm. The vagina and the endopelvic fascia, which is connected to the levator ani muscle, is the part that is very difficult to dissect during vaginectomy. You are right that the supporting tissues don't attach to the urethra itself, or the area between the urethra and the pubic bones, or even necessarily behind the urethra. Support has to do with the overall body of endopelvic connective tissue and its attachments to the vagina. The previous concept that it was a pubo-urethral ligament going from the pubic bone to the urethra that held the urethra up was looking in the wrong area for the support.

Are you saying that the vagina and the more posterior tissues are also flimsy? That has not been my experience.

Blaivas: No, it's not flimsy. If anything, the support is more like a sling.

DeLancey: Exactly. And the urethra exists within an environment that influences it, rather than the urethra itself being attached to the pelvic bones.

On the rapid contraction of the pelvic floor when somebody is asked to stop urinating, I have the same impression that the response of the pelvic floor is very quick. There are two different striated muscles that could be responsible. One has been described as being slow-twitch, which is the urethral sphincter. The other, the levator ani, is equally divided between slow-twitch and fast-twitch fibres, which suggests that that may be a portion of the levators responsible for urethral closure. I don't know any way of deciding which it is, but I agree that is not the slow, gradual increase in pressure that would be expected with smooth muscle, or smooth muscle-like, contractions.

The descent of the bladder neck in voiding is a very interesting question. I have also looked at a number of studies to see how often this occurs, and it is certainly not the only way that people void; I think it is the minority. Paul Hodgkinson pointed out that women void differently, and that this may be *one* feature of some but not others (Hodgkinson & Morgan 1969).

Blaivas: Would you agree that in order to void by straining, something has to be wrong with the urethra (without having a bladder contraction)?

DeLancey: That I don't know.

Blaivas: I think the normal urethra stays closed all the time, except during abnormalities of stress incontinence or during detrusor contraction, and that in some way this micturition reflex is integrated in a way to open the urethra and have the bladder contract. The bladder can contract without causing any rise in pressure at all, if the urethra opens widely enough. The concept of urethral instability, which is a controversial topic, I think is just a micturition reflex which occurs with a urethra that is so wide that you don't measure the pressure.

DeLancey: Yes. By talking about the suspensory mechanism I did not mean to suggest that nothing else is involved in voiding. I was trying to explore the nature of the voluntary beginning of micturition, and why it is that although the urethra doesn't descend necessarily at the onset of micturition, in fluoroscopic evaluations of almost all subjects who are asked to interrupt voiding, there is an elevation of the vesical neck at the time they interrupt.

Blaivas: When the urethra closes, it looks as if it is going up because it is closing circumferentially, and it becomes narrow whenever the skeletal muscle contracts. The proximal extent of striated muscle in the urethra is variable, in both sexes.

DeLancey: Two camps have described urethral closure. One has said that it stops at the distal urethra and slowly works its way back up. The second maintains that it stops at the vesical neck. If it were only the striated sphincter, then the proximal 1.5 cm of the urethra should stay open, because it doesn't start until that point.

Blaivas: We have looked at many videos, and it appears as if you put a constricting band around the mid portion of the urethra; the constriction extends in both directions in almost everyone.

Stanton: What kind of women were you reviewing, Dr Blaivas? Were these normal women, or preoperative or postoperative patients?

Blaivas: I was describing a great variety of cases of stress incontinence, voiding dysfunction, neurological conditions, and so on.

Stanton: If you are not looking at normal subjects, we cannot use these data. I think that in normal women, when we ask them to cough, there is some descent of the bladder neck and sometimes some opening of the bladder neck. If you then ask them to void, the pelvic floor really does come down. You won't necessarily find this in your group of women with incontinence. One has to draw a distinction between those with and those without symptoms.

Blaivas: They are not all abnormal. There are many people who are nearly normal but are complaining of one thing—a little frequency and urgency, perhaps—but do not have any overt abnormalities.

Stanton: The statement was made that there is a group of women who appear to relax their pelvic floors when they void, and you say that they should have a destrusor contraction but, because the urethra is wide open, you don't see this. I would refute that by saying that if you ask these women to stop, and the striated muscle will shut off quickly, if that detrusor is contracting you would expect to see an isometric contraction, which you don't. I suspect that this group of women are not voiding with a detrusor contraction; they are voiding by gravity, or with some abdominal straining.

Blaivas: You are absolutely correct, if that happens; if you ask them to stop and there's no rise in pressure, there probably is no detrusor contraction.

Stanton: In this concept of the mechanism of continence, Dr DeLancey, where does the main defence mechanism lie? People talk about the bladder neck as the main mechanism, but I don't agree. The main mechanism really resides in the mid urethra, and perhaps the bladder neck acts there as a standby, because, when stress continence occurs, that is often the mechanism that fails first.

DeLancey: Most people would agree that in the majority of healthy young women during a cough, urine does not get into the urethra. In continent multiparous women, who are older, there are a group (roughly 50%) in whom urine gets past the internal urinary meatus and must be stopped by the urethra. So I suppose the ideal would be that the level of continence is at the vesical neck. There are certainly some continent multiparous women in whom the distal sphincter mechanism has good reason to be there, to act as a backup mechanism in those individuals in whom urine passes the internal meatus. They are still continent although not perfectly so. Thus there may be two different groups, one group of women who are continent at the vesical neck, and another of women who episodically need to depend on the external sphincter.

Stanton: Your data would suggest that the bulk of that sphincter is really in the mid urethra?

DeLancey: The largest quantity of striated muscle within the urethra itself is just at and below the mid-point.

Kirby: I agree with what you say about the striated muscle and about the collagenous ligamentous supports, but you may have underestimated the role of the smooth muscle, which may act at the bladder neck, or in the mid urethra or a little below, and which I think is under sympathetic control. It's well documented by Donker and colleagues (1972) that phentolamine causes the urethral pressure to fall. And clinically, if you give an α-adrenergic-blocking agent, the patient can develop stress urinary incontinence. How important is that component of continence? Is it mainly a passive component, or is it involved in active continence?

DeLancey: Anatomically there is no way of resolving that. I certainly don't think that the smooth muscle is less important than striated muscle. In the myelodysplastic individual, who is incontinent, or in someone on α-adrenergic blockers, when the vesical neck is open, it's that portion for that individual that makes the difference between stress incontinence and normality. But anatomically one cannot say which structure is most or least important; they are all there, and presumably they are there for a reason. Maybe in different patients there are different dysfunctions in each of these areas. We clinically recognize that patients with stress incontinence are not all alike, and that in defining the different structures involved in the continence mechanism our role is simply to make a list of the structures which can contribute to continence. But I can say that there is a visible area in the proximal urethra that is sphincteric in orientation, at least.

Christensen: This discussion reminds me of the debate that went on 25 years ago about the role of the lower oesophageal sphincter, the very existence of which was being debated then. The evidence that firmly established its existence consisted of cutting the region into small strips of smooth muscle, putting them in organ baths and showing that strips of muscle from one region behaved differently from those above and below it by maintaining a high degree of tone and relaxing with nerve stimulation. Thus, it was physiologically shown to be a different muscle (Christensen et al 1973). We now also know that it is an ultrastructurally different muscle, containing more mitochondria than muscle from above and below the sphincter, and the mitochondria are in entirely different positions in the muscle cells (Christensen & Roberts 1983). Also, the sphincter muscle is metabolically distinct (Robison et al 1984). Has that sort of work been done on the presumed smooth muscle sphincter at the bladder neck? Can we define it in those precise terms?

DeLancey: I don't know that strips have been studied from different locations in the urethra and vesical neck. The difficulty in this area is in separating out the relevant muscle fibres from one another. In order to see the differences in function one would need to take serial histological sections. This would preclude a functional analysis. I suppose you could harvest tissue and use some samples for organ bath studies and others for histological study, but this is a very small area (about 4 cm long by 2 cm in diameter).

Christensen: Those are about the same dimensions as those of the lower oesophageal sphincter, where I was able to do the studies I mentioned.

de Groat: Where is the functional sphincter located? In normal subjects, during a cough, urine doesn't enter the urethra. Thus it would appear that the functional sphincter is at the bladder neck. Jerry Blaivas has pointed out that patients who have damage to the pudendal nerves are still continent; urine is held in the bladder. Thus it is not the distal urethra or the striated muscle sphincter but rather the bladder neck (the smooth muscle, or elastic tissue or neural input) which maintains continence.

DeLancey: Part of the difficulty in ascribing the level of continence to the vesical neck in all women was that when we excised 1 cm of the distal urethra in women undergoing radical vulvectomy, they became incontinent. The resting pressures in their urethras didn't change, or their urethral mobility. We were left with the idea that perhaps these women didn't have perfect continence beforehand (and many women, even nulliparous women, say that they occasionally lose urine). These were older women, who perhaps already had an inadequate internal sphincteric mechanism and had been relying on the distal mechanism to stay dry during a cough. So that in a normal healthy young woman, the vesical neck may be the normal mechanism and perhaps only in these older women would incontinence after distal urethral excision occur. We would say that the striated uro-genital sphincter is a backup mechanism and may have a role in certain individuals.

de Groat: Another possibility is that the pelvic floor musculature has an afferent system, and when the muscles are stretched, the afferents are activated and trigger sympathetic reflexes back to the bladder neck and to the urethra, which cause closure. If this reflex pathway were damaged, it might reduce the safety factor for maintenance of continence.

Andersson: We have done experiments that may be relevant. In cystourethrectomy specimens from women, we dissected out ring preparations from the whole urethra, opened up the rings and examined contractility in an organ bath (Ek et al 1977). We found uniform contractile activity; we couldn't identify a specific smooth muscle sphincter area.

Staskin: I believe there is also a significant contribution to urethral resistance from the urethral mucosa and submucosal vasculature, which provide coaptation and compression. In post-menopausal women the spongy layer atrophies (it is oestrogen dependent) and the resting closure pressure of the urethra decreases. The function of the smooth muscle which surrounds the urethra is also oestrogen dependent.

Secondly, it is important to differentiate between the resting urethral closure pressure and the dynamic events associated with increases in intra-abdominal pressure. The transmission pressures during 'stress' to the bladder neck and proximal urethral areas provide a compensatory mechanism for the pressure which is transmitted intravesically. In fact, with the surgical correction of stress incontinence in women, we re-support the bladder neck within the zone of intra-abdominal pressure transmission and often create above-normal transmission ratios in the proximal urethra. There is also active contraction of the external sphincter muscle in the mid-urethral area. It is not the highest level of resting closure pressure that we are interested in, but the combination of passive closure pressure, dynamic pressure transmission, and active muscular contraction that contributes to urethral resistance during activity.

References

Bartolo DCC, Roe AM, Locke-Edmunds JC, Virgee J, Mortensen NJMcC 1986 Flap valve theory of anorectal continence. Br J Surg 73:1012–1014

Christensen J, Roberts RL 1983 Differences between esophageal body and lower esophageal sphincter in mitochondria of smooth muscle in opossum. Gastroenterology 85:650–656

Christensen J, Conklin JL, Freeman BW 1973 Physiologic specialization at esophagogastric junction in three species. Am J Physiol 225:1265– 1270

Donker PJ, Ivanovich IF, Noach EC 1972 Analysis of urethral pressure profile by means of EMG and the administration of drugs. Br J Urol 44:180–193

Duthie HL 1971 Progress report. Anal continence. Gut 12:844-852

Ek A, Alm P, Andersson K-E, Persson CGA 1977 Adrenoceptor and cholinoceptor mediated responses of the isolated human urethra. Scand J Urol Nephrol 11:97–102

Hodgkinson CP, Morgan JE 1969 Basic pressures of voiding in the adult female. Am J Obstet Gynecol 103:755–772

Phillips SF, Edwards DAW 1965 Some aspects of anal continence and defaecation. Gut 6:396–406

Robison BA, Percy WH, Christensen J 1984 Differences in cytochrome C oxidase capacity in smooth muscle of opossum esophagus and lower esophageal sphincter. Gastroenterology 87:1009–1013

The dual function of capsaicin-sensitive sensory nerves in the bladder and urethra

Carlo Alberto Maggi

Pharmacology Department, A. Menarini Pharmaceuticals, Via Sette Santi 3, 50131 Florence, Italy

Abstract. The sensory innervation of the urinary bladder and urethra plays a key role in a variety of reflexes involved in urine storage and voiding. Dysfunction of these systems is a possible cause of many disturbances related to urine continence but basic knowledge in this field has been hampered by the lack of tools for studying sensory nerves. The use of capsaicin, the pungent ingredient of red peppers, allowed us to investigate the anatomical and functional properties of a specific subset of sensory neurons in the lower urinary tract. These 'capsaicin-sensitive' neurons play a dual sensory and 'efferent' function, determined by transmitter release from their central and peripheral nerve endings. Tachykinins, including substance P, and other neuropeptides such as calcitonin gene-related peptide, mediate the functions of these sensory neurons. The 'sensory' function includes regulation of micturition threshold, activation of cardiovascular reflexes and perception of pain from the urinary bladder. The 'efferent' function includes local regulation of muscle cell activity, nerve excitability, blood flow and plasma protein extravasation. Recent data suggest that capsaicin-sensitive sensory nerves could be present in the human bladder.

1990 Neurobiology of Incontinence. Wiley, Chichester (Ciba Foundation Symposium 151) p 77–90

Sensory impulses arising from the urinary tract provide the basis for the reflex regulation of vesico-urethral motility necessary for efficient urine storage and voiding. Theoretically, dysfunction of sensory nerves might be involved in various disturbances of vesico-urethral motility as well as in pain arising from the bladder and urethra. In recent years the study of sensory nerves in the lower urinary tract has been greatly facilitated by the use of capsaicin, the pungent ingredient of many red peppers, which possesses a selective action on certain primary sensory neurons (see Szolcsányi 1984, Maggi & Meli 1986, 1988 and Holzer 1988 for reviews). The available evidence indicates that the capsaicin-sensitive nerves not only transmit sensory impulses from the periphery to the central nervous system but also have an 'efferent' function which is determined by the local release of transmitters in the periphery (Szolcsányi 1984, Maggi & Meli 1986, 1988, Holzer 1988).

Capsaicin as a tool for the study of bladder function

The function of capsaicin-sensitive primary sensory neurons in the lower urinary tract of experimental animals has been investigated using capsaicin itself in two ways. With the first approach, the *acute* effect of capsaicin was studied, either *in vivo* or *in vitro*. The consequent functional responses are assumed to be dependent upon sensory nerve stimulation. In *in vivo* conditions, the application of capsaicin to the receptive field of sensory neurons activates the reflex responses which are mediated by these nerves (Maggi et al 1984, 1986, Giuliani et al 1988). Further, local effects can also be observed which persist after acute but not chronic extrinsic denervation (Maggi et al 1986). Acute effects of capsaicin are also observed in *in vitro* experiments, reflecting the ability of this drug to induce transmitter release from sensory nerve terminals (Szolcsányi 1984, Maggi & Meli 1988).

Like many other pharmacological tools, capsaicin can exert unspecific effects (those not involving sensory nerves). The hallmark of the specific action of capsaicin on sensory nerves is desensitization (Maggi & Meli 1988). This is a complex phenomenon which encompasses several stages and presumably several mechanisms of action (Szolcsányi 1985). From a descriptive point of view, capsaicin desensitization means that after exposure to high concentrations of capsaicin, the sensory neurons become inexcitable by capsaicin itself. Thus, the specificity of the acute effects of capsaicin can be checked by comparing the effect of capsaicin in vehicle-pretreated and capsaicin-pretreated (desensitized) animals or preparations.

The second approach takes advantage of the fact that after capsaicin desensitization, sensory nerves become inexcitable not only by capsaicin but also by other stimuli such as distension or chemicals, including mediators of inflammation (prostaglandins, bradykinin etc.). Therefore, when this approach is used, animals are treated with large doses of capsaicin in order to desensitize or inactivate the sensory nerves. Natural stimuli thought to be relevant for the function under study (such as volume-evoked distension in the case of the urinary bladder) are then applied in both vehicle- and capsaicin-pretreated animals. Differences between the groups are ascribable to chemical sensory denervation produced by capsaicin pretreatment.

Capsaicin-sensitive innervation of the bladder and urethra

The cell bodies of capsaicin-sensitive primary sensory neurons are located in dorsal root ganglia and send fibres in both central and peripheral directions.

In rats, two distinct groups of primary sensory neurons innervate the urinary bladder, located in dorsal root ganglia T12–L3 and L6–S1 (Sharkey et al 1983, Su et al 1986, Jancsó & Maggi 1987).

Immunohistochemistry has shown that a variety of neuropeptides are stored in capsaicin-sensitive primary sensory neurons (Holzer 1988). Among these, a transmitter role seems likely for substance P (SP) and other tachykinins (TKs) such as neurokinin A (NKA), and also for the calcitonin gene-related peptide (CGRP). The possible functional significance of other neuropeptides shown to be present in these sensory neurons is, at present, unsettled. TKs and CGRP, synthesized at neuronal body level, are transported to both central and peripheral endings from where they are released to stimulate postsynaptic (in the central nervous system and autonomic ganglia) and postjunctional (in the periphery) receptors.

The central projections of sensory nerves of the bladder have been investigated in rats, cats and monkeys by using axonal tracing techniques (de Groat 1987). By combining the retrograde transport of tracers and systemic capsaicin pretreatment (which, at high doses, produces neurotoxic effects on these primary sensory neurons), Jancsó & Maggi (1987) determined the central projections of capsaicin-sensitive bladder afferents in rats.

The peripheral distribution of the capsaicin-sensitive nerves in the bladder and urethra has been studied by immunohistochemistry. Nerve profiles containing TK- and CGRP-like immunoreactivity (LI) have been observed beneath and within the urothelium and in association with blood vessels and muscle layers (Sharkey et al 1983, Su et al 1986). In various species, these nerves are more abundant in the trigone and bladder base than in the body or the dome. TK- and CGRP-LI has also been detected in the urinary bladder of rats and guinea pigs by radioimmunoassay (Maggi et al 1988, Abelli et al 1988). Peptide-containing nerve fibres can no longer be observed immunohistochemically in the bladders of capsaicin-treated animals. Likewise, tissue levels of TKs and CGRP are reduced by systemic capsaicin pretreatment (Sharkey et al 1983, Su et al 1986, Maggi et al 1988, Abelli et al 1988).

Sensory functions of capsaicin-sensitive nerves

The sensory function of capsaicin-sensitive nerves has been studied by assessing the acute effect of capsaicin application on the bladder and urethra as well as changes in responses to natural stimuli after systemic capsaicin pretreatment. The available evidence indicates that these sensory nerves modulate the volume threshold for eliciting reflex micturition in both rats and guinea pigs (Maggi et al 1986, 1987). In the former species the functional deficit in reflex micturition produced by capsaicin desensitization was quantitatively more severe when newborn rats were pretreated with capsaicin than when adults were pretreated. After systemic capsaicin desensitization of adult rats (threshold dose 25 mg/kg s.c., maximal effects at 50 mg/kg s.c.), larger volumes of fluid are required to elicit reflex micturition, but only when the bladder is filled at a low, physiological rate (Figs. 1 and 2; Maggi & Meli 1988). At a high filling rate no difference between rats treated with capsaicin as adults and controls was observed in the volume threshold to elicit micturition. By contrast, in rats desensitized to capsaicin as newborns, reflex micturition is virtually abolished at both low and high filling rates. As a consequence a marked enlargement of the bladder occurs in these animals (Sharkey et al 1983, Santicioli et al 1985, Su et al 1986).

Anatomical data have shown that the degree of neurotoxic activity of capsaicin on primary sensory neurons varies when the drug is administered to adult rather than newborn rats (Jancsó et al 1985). In adults, no more than 20% of elements in dorsal root ganglia are affected by capsaicin, whereas in newborn rats a permanent loss of about 50% of primary afferents occurs. Capsaicin pretreatment of adult rats with 50 mg/kg s.c. capsaicin depleted the bladder of SP-, NKA- and CGRP-LI (Abelli et al 1988). On the basis of these results we proposed (Maggi & Meli 1988) that multiple populations of bladder sensory nerves exist, subserving different functional roles. In particular, those bladder sensory nerves which are fully sensitive to the action of capsaicin in adult rats seem to have the following characteristics:

Sensory functions: modulatory influence on micturition threshold, activation of cardiovascular sympathetic reflexes, mediation of visceral pain.
Transmitter content: SP-LI, NKA-LI and CGRP-LI.

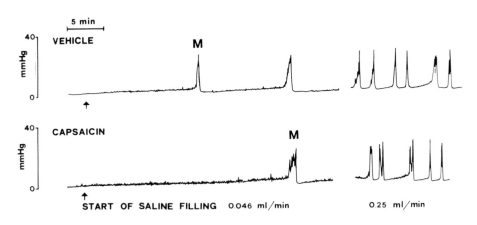

FIG. 1. Cystometric recordings showing the micturition reflex elicited by transvesical saline filling in vehicle- and capsaicin-pretreated adult rats (50 mg/kg s.c.). M, micturition. Note the marked increase in bladder capacity of capsaicin-treated rats when cystometry was performed at a low, physiological filling rate. Note that at a high filling rate (right panels) differences are no longer evident between vehicle- and capsaicin-treated animals.

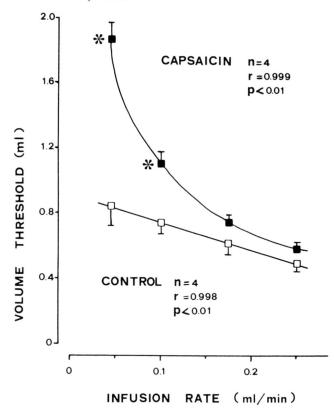

FIG. 2.   Quantitative data showing the increase in bladder capacity (volume threshold for reflex micturition) produced by systemic capsaicin desensitization in adult rats (50 mg/kg s.c., four days previously). In both groups a signficant inverse relationship exists between infusion rate and volume threshold for reflex micturition. Each value is mean ± SE of eight experiments.
*Significantly different from controls, $P < 0.05$.

'Efferent' functions of capsaicin-sensitive nerves

One peculiar feature of capsaicin-sensitive nerves is their ability to release stored transmitters from peripheral endings. This can occur in two ways (Szolcsányi 1984, Maggi & Meli 1988), namely (a) from the same sensory receptor that has been activated by the environmental stimulus, and (b) by antidromic invasion of other peripheral terminals of the same sensory neurons (axon reflex arrangement). Released transmitters have been shown to exert a variety of local effects in the urinary bladder and urethra, including smooth muscle contraction and/or relaxation, the modulation of nerve excitability, and an increase in vascular permeability (neurogenic inflammation).

Capsaicin and the human bladder

SP-, NKA- and CGRP-like immunoreactivity is present in human bladder muscle and mucosa, as determined by radioimmunoassay (C. A. Maggi, P. Geppetti & E. Theodorsson, unpublished data). Further, nerve fibres containing SP-LI have been observed in the human bladder (Gu et al 1984). TKs exert a potent contractile effect on human bladder muscle by activating NK-2 receptors, although no evidence for specific motor responses to capsaicin was obtained on bladder strips from the dome of the human bladder (Maggi et al 1989a).

Intravesical infusion of capsaicin (1–10 µM) in humans produces a warm to burning sensation, paralleled by anticipation of the first desire to void and by decreased bladder capacity (Maggi et al 1989b). Repeated administration of the same concentration of capsaicin produced effects of progressively decreasing efficacy, suggesting ongoing desensitization (G. Barbanti et al, unpublished). On this basis the hypothesis was advanced that capsaicin-sensitive sensory nerves might be present in the human bladder and that capsaicin itself, or substances related to it, might be used in urological practice for diagnostic or therapeutic purposes. Clearly, much work is still needed to substantiate this hypothesis.

Conclusions

In conclusion, capsaicin has proved to be an extremely useful pharmacological tool for establishing the presence, distribution and function of primary afferents innervating the mammalian urinary bladder. Definition of the properties and pathophysiological relevance of this system is expected to suggest new methods for the diagnosis and treatment of human disorders of the lower urinary tract.

References

Abelli L, Conte B, Somma V et al 1988 The contribution of capsaicin-sensitive sensory nerves to xylene-induced visceral pain in conscious, freely moving rats. Naunyn-Schmiedeberg's Arch Pharmacol 337:545–551
de Groat WC 1987 Neuropeptides in pelvic afferent pathways. Experientia (Basel) 43:801–813
Giuliani S, Maggi CA, Meli A 1988 Capsaicin-sensitive afferents in the rat urinary bladder activate a spinal sympathetic cardiovascular reflex. Naunyn-Schmiedeberg's Arch Pharmacol 338:411–416
Gu J, Blank MA, Huang WM et al 1984 Peptide-containing nerves in human urinary bladder. Urology 24:353–360
Holzer P 1988 Local effector function of capsaicin-sensitive sensory nerve endings: involvement of tachykinins, calcitonin gene-related peptide and other neuropeptides. Neuroscience 24:739–768
Jancsó G, Maggi CA 1987 Distribution of capsaicin-sensitive urinary bladder afferents in the rat spinal cord. Brain Res 418:371–376
Jancsó G, Kiraly E, Joo F, Such G, Nagy A 1985 Selective degeneration by capsaicin of a subpopulation of primary sensory neurons in the adult rat. Neurosci Lett 59:209–214

Maggi CA, Meli A 1986 The role of neuropeptides in the regulation of the micturition reflex. J Autonom Pharmacol 6:133–162

Maggi CA, Meli A 1988 The sensory-efferent function of capsaicin-sensitive sensory neurons. Gen Pharmacol 19:1–43

Maggi CA, Santicioli P, Meli A 1984 The effects of topical capsaicin on rat urinary bladder motility *in vivo*. Eur J Pharmacol 103:41–50

Maggi CA, Santicioli P, Borsini F et al 1986 The role of the capsaicin-sensitive innervation of the rat urinary bladder in the activation of micturition reflex. Naunyn-Schmiedeberg's Arch Pharmacol 332:276–283

Maggi CA, Giuliani S, Santicioli P et al 1987 Species-related variations in the effects of capsaicin on urinary bladder functions: relation to bladder content of substance P-like immunoreactivity. Naunyn-Schmiedeberg's Arch Pharmacol 336:546–555

Maggi CA, Geppetti P, Santicioli P et al 1988 Tachykinin-like immunoreactivity in the mammalian urinary bladder: correlation with the functions of capsaicin-sensitive sensory nerves. Neuroscience 26:233–242

Maggi CA, Patacchini R, Santicioli P et al 1989a Further studies on the motor response of the human isolated urinary bladder to tachykinins, capsaicin and electrical field stimulation. Gen Pharmacol 20:663–670

Maggi CA, Barbanti G, Santicioli P et al 1989b Cystometric evidence that capsaicin-sensitive nerves modulate the afferent branch of micturition reflex in humans. J Urol 142:150–154

Santicioli P, Maggi CA, Meli A 1985 The effect of capsaicin pretreatment on the cystometrograms of urethane-anaesthetized rats. J Urol 133:700–703

Sharkey KA, Williams RG, Schultzberg M, Dockray GJ 1983 Sensory substance P innervation of the urinary bladder: possible site of action in causing urine retention in rats. Neuroscience 10:861–868

Su HC, Wharton J, Polak JM et al 1986 CGRP immunoreactivity in afferent neurons supplying the urinary tract: combined retrograde tracing and immunohistochemistry. Neuroscience 18:727–747

Szolcsányi J 1984 Capsaicin-sensitive chemoceptive neural system with dual sensory-efferent function. In: Chahl LA et al (eds) Antidromic vasodilatation and neurogenic inflammation. Akademiai Kiado, Budapest, p 26–52

Szolcsányi J 1985 Sensory receptors and the antinociceptive effects of capsaicin. In: Hakanson R, Sundler F (eds) Tachykinin antagonists. Elsevier Science Publishers, Amsterdam, p 45–56

DISCUSSION

Burnstock: Can I press you, Dr Maggi, on the distribution of substance P and the calcitonin gene-related peptide (CGRP) in the bladder? You found both transmitters in the dome and the neck of the bladder. There are examples where substance P and CGRP are known to co-exist in the same sensory nerve, but this is not always the case. Many sensory nerves in the brain and elsewhere contain *either* CGRP *or* substance P, often together with other transmitters. Some reports suggest that CGRP is associated with pain fibres in some areas, and substance P less so. It would be nice to know the exact distribution of these two sensory neuropeptides and whether there is co-localization in all regions of the bladder, or whether in some areas one of them is dominant. Can you tell us whether they exist in the urethra, in the vesical neck, and so on?

Maggi: The distribution of capsaicin-sensitive afferents has not been much investigated in the bladder and urethra, at least in terms of possible regional differences in density of innervation. For CGRP the density of fibres is for some reason greater in the bladder base than in the dome (Su et al 1986). Some studies have shown co-localization of substance P (or other tachykinins) and CGRP in the *same* nerve fibres of the bladder which are capsaicin sensitive (Sundler et al 1985, Gibbins et al 1985, Franco-Cereceda et al 1987), but there is not much detailed information as to whether co-localization of these peptides is homogeneous throughout the bladder or urethra. It would also be interesting to know whether there is a differential expression of these peptides in different layers of the bladder—for example, the mucosa as compared to the muscle. This does not seem to occur in the guinea pig bladder, at least for substance P and CGRP, which were detected by radioimmunoassay in similar relative amounts in the dome and neck as well as in the mucosa and the muscle in this species (Maggi et al 1988).

de Groat: We have not done much on this topic in the rat, but in cat we have used dye-tracing techniques to label specific populations of dorsal root ganglion cells and then have examined the co-localization of neuropeptides in the cells. About 50% of the VIP neurons contained substance P, for example. In general there was considerable overlap between these peptides in bladder afferents, in colon afferents and in afferents in the pudendal nerve. However, co-localization has not been examined in the peripheral terminals, only in the cell bodies in the dorsal root ganglia.

Dr Maggi, does distension of the bladder release peptides from the capsaicin-sensitive afferents?

Maggi: We have never found release when applying stretch, for example. This may simply mean that their 'efferent' function is activated only with intense stimulation of the sensory fibres. But there is the problem that the maximal amount of transmitter released by capsaicin, which is a very strong stimulus, is no more than 5–15% of the total peptide content of the tissue. We cannot exclude that there is a 'microrelease' of peptides produced by stretch that we cannot detect with the present radioimmunoassay techniques.

de Groat: So there is no evidence that distension of the kind that occurs during a normal cystometrogram (CMG) releases neuropeptides; however, there may be an undetectable microrelease.

Maggi: If we look at other tissues, such as the skin, even a single nerve impulse, conducted antidromically, can activate the 'efferent' function of sensory nerves, producing, for example, vasodilatation (Szolcsányi 1988). So the feeling of some people working in this field is that there is an 'efferent' function of capsaicin-sensitive sensory nerves, which is probably physiological; that is to say, it may occur every time the fibre is activated. But a direct demonstration of sensory peptide release by a physiological stimulus such as a stretch of the tissue is still lacking.

de Groat: It would be important to identify the site where the capsaicin-sensitive afferents act during a normal CMG, to facilitate the micturition reflex. For example, do they act in the periphery, to release neuropeptides which then facilitate the firing of the larger afferents which induce the micturition reflex, or do they act centrally to facilitate the micturition reflex in the central nervous system? Have you any data which would indicate whether this is a peripheral or central site of action?

Maggi: Peripheral administration of tachykinins can certainly activate or facilitate the micturition reflex, at least in rats (see Maggi et al 1987). On the other hand, there are no data on the effect of central (e.g. intrathecal) administration of sensory neuropeptides on bladder motility. When looking at capsaicin, we have shown that its local application to the rat bladder, with modalities which did not determine widespread desensitization throughout the body, increased bladder capacity in the same manner as produced by systemic treatment (Maggi et al 1989a). This seems logical, because blockade or desensitization of the sensory fibres in the periphery renders them unresponsive to physiological stimuli, such as distension. On the other hand, Durant & Yaksh (1988) showed that intrathecal administration of capsaicin blocked micturition in rats. This might have involved blockade of the central endings of these sensory nerves.

Tiseo: Blockade of micturition occurred in only about 50% of the rats and it was also transient, with most animals recovering within 4–7 days. In relation to the recurring C fibre reflex arc, we found that in the intact rat, intrathecally infused capsaicin had little effect on the volume-evoked micturition reflex. As I shall discuss in my paper, in spinally transected rats we were able to modify recovery of the reflex with capsaicin.

Burnstock: In the intramural ganglia of the guinea pig bladder there is a subpopulation of neurons that are extremely sensitive to substance P, which produces a long-lasting depolarization. So substance P could be acting at ganglion level. We certainly see substance P immunofluorescent fibres round the ganglion cells. Therefore one site for these sensory-motor fibres to bladder might be the intramural ganglia. Another might be the blood vessels, where (as you pointed out) CGRP is often an extremely potent vasodilator.

Toson: Dr Maggi, you have demonstrated that the substance P antagonist [D-Pro[4], D-Trp[7,9,10], Phe[11]]SP(4–11) is able to antagonize the contractile effect of capsaicin in guinea pig bladder *in vitro*. Have you tested this antagonist in an *in vivo* animal model, to study its effect on micturition?

Maggi: No, we have not. The problem is that the available tachykinin antagonists are not good enough for *in vivo* studies, in my view. They have very low affinity and may have unspecific side-effects. In *in vitro* experiments you can easily check for unspecific effects of the antagonists, such as response to electrical stimulation, but if you give them *in vivo*, by the intrathecal route, for example, there are many problems, including the possible vasoconstrictor or neurotoxic effects of tachykinin antagonists and also local anaesthetic activity. So if you put the antagonists peripherally onto the bladder there may be an action on other nerves as well as on sensory nerves. This is an important experiment to do, but we need better tools.

A further problem is that the capsaicin-sensitive sensory neurons contain and release not only tachykinins, but also CGRP and probably other transmitters as well. So you could equally well give a tachykinin antagonist and see nothing. One might conclude that substance P is not involved in micturition, but other substances may be co-released along with tachykinins and sustain a functional response even when tachykinin receptors are blocked.

de Groat: There is an interesting discrepancy between your capsaicin studies in the rat, where it appeared that the neurotoxin affected C fibre afferent pathways and shifted the micturition reflex threshold, and other studies by Jänig in the cat, where C fibre afferents were not activated by bladder distension under normal conditions. Your data suggest that C fibres are activated by slow bladder distension and have some effect on micturition. Jänig's results suggest that C fibres would *not* be activated by distension. Is there some way to reconcile the findings?

Maggi: Capsaicin is selective for sensory nerves but is not specific for C fibres. This has been clearly shown by Szolcsányi et al (1988) who studied the excitatory effect of capsaicin on single afferent fibres of the saphenous nerve in adult rats. They showed that capsaicin excites only the polymodal nociceptors. These latter have fibres which conduct in the C and the Aδ range. At the same time, many other types of C fibres were not excited by capsaicin in adult rats (Szolcsányi et al 1988). Therefore, in adult rats, capsaicin is specific, at the somatic level, for polymodal nociceptors. On the other hand, there is evidence that when capsaicin is administered to a newborn rat you can get an effect on a much larger fraction of afferents. Lawson & Harper (1984) showed that this type of treatment destroys about 85% of C fibres and also some myelinated afferents.

At this stage it is difficult to make meaningful correlations between neurophysiological experiments, either in cats or rats, and the effect of capsaicin pretreatment on the micturition reflex. The questions are: (a) which type of bladder afferents are affected by the capsaicin treatment, and (b) are capsaicin-sensitive bladder afferents mechanosensitive? We need a neurophysiologist— perhaps you!—to identify which bladder afferent fibres are excited by capsaicin in rats or cats and whether the same fibres are mechanosensitive or not.

de Groat: My conclusion from these observations is that capsaicin-sensitive afferents represent a somewhat undefined population of axons that could be composed of C fibres as well as A fibres. One way of interpreting the changes is that low doses of capsaicin are selective for C fibres, but that in a high enough dose the neurotoxin starts to act on other fibres as well, so it may be destroying a variety of fibre types.

Marsden: What determines the toxicity of capsaicin to different classes of nerve fibres, apart from age?

Maggi: Administration of a high dose of capsaicin (e.g. 50 mg/kg, s.c.) to newborn rats determines a lifelong loss of about 50% of sensory neurons in dorsal root ganglia. As I said, there is a massive but not complete loss of C fibres (Lawson & Harper 1984). On the other hand, high doses of capsaicin administered to adult rats do not affect more than 20% of sensory neurons in dorsal root ganglia (Jancsó et al 1985). Therefore there is a big quantitative difference in the number of sensory neurons which are capsaicin sensitive in newborn and adult animals. It appears likely that sensitivity to capsaicin is due to expression of a capsaicin 'receptor' on the cell membrane of these primary sensory neurons (Szolcsányi & Jancsó-Gabor 1975, James et al 1988). The mechanism through which capsaicin kills these cells probably depends on the fact that they become poisoned by large amounts of calcium ions which enter the cells through a channel whch is opened by stimulation of the capsaicin receptor (Jancsó et al 1984, Wood et al 1988). At this stage there is no definitive explanation for the different effect of capsaicin in adult and newborn rats. One working hypothesis is that the proposed capsaicin receptor is expressed on a larger fraction of sensory neurons at birth than in adult rats or, to put it in another way, that some sensory neurons have the receptors in the early postnatal period and lose them during postnatal development.

Marsden: If the differential toxicity is related to the presence or absence of capsaicin receptors in the normal animal, one would have to determine the distribution of those receptors in pathological states if one wanted to predict what capsaicin would do in human disease states.

Maggi: Recent data indicate that it is possible to study the capsaicin receptor with binding techniques. This has been done using tritiated resiniferatoxin (RTX). This is an ultrapotent capsaicin analogue of natural origin (Szallasi & Blumberg 1989a). Szallasi & Blumberg (1989b) reported that specific RTX-binding sites can be detected on dorsal root ganglia but not in brain areas, and the binding of labelled RTX was prevented by capsaicin. These binding sites could correspond to the capsaicin 'receptor' that I mentioned.

Andersson: On the efferent functions of these sensory nerves, if you release from those neurons peptides such as substance P, or CGRP, you can get direct effects on smooth muscle of different types. Do these direct smooth muscle effects correlate with the effects of the neuropeptides on the micturition reflex?

Maggi: No! As an example, if you apply capsaicin to isolated strips of bladder muscle from rats and guinea pigs, taken from the dome and the neck of the bladder, you will get a contraction in the rat bladder, both in the dome and in the neck, whereas in the guinea pig you will get contraction in the dome but relaxation in the bladder neck.

When we give capsaicin to rats and guinea pigs we see an increase in bladder capacity in both species, but the local motor responses are different. Tachykinins and CGRP are released in similar relative amounts in the guinea pig bladder, and differences in the motor response originate at postjunctional level. In the guinea pig bladder the tachykinins are potent contractile agents but CGRP has a relaxant effect. When we compare responses to the exogenous peptides, substance P has more potent contractile effects on the dome than on the neck in guinea pigs, whereas CGRP relaxes the neck more than the dome. In the rat bladder, tachykinins produce a contraction while CGRP has no motor effect, either contractile or relaxant. So there are differences between species, and between different parts of the bladder in the same species, in the local motor response to capsaicin, but the effect of systemic capsaicin administration on bladder capacity is just the same.

Andersson: Is your conclusion that the efferent function of these peptides is not as important as their activating effect on the micturition reflex?

Maggi: You have to consider that the released neuropeptides can do several things. They not only contract or relax the smooth muscle, but can also facilitate transmission from other nerves. Release of tachykinins also induces vasodilatation and plasma extravasation. It thus may be important in inflammatory conditions. So you have a cascade of effects, which can affect sensory nerves indirectly.

Andersson: Do you believe that any of these peptides could induce an emptying contraction of the bladder smooth muscle?

Maggi: I don't think that the local motor response to sensory peptides is big enough to produce an emptying contraction of the bladder muscle. In addition, such a contraction, either big or small, is most likely not accompanied by sphincter opening. I think that these local motor changes could perhaps produce some detrusor instability.

Marsden: You persuaded your surgeons to infuse capsaicin into the bladders of human subjects; was micturition very painful?

Maggi: The patients who agreed to do this were all except one suffering from hypersensitive bladder disorders, very severe conditions not responding to other treatments such as intrathecally injected morphine. They had about 15–20 micturition episodes during the day, or at night, many of them very painful. They accepted this experimental intravesical infusion of capsaicin and reported a transient burning sensation during the infusion (referred to the suprapubic area) and, in males, along the urethra during and after micturition. The sensation persisted for 10–120 min after micturition and its intensity varied greatly between subjects. On the other hand, all the patients were very happy, because they got relief of their symptoms for four to 16 days after capsaicin instillation, and asked for a new treatment when symptoms reappeared. These observations have been made on a very small group of patients (Maggi et al 1989b), and much work still needs to be done to define the possible role of capsaicin as diagnostic or therapeutic aid in this field.

References

Durant PAC, Yaksh TL 1988 Micturition in the unanesthetized rat: effects of intrathecal capsaicin, N-vanillylnonanamide, 6-hydroxydopamine and 5,6-dihydroxytryptamine. Brain Res 451:301–308

Franco-Cereceda A, Henke H, Lundberg JM, Petermann JB, Hökfelt T, Fischer JA 1987 CGRP in capsaicin-sensitive substance P immunoreactive sensory neurons in animals and man: distribution and release by capsaicin. Peptides 8:399–410

Gibbins IL, Furness JB, Costa M, Mac Intyre I, Hillyard CJ, Girgis S 1985 Co-localization of CGRP-like immunoreactivity with substance P in cutaneous, vascular and visceral sensory neurons of guinea-pigs. Neurosci Lett 57:125–130

James IF, Walpole CSJ, Hixon J, Wood JN, Wrigglesworth R 1988 Long-lasting agonist activity produced by a capsaicin-like photoaffinity probe. Mol Pharmacol 33: 643–649

Jancsó G, Karcsú S, Kiraly E et al 1984 Neurotoxin-induced nerve cell degeneration: possible involvement of calcium. Brain Res 295:211– 216

Jancsó G, Kiraly E, Joo F, Such G, Nagy A 1985 Selective degeneration of a subpopulation of primary sensory neurons in the adult rat. Neurosci Lett 59: 209–214

Lawson SN, Harper AA 1984 Neonatal capsaicin is not a specific neurotoxin for sensory C fibres or small dark cells of rat dorsal root ganglia. In: Chahl LA et al (eds) Antidromic vasodilatation and neurogenic inflammation. Akademiai Kiado, Budapest, p 111–118

Maggi CA, Giuliani S, Santicioli P, Abelli L, Regoli D, Meli A 1987 Further studies on the mechanisms of the tachykinin-induced activation of micturition reflex in rats: evidence for the involvement of the capsaicin-sensitive bladder mechanoreceptors. Eur J Pharmacol 136:189– 205

Maggi CA, Santicioli P, Patacchini R et al 1988 Regional differences in the motor response to capsaicin in the guinea-pig urinary bladder: relative role of pre- and post-junctional factors related to neuropeptide-containing sensory nerves. Neuroscience 27:675–688

Maggi CA, Lippe ITH, Giuliani S et al 1989a Topical versus systemic capsaicin desensitization: specific and unspecific effects as indicated by modification of reflex micturition in rats. Neuroscience 31:745– 756

Maggi CA, Barbanti G, Santicioli P et al 1989b Cystometric evidence that capsaicin-sensitive nerves modulate the afferent branch of micturition reflex in humans. J Urol 142:150–154

Su HC, Wharton J, Polak JM et al 1986 CGRP immunoreactivity in afferent neurons supplying the urinary tract: combined retrograde tracing and immunohistochemistry. Neuroscience 18:727–747

Sundler F, Brodin E, Ekblad E, Hakanson R, Uddman U 1985 Sensory nerve fibers: distribution of substance P, neurokinin A and CGRP. In: Hakanson R, Sundler F (eds) Tachykinin antagonists. Elsevier, Amsterdam, p 3–14

Szallasi A, Blumberg PM 1989a Resiniferatoxin, phorbol-related diterpene acts as an ultrapotent analog of capsaicin, the irritant constituent in red pepper. Neuroscience 30:515–520

Szallasi A, Blumberg PM 1989b Specific binding of resiniferatoxin, an ultra-potent capsaicin analog to dorsal root ganglia membranes. Pharmacologist 31: 183

Szolcsányi J 1988 Antidromic vasodilatation and neurogenic inflammation. Agents Actions 23:4–11

Szolcsányi J, Jancsó-Gabor A 1975 Sensory effects of capsaicin congeners. I. Relationship between chemical structure and pain- producing potency of pungent agents. Arzneim Forsch 25:1877–1881
Szolcsányi J, Anton F, Reeh PW, Handwerker HO 1988 Selective excitation by capsaicin of mechano-heat sensitive nociceptors in rat skin. Brain Res 446:262–268
Wood JN, Winter J, James IF, Rang H, Yeats J, Bevan S 1988 Capsaicin- induced fluxes in dorsal root ganglion cells in culture. Neuroscience 8:3208–3220

The spinal pharmacology of urinary function: studies on urinary continence in the unanaesthetized rat

Paul J. Tiseo and Tony L. Yaksh

University of California, San Diego Medical Center, Department of Anesthesiology, T-018, La Jolla, CA 92093, USA

Abstract. The volume-evoked micturition reflex (VEMR) is under the control of a complex vesico-spino-bulbo-spino-vesical reflex arc. When functional this system provides for the storage and retention of urine and its subsequent efficient expulsion by virtue of a joint contraction of the bladder and synergic relaxation of the urethral sphincter. Transection of the spinal cord results in an initial disruption of this organization (areflexia) followed by a time-dependent change in the characteristics of the functioning of this reflex system. The growth of knowledge of the pharmacology of spinal systems has yielded considerable information on the potential spinal neurotransmitter systems and their associated receptors. Given the possible role of such systems in mediating and modulating the VEMR, a reasonable approach has been to investigate the effects of spinally administered agonists and antagonists in unanaesthetized animals in which the VEMR can be examined. Thus, it appears that the initial state of bladder distension is signalled by larger (A type) afferent fibres. After spinal injury and the loss of this supraspinal control, smaller unmyelinated C fibres play a predominant role in controlling this reflex. On stimulation these C fibres release peptides (VIP, CCK, substance P, CGRP) and excitatory amino acids (glutamate). Studies in this laboratory have shown that whereas administration of these peptides is without effect in normal intact rats, the antagonists for glutamate and VIP receptors (but not CCK) produce a dose-dependent increase in spontaneous bladder contractions with a corresponding decrease in the volume required to evoke a VEMR. Other spinal systems, such as those for opioids and GABA, are known to exert modulatory effects upon spinal somatomotor reflex arcs. In the spinal cord these agonists (μ/δ and $GABA_{A/B}$) produce discrete changes in the VEMR in intact and spinally transected animals. Thus these studies may provide insight into the coordinated mechanisms which govern the VEMR and may also allow the development of pharmacological approaches to managing the dysfunctional bladder.

1990 Neurobiology of Incontinence. Wiley, Chichester (Ciba Foundation Symposium 151) p 91–109

The bladder functions to collect and retain urine under low intravesical pressures. Mechanistically this reflects a filling-evoked relaxation of the smooth muscle and an increase in the tone of the external urethral sphincter. On sufficient distension a micturition reflex mediated by the activation of afferents passing through the pelvic nerve to the L6–S1 spinal segment is initiated (Jancsó & Maggi 1987). This volume-evoked micturition reflex (VEMR) represents, in its simplest form, an increased parasympathetic outflow to the vesical smooth muscle and a concurrent reduction in the somatomotor outflow to the striated musculature of the external sphincter. The classic lesion studies of Barrington emphasized the importance of the spino-bulbo-spinal component in this reflex arc (Barrington 1925). It is now appreciated that for the supraspinal component at least two spinobulbar pathways convey information on bladder fullness from the spinal cord to the pontine micturition centre: a ventrolateral component originating in the marginal zone of the sacral dorsal horn (spinothalamic tract), and a component which is thought to consist of large afferent collaterals travelling in the dorsal column. Bulbospinal projections arising from the region of the pontine micturition centre travel via the lateral spinal funiculi to the sacral parasympathetic nucleus.

From our perspective an important question relates to the pharmacology of the neurotransmitter and receptor systems which mediate the excitation and inhibition exerted by the primary afferent and bulbospinal/intrinsic terminal systems which potentially mediate the VEMR. Histochemical studies have emphasized the presence of a variety of potential neurotransmitter systems which characterize various bulbospinal, intrinsic and primary afferent systems. These are partially summarized in Table 1.

Electrophysiological studies have suggested that the afferent limbs relevant to bladder contraction consist of relatively rapidly conducting A fibres (de Groat et al 1981). The micturition reflex pathway activated by this input appears to involve an obligatory spinobulbospinal substrate because the efferent reflex evoked by A fibre stimulation is lost on spinal transection. At intervals after transection the reflex reappears but, electrophysiologically, the afferent limbs involved in this reflex appear now to be mediated by afferents having a high electrical threshold and conduction velocity normally associated with C fibres

TABLE 1   Spinal neurotransmitter systems that may mediate the micturition reflex

Primary afferents	Bulbospinal pathways	Interneurons
Substance P	Noradrenaline ($\alpha 1$, $\alpha 2$)	Enkephalins (μ, δ)
Cholecystokinin ($CCK_{A,B}$)	Serotonin ($5\text{-}HT_{1,2,3}$)	Glycine
Somatostatin	Neuropeptide Y (Y_1, Y_2)	GABA (A, B)
Dynorphin (κ)	Dopamine (D_1, D_2)	Neurotensin
Vasoactive intestinal peptide (VIP)	Oxytocin	
Calcitonin gene-related peptide (CGRP)	Vasopressin	

(de Groat et al 1981). This C fibre afferent-evoked reflex arc, although present, is weak or undetectable in animals with an intact neuraxis and is seen to play a significant role in micturition only after loss of the supraspinal reflex arc. The mechanism of this synaptic reorganization is not known, but the delay in recovery suggests the possibility of trophic changes such as axonal sprouting or the formation of new reflex connections within the sacral parasympathetic nucleus. These electrophysiological results suggesting a role of large diameter afferents in intact animals are in accord with evidence showing that spinally administered capsaicin, a neurotoxin acting on small afferents, has only transient effects on the VEMR in intact animals (Durant & Yaksh 1988; see also Maggi 1990).

The significance of this synaptic reorganization is that although the identity of the transmitter(s) contained in A fibres is not known, the neurotransmitters contained in C fibres have been widely studied. Subpopulations of C fibre axon/ganglia cells have been identified which contain a variety of peptides having postsynaptic excitatory effects. Among these peptides are substance P, cholecystokinin (CCK), bombesin, calcitonin gene-related peptide (CGRP), somatostatin (SST), and vasoactive intestinal peptide (VIP) (see Jessell & Dodd 1989). Substance P, CCK, bombesin and CGRP are known to exist in afferent populations which are capsaicin sensitive, while VIP does not. In addition, recent evidence has suggested that glutamate, an excitatory amino acid which is widely distributed, may also be contained in and released from small primary afferents.

The excitation of parasympathetic neurons must be accompanied by a decrease in the activity of somatomotor neurons to the external sphincter for a synergic response to be achieved. Not surprisingly, therefore, such afferent activation evoked by the distension of the bladder must evoke modulatory systems which inhibit somatomotor activity. Electrophysiological studies have indeed demonstrated such a reciprocal organization. The origin of such inhibition is not precisely known but can potentially arise from bulbospinal systems arising from the medial and lateral medulla or intrinsically from local sacral systems. Considerable insight into the functional organization of the vesico-spino-bulbo-spino-vesical reflex arc may be derived from the investigation of spinally transected animals. Routinely, such intervention results in a loss of parasympathetic outflow to the bladder and acutely in the loss of sphincter tone. With time, sphincter tone reappears and there is a return of spontaneous bladder activity. Though other factors may be relevant, one interpretation of these events is that in the intact animal a bulbospinal physiological system governs sphincter relaxation (which is either directly inhibitory on preganglionic parasympathetic neurons or excites a local inhibitory interneuron) and that in the spinally transected animal a local sacral inhibitory element is relevant.

Bulbospinal systems, releasing noradrenaline and serotonin and acting upon dorsal horn systems, may exert inhibitory (α_2 and 5-HT$_1$) and excitatory (α_1 and 5-HT$_{2-3}$) effects. A variety of intrinsic neurotransmitter systems have also been identified, including those which are excitatory (neurotensin), and those which are predominantly inhibitory (enkephalin: μ, δ and κ receptors; GABA: $GABA_A$ and $GABA_B$ receptors; and glycine). The role played by these various spinal neurotransmitter receptor systems has not been elucidated.

The studies reported here were designed to address specifically the role played by these various primary afferent and bulbospinal/intrinsic terminal systems on the VEMR. By studying the agents given directly into the spinal space, we can examine more closely the effects of activating receptors that are postsynaptic to that input. Though the mechanism mediating synchronous contraction of the bladder and relaxation of the sphincter is not known, our investigations should allow us to assess which agents can evoke the appropriate parasympathetic outflow. Such information does not currently exist and these experiments will provide fundamental insights into the pharmacology of the synapses modulating this outflow.

We are also interested in the characteristics of these agents in spinally injured and incontinent animals. Given the change in the presumed identity of the afferents which occurs after spinal injury, it is not unreasonable to suspect that the effects of a given spinally administered neurotransmitter on the micturition reflex will also change. It thus seems reasonable to speculate that we shall be able to drive the micturition reflex in the areflexic bladder with one of several agonists. Such results would provide important insights into the mechanism of the micturition reflex and would suggest possible alternatives for the therapeutic management of the areflexic bladder after spinal injury. Two points should be stressed. First, this approach differs from the systemic administration of drugs which act only on peripheral ganglionic transmission or directly stimulate smooth muscle contractions. In addition to evoking bladder contractions, we aim to evoke a synchronous relaxation of the sphincter. As such, this approach differs from studies in which afferent and efferent tracts are electrically stimulated, yielding activation of all systems. Secondly, none of the primary afferent transmitters passes the blood–brain barrier. Treatment with such drugs would require direct spinal administration, as we are employing in these animal studies. We note that such repeated spinal administration in man is eminently practical and involves methods that have been used extensively. The present experiments thus not only may enhance our fundamental knowledge of the micturition reflex, but suggest potentially novel approaches to managing bladder dysfunction in the spinally transected human.

The spinal pharmacology of the micturition reflex can be studied in a chronic unanaesthetized rat model which utilizes a continuous infusion of saline into the bladder and cystometrography. Because anaesthetics alter synaptic transmission, an unanaesthetized animal offers the advantage of a system that mimics the normal physiological state more closely than other models. Intravesical pressure during saline infusion and voiding is measured using a catheter implanted surgically through the bladder wall and connected to a pressure transducer. Chronically implanted intrathecal catheters allow drugs to be injected into the spinal space, so that the effects of activating receptors postsynaptic to that input can be studied. This approach can similarly be used to characterize the pharmacology of the VEMR in the spinally transected animal.

Methods

Much effort has been devoted to developing a suitable model for quantitative studies on the physiology and pharmacology of micturition in animals. Several models have been reported using the rat (Sato et al 1975, Sillen 1980, Dray & Metsch 1984a, b, Maggi et al 1984, Conte et al 1988), the cat (Barrington 1925, de Groat & Ryall 1969) and the dog (Jonas et al 1975, Moreau et al 1983). However, most studies on bladder function have used anaesthetics, urethral catheterization, or electrical stimulation. Anaesthetics alter synaptic transmission, as already stated. Urethral catheterization precludes study of the synergism between bladder contraction and sphincter relaxation, and electrical stimulation activates afferent and efferent pathways simultaneously, yielding activation of all systems. To avoid these limitations we have developed a chronic unanaesthetized rat model (Yaksh et al 1986) in which a catheter (PE-90) is implanted through the bladder wall, secured with a purse-string suture and externalized percutaneously to allow for infusion of saline and measurement of intravesical pressure. These animals are also implanted with a chronic intrathecal catheter (PE-10) to allow delivery of drugs into the lumbar intrathecal space.

The VEMR was studied during a constant infusion of saline (200 µl/min) into the bladder before and after intrathecal injection of an agent. The testing protocol was the same for both intact and spinally transected animals. For cystometrography the rat was placed in a restraining cage sufficiently large enough to allow the animal to adjust itself in a normal crouched position. Under the rear of the animal was placed a stainless steel collecting funnel opening into a strain gauge-mounted cup for measuring urine volumes. The bladder catheter was connected to a Harvard Apparatus pump for continuous infusion of saline and to a transducer for bladder pressure monitoring. Transducer and strain-gauge outputs were recorded simultaneously on a two-channel chart recorder (see Fig. 1). The parameters measured were intravesical baseline pressure, bladder opening pressure, peak pressure, the volume of urine emitted at the time of micturition, and time to micturition. A typical VEMR for an unanaesthetized rat is shown in Fig. 2.

To study the VEMR in spinally transected animals we anaesthetized rats bearing chronic intrathecal and bladder catheters with halothane. A laminectomy was performed and the cord was transected at level T10, care being taken to spare the catheters. After spinal transection the rat was given extensive support maintenance, including a daily regimen of bladder emptying, subcutaneously

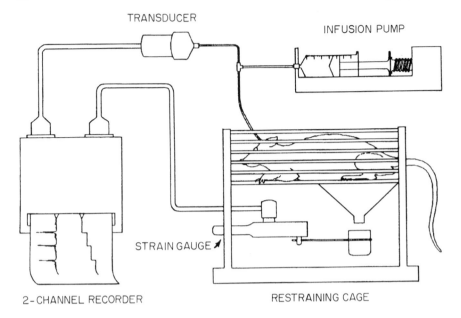

FIG. 1.   The equipment required to perform cystometry in an unanaesthetized rat. An infusion pump delivered saline through a chronically implanted catheter. The pressure in-line was monitored by a transducer. The animal was relatively restrained and the tail end was located over a stainless steel funnel which emptied into a strain gauge-mounted cup. Outputs of transducer and strain gauge were simultaneously monitored on a strip chart recorder. (By permission of the *American Journal of Physiology*.)

administered fluids (5% dextrose, lactated Ringer solution), and antibiotics. In the days immediately after surgery there was a total loss of the micturition reflex, but from around Day 7 after transection a time-dependent spontaneous recovery in detrusor muscle function was reliably observed.

Results

We set out to investigate systematically the role of receptors for neurotransmitters found in C fibre primary afferents as well as selective antagonists for these agents in the VEMR. We have also looked at the effects of transmitters released from bulbospinal pathways (noradrenaline, dopamine, 5-HT), as well as those released from intrinsic interneurons (enkephalins, GABA, glycine).

Primary afferent neurotransmitters

To assess the role of endogenous terminal activity on the micturition reflex, putative C fibre primary afferent neurotransmitters were administered

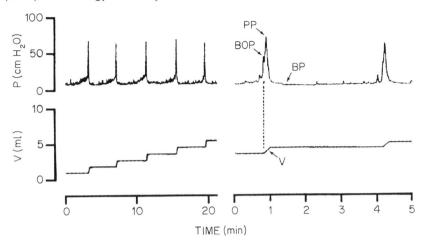

FIG. 2. A typical normal cystometrogram was obtained in an unanaesthetized male rat during continuous infusion of saline (200 μl/min). *Top tracing:* intravesical pressure (cmH₂O). *Lower tracing:* volume of urine in collection cup (ml) as a function of time (min). *Left tracing:* made at an infusion rate of 5 mm/min. *Right tracing:* from same animal made at a five-fold faster rate to show relationship between notch observed in rising phase of bladder contraction and expression of urine (vertical dashed line). BP, baseline pressure; BOP, bladder opening pressure; PP, peak pressure; V, volume of urine expressed per bladder contraction.

intrathecally and their effect on VEMR parameters was measured. We tested glutamate, substance P, VIP, SST and CCK in the intact rat. In no animals tested were these agents found to produce a change in either the intravesical pressure profiles of the VEMR or the rate and amplitude of bladder contractions.

Administration of *antagonists* for glutamate receptors of the N-methyl-D-aspartate type (MK-801, AP-5), and also VIP ([4-Cl-D-Phe[6], Leu[17]]VIP), produced a dose-dependent increase in the frequency of detrusor muscle contraction and sphincter opening pressure with a corresponding decrease in the time/volume to VEMR. The CCK antagonist (L-364, 718-000) produced *no* change in VEMR parameters. Spantide, a putative substance P antagonist, produced a dose-related blockade of sphincter function with a corresponding increase in intravesical pressure and overflow incontinence. This blockade, however, was reliably associated with a motor dysfunction involving the hind limbs. At lower doses (3 or 10 μg, intrathecally) this dysfunction was observed to be transient, but at the higher dose (30 μg) the paralysis was permanent.

The administration of primary afferent neurotransmitters into the lumbar spinal space of spinally transected rats produced changes in VEMR parameters that were not seen in the intact animal. In general, the transected animals displayed spontaneous recovery of detrusor muscle or urethral sphincter function between five and 10 days after spinal transection. Before the onset of recovery, a constant infusion of saline would result only in high intravesical pressures and overflow incontinence. Any agent administered before spontaneous recovery began was unable to generate detrusor muscle contractions or relaxation of the sphincter.

In spontaneously recovering animals with hyperreflexic bladders, the excitatory amino acid glutamate (10 or 30 µg) was found to produce a *decrease* in the rate and amplitude of detrusor muscle contractions, with no effect on sphincter function. However, in several animals glutamate was also found to produce no effect on the bladder at these same doses. Although an inhibition of detrusor muscle contractions was not what we expected from an excitatory transmitter such as glutamate, it does correlate with the dose-related excitatory effects produced by the NMDA antagonists in the intact animals.

The VIP antagonist [4-Cl-D-Phe[6], Leu[17]] VIP also produced a dose-related excitatory effect on detrusor muscle contractions in the intact animal. Preliminary studies with VIP in transected rats, however, have shown that this peptide produces no real change in VEMR parameters during spontaneous recovery. Many laboratories have shown that VIP plays a role in the transmission of visceral afferent information, as well as a modulatory role in the pelvic ganglia and as a neurotransmitter released from postganglionic nerves in the bladder wall (for review see Maggi & Meli 1986), and we are unable to explain the lack of effect of VIP in our model. Further studies are currently under way.

Administration of substance P (3, 10 and 30 µg intrathecally) reliably produced a blockade of urethral sphincter function in spontaneously recovering animals. Interestingly, hyperreflexive detrusor muscle contractions seemed to be unaffected by the intrathecal administration of substance P but were eventually limited as a result of the high intravesical pressures produced by the sphincter blockade (see Fig. 3). The role of substance P in the sensory innervation of the bladder is well documented (Maggi et al 1984, Kawatani et al 1985; for review see Maggi & Meli 1986). It has been reported, however, that the distribution of substance P innervation of the bladder is uneven, with the highest density being observed in the neck and trigonal areas (Yokokawa et al 1985). The sphincter blockade produced by intrathecally administered substance P in the transected animal, with a lack of effect on the bladder body, may be interpreted in the light of this uneven distribution of substance P afferent fibres.

Bulbospinal systems

Bulbospinal projection systems containing a variety of neurotransmitters have been identified, of which the principal elements are thought to be noradrenaline and serotonin. These systems arise from cell bodies in the caudal midline raphe of the medulla and several medullary and pontine nuclei (including the locus ceruleus and the lateral tegmentum), respectively. In addition, dopamine-containing pathways originating from cell bodies in the ventral brainstem are

substance P CMG, Intact Animal

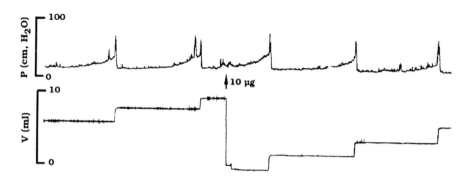

substance P CMG, Transected Animal, Day 16

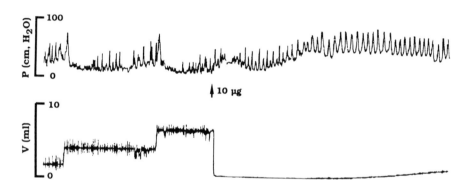

FIG. 3. The effect of substance P given intrathecally (10 µg) on the VEMR in intact and spinally transected rats. Substance P produces no change in VEMR parameters in a normal rat but reliably produced a blockade of urethral sphincter function in rats recovering spontaneously after spinal transection.

known to project into the spinal grey matter (Dahlström & Fuxe 1965, Bjorklund & Skageberg 1979). These bulbospinal systems have been shown to exert a powerful modulatory influence over activity in dorsal and motor horn neurons, as well as outflow from the intermediolateral cell columns. Thus, the iontophoretic administration of dopamine, α_2 and 5-HT$_1$ agonists can exert an inhibitory influence on dorsal horn wide dynamic range neurons. α_1 and other 5-HT agonists appear to exert an excitatory effect.

The intrathecal administration of 5-HT in a dose range which obtunds nociceptive reflexes (100–200 µg) has no detectable effect on any phase of the

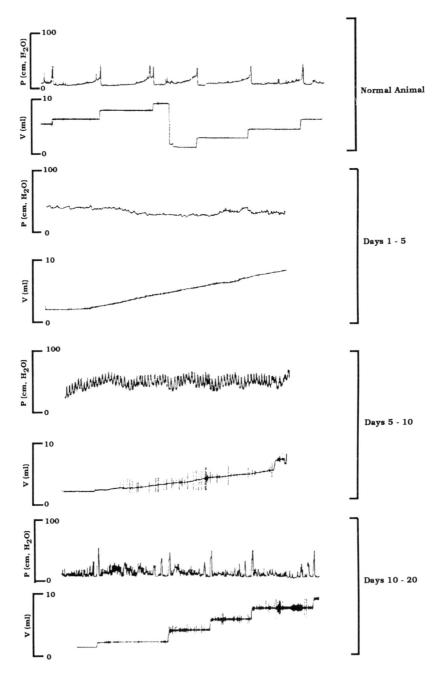

FIG. 4 (*caption opposite*)

cystometrogram in the unanaesthetized model. Similarly, the mixed 5-HT receptor antagonist methysergide was without effect on the spontaneous VEMR (P. A. C. Durant & T. L. Yaksh, unpublished observations).

The activation of spinal α_2 receptors by the polar agent ST-91 yields a dose-dependent decrease in the volume necessary to evoke a micturition reflex. Transient blockade of sphincter function was observed in the face of increased bladder pressure. The spinal α_1 agonist, methoxamine, was without effect. The intrathecal dopamine agonist, apomorphine, results in a reduction in the volume necessary to evoke a VEMR with a slight reduction in the sphincter opening pressure (Durant & Yaksh 1988).

The role of spinal receptors for the bulbospinal neurotransmitters in the VEMR of the chronic spinal animal has not yet been examined. This should represent an important line of investigation, in view of the disability associated with the transection.

Interneuron neurotransmitters

Evidence suggests that GABA receptors may be involved in the regulation of reflexly activated bladder motility by acting at the level of the pelvic ganglia (de Groat 1970, Maggi et al 1985) and the sacral parasympathetic nucleus (de Groat et al 1981), as well as on centres regulating activation at supraspinal levels (Sillen 1980, Sillen et al 1985). The effect of the spinal GABA system on micturition was investigated using the GABA$_A$ receptor agonist, muscimol, and the GABA$_B$ receptor agonist, baclofen.

Previous studies in anaesthetized animals have shown the ($-$)-baclofen and the racemic mixture ($\pm$)-baclofen can markedly reduce voiding efficiency on systemic administration (Sillen et al 1985, Maggi et al 1987, Kontani et al 1988), as well as central administration (Sillen et al 1985, Kontani et al 1988). The intrathecal administration of a low dose of ($-$)-baclofen (0.1 µg) generally had little effect on the VEMR. Doses of 1 µg reliably produced flaccidity of the hindlimbs, but only occasionally (20%) caused a blockade of sphincter function and an inhibition of the VEMR. At 10 µg, a long-lasting inhibition of the VEMR was observed in all rats tested. This blockade of the VEMR was always accompanied by hindlimb paresis.

FIG. 4.   Time course of spontaneous recovery after spinal transection in the rat. *Normal animal:* cystometrogram showing bladder contractions corresponding to synergic sphincter relaxation (increase in volume = emission of urine). *Days 1–5 after transection:* characterized by a complete loss of bladder function, high intravesical pressures, overflow incontinence. *Days 5–10 after transection:* appearance of random detrusor muscle function and sphincter dyssynergia with continued overflow incontinence. *Days 10–20 after transection:* appearance of more controlled detrusor contractions as well as synergic sphincter relaxation.

The inactive isomer, (+)-baclofen, was also tested in the same dose range. Intrathecal administration of 0.1, 1 or 10 µg of (+)-baclofen produced no change in any VEMR parameters, nor did it cause any muscle weakness in any of the animals tested.

Although it has been suggested that GABA$_A$ receptors modulate reflex micturition by acting at both spinal and supraspinal sites in the CNS (Sillen 1980, Maggi et al 1987), we have found in this study that intrathecally injected muscimol in an unanaesthetized rat produces no significant change in the VEMR. This is interesting in light of the fact that muscimol (10 or 30 µg) produces the same hindlimb muscle weakness that we observed with baclofen, but has no effect on sphincter function or detrusor muscle contractions.

Spontaneous recovery after spinal injury

As shown in Fig. 4, vesicular infusion of saline (200 µl/min) in an intact rat resulted in a reliable increase in vesical pressure, along with a relaxation of the sphincter and a corresponding emission of urine. Transection of the spinal cord produced an acute loss of bladder contractions and resulted in high intravesical pressures and overflow incontinence. This overflow incontinence occurred at vesical pressures greater than the sphincter opening pressures observed in the intact animal, suggesting a failure of the external sphincter to relax. Over the ensuing period there was a progressive return of function, with spontaneous detrusor contractions first appearing around 5–10 days. Sphincter responses were consistently delayed in comparison and usually appeared only after Day 10 post-transection. Synergic sphincter function and some degree of continence followed several days later. Characteristically, there were extended periods during recovery in which the bladder displayed an increased rate and amplitude of spontaneous contractions which did not result in an appropriate VEMR. This activity was often accompanied by a pronounced hindlimb clonus.

Conclusion

Although the afferent fibre types which predominate in man after spinal injury remain unknown, we have shown in this report that it is possible to produce changes in the VEMR of chronic spinal rats with the intrathecal administration of peptide neurotransmitters which are known to be released from C fibre afferents in intact rats.

In theory, a major advantage of the intrathecal administration of drugs in this situation is that it allows us the opportunity to try to replace or *mimic* the neurotransmitter environment that is lost after spinal injury by delivering agents directly into the lumbosacral spinal space in the area of the parasympathetic nucleus. As the identity of Aδ fibre neurotransmitters remains unknown, we have concentrated our efforts on those neurotransmitters known to be contained in C fibre afferents, descending bulbospinal pathways, and local interneurons. The results presented here show that such an approach is feasible. We also note that similar spinal administration in man is eminently practical and involves methods that have been used extensively. These experiments, and this animal model, not only provide promise of enhancing our fundamental knowledge of the micturition reflex, but also suggest a potentially novel approach to managing bladder dysfunction in spinally injured patients.

References

Barrington FJF 1925 The effect of lesions of the hind- and midbrain on micturition in the cat. QJ Exp Physiol 15:181

Bjorklund A, Skageberg G 1979 Evidence for a major spinal cord projection from the diencephalic A11 dopamine cell group in the rat using transmitter specific fluorescent retrograde tracing. Brain Res 177:170

Conte B, D'Aranno V, Santicioli P et al 1988 New method for recording cystometrograms in conscious, freely moving rats. J Pharmacol Methods 19:57–61

Dahlström A, Fuxe K 1965 Evidence for the existence of monoamine neurons in the central nervous system. Acta Physiol Scand 64 (Suppl 247)

de Groat WC 1970 The action of GABA and related aminoacids on mammalian autonomic ganglia. J Pharmacol Exp Ther 172:384–386

de Groat WC, Ryall RW 1969 Reflexes to sacral preganglionic parasympathetic neurones concerned with micturition in the cat. J Physiol (Lond) 200:87–108

de Groat WC, Nadelhaft I, Milne RJ, Booth AM, Morgan C, Thor K 1981 Organization of the sacral parasympathetic reflex pathways to the urinary bladder and large intestine. J Auton Nerv Sys 4:135–160

Dray A, Metsch R 1984a Morphine and the centrally mediated inhibition of urinary bladder motility in the rat. Brain Res 297:191–195

Dray A, Metsch R 1984b Opioid receptor subtypes involved in the central inhibition of urinary bladder motility. Eur J Pharmacol 104:47–53

Durant PAC, Yaksh TL 1988 Micturition in the unanesthetized rat: effects of intrathecal capsaicin, N-vanillylnonanamide, 6-hydroxydopamine and 5,6-dihydroxytryptamine. Brain Res 451:301–308

Jancsó G, Maggi CA 1987 Distribution of capsaicin-sensitive urinary bladder afferents in the rat spinal cord. Brain Res 418:371–376

Jessell TM, Dodd J 1989 Functional chemistry of primary afferent neurons. In: PD Wall, R Melzack (eds) Textbook of pain, 2nd edn. Churchill Livingstone, Edinburgh, p 82–102

Jonas U, Jones LW, Tanagho EA 1975 Spinal cord vs detrusor stimulation. A comparison study in six acute dogs. Invest Urol 13:171–178

Kawatani M, Erdman SL, de Groat WC 1985 VIP and substance P in primary afferent pathways to the sacral spinal cord of the cat. J Comp Neurol 241:327–347

Kontani H, Kawabata Y, Koshiura R 1988 The effect of baclofen on the urinary bladder contraction accompanying micturition in anesthetized rats. Jpn J Pharmacol 46:7–15

Maggi CA 1990 The dual function of capsaicin-sensitive sensory nerves in the bladder and urethra. In: Neurobiology of incontinence. Wiley, Chichester (Ciba Foundation Symposium 151) p 77–90

Maggi CA, Santicioli P, Meli A 1984 The effects of topical capsaicin on rat urinary bladder motility in vivo. Eur J Pharmacol 103:41–50

Maggi CA, Santicioli P, Meli A 1985 GABA inhibits excitatory neurotransmission in rat pelvic ganglia. J Pharm Pharmacol 37:349–351

Maggi CA, Meli A 1986 The role of neuropeptides in the regulation of the micturition reflex. J Auton Pharmacol 6:133–162

Maggi CA, Furio M, Santicioli P, Conte B, Meli A 1987 The spinal and supraspinal components of GABAergic inhibition of the micturition reflex in rats. J Pharmacol Exp Ther 240:998–1006

Moreau PM, Lees GE, Gross DR 1983 Simultaneous cystometry and uroflowmetry for evaluation of the caudal part of the urinary tract in dogs: reference values for healthy animals sedated with xylazine. Am J Vet Res 44:1774–1781

Sato A, Sato Y, Shimada F, Torigata Y 1975 Changes in vesical function produced by cutaneous stimulation in rats. Brain Res 94:465–474

Sillen U 1980 Central neurotransmitter mechanisms involved in the control of urinary bladder function. Scand J Urol Nephrol Suppl 58:1–45

Sillen U, Persson B, Rubenson A 1985 Central effects of baclofen on the L-dopa induced hyperactive urinary bladder of the rat. Naunyn-Schmiedeberg's Arch Pharmacol 330:175–178

Yaksh TL, Durant PAC, Brent CR 1986 Micturition in rats: a chronic model for study of bladder function and effect of anesthetics. Am J Physiol 251:1177–1185

Yokokawa K, Sakanaka M, Shiosaka S, Tohyama M, Shiotani Y, Sonada T 1985 Three dimensional distribution of substance P-like immunoreactivity in the urinary bladder of the rat. J Neural Transm 63:209–222

DISCUSSION

Brading: Do you have any problems with maintaining the spinally transected rats in a healthy state?

Tiseo: We had problems initially, but now post-operatively the rats are given 5% dextrose plus electrolytes; their bladders are expressed daily, and they receive antibiotics daily.

Staskin: The larger spikes in your records appear to represent bladder contractions. Are the smaller spikes also bladder contractions, or is it abdominal spasticity? If so, you would need a rectal catheter, to make sure that what you call detrusor activity isn't abdominal pressure transmitted to the bladder.

Secondly, from a urodynamic point of view, I wonder whether one can correlate urine *flow* patterns with sphincter function, without measuring the bladder and sphincter interactions.

Tiseo: I can't rule out that the spontaneous activity between detrusor contractions is abdominal spasms, although we see a similar 'noisy' effect with several agents in the intact animal, where I wouldn't expect abdominal spasm to play a role.

Staskin: Any activity that increases abdominal pressure will increase intravesical pressure, so that respirations or even moving around the cage could cause small spikes.

Tiseo: The rats can only move in a very limited way in the cage. We would need to do an EMG on the abdominal muscles to rule spasticity out, but we don't see the rats straining or twitching, so it does not seem that abdominal spasms are responsible for the activity that we see on the CMGs.

Staskin: The bladder activity correlates well with what you call clonus measurements, in the transected rats; every time you gave some medication that looked as if it might decrease bladder activity, it also decreased the urine flow, and that also correlated with the disappearance of the small spikes which I suggest might *not* be bladder activity. It may also have relaxed the sphincter, allowing overflow voiding.

Blaivas: I gather that you measured the *volume* of urine emitted but did not calculate the flow rate. We have developed a urine flow meter for rats that seems to be accurate over voided volumes from 100 ml down to less than 0.01 ml. The flow meter consists of a small collecting cup which has two wire electrodes. The rate at which urine goes in the collecting cup changes the resistance in two wires. It may be a useful way of looking at flow rates. I raise this because in your tracings of bladder pressure, the maximum pressure seemed so much higher than the opening pressure. Is that a normal phenomenon in the rat? It implies that either the bladder is continuing to contract, and more strongly, or there is increasing resistance to flow.

Tiseo: We see this in all our tracings in both the normal and chronic spinal rats. It appears that the bladder is contracting more strongly as the sphincter opens.

Blaivas: Most of the time, rabbits do not do this, and most humans don't, not to that degree.

Tiseo: On the tracings, what looks like a large increase is only a pressure difference of a few centimetres of water.

Blaivas: The scale went up to 100 cm of water?

Tiseo: Yes, but generally the range covers between zero and 50 cmH$_2$O.

Blaivas: How did you determine the interaction between detrusor and sphincter? You referred to the fact that the sphincter was opening or closing, but how did you know that, from the tracings?

Tiseo: We felt that as we were constantly infusing the bladder with saline, if we saw a constant increase in intravesical pressure, then the sphincter was probably not functioning, and not opening; because the bladder was continuously filling, intravesical pressure was becoming greater.

Blaivas: That is not necessarily true if the bladder isn't contracting. Dr Staskin suggested measuring rectal pressure, and this would clearly be useful. You don't ordinarily need to measure it in an animal preparation when the animal is anaesthetized, but in an awake animal with the ability to make some movements or to have clonus, rectal pressure measurements would help.

de Groat: We have recently done electrophysiological studies on the normal and the chronic spinally transected rat (Mallory et al 1989). The normal rat has a supraspinal pathway controlling micturition. The chronically transected rat has a spinal pathway, but the afferent limb for *both* pathways in the rat consists of *myelinated* afferent fibres. So the concept that emerged from studies on cats, and which you are using to interpret your results in rats, namely that C fibre afferents trigger micturition in spinal animals, does not apply to the rat.

Tiseo: The afferents from the bladder have not changed after transection, but whereas the second-order neuron that the afferents were synapsing on may have been an A fibre in the intact rat, they are now synapsing onto a C fibre in the transected spinal cord. Is this correct?

de Groat: The second-order neurons have not been identified in the rat, and are not well identified in the cat. We don't know anything about the interneuronal pathways in the spinal cord which process the C fibre afferent evoked reflex in the chronic spinal animal. What we have shown (as described in my paper) is that in the normal cat the supraspinal pathway is triggered by Aδ type myelinated afferents and in the chronic spinal, paraplegic cat it is triggered by C fibre, unmyelinated afferents.

The rat is different: both the spinal pathway and the supraspinal pathway seem to be triggered by myelinated fast-conducting fibres. We measured this electrophysiologically and were surprised to find that rat and cat are different. It is however consistent with our capsaicin experiments, where we showed that capsaicin does not block micturition in the spinal rat but does block in the spinal cat. So the neurotoxin studies correlate with the electrophysiological studies. Thus the cat data do not apply to the rat.

Tiseo: We compared the effects of capsaicin in intact and transected rats. As Dr Maggi said earlier, in the intact rat, capsaicin has little effect.

de Groat: We find that also.

Tiseo: When we administer capsaicin to the spontaneously recovering rat, after spinal transection, we can modify the recovery that we see.

de Groat: How long does that effect of capsaicin last?

Tiseo: It is a very acute effect and lasts perhaps 1–2 hours.

de Groat: We have different results. We find an acute depressant effect of capsaicin which lasts for about 12 h. This effect occurs with large doses of capsaicin and is similar to what Lembeck described in his initial studies with systemic administration of capsaicin. We attribute the depression to block of axonal conduction in the Aδ fibre pathway. We detected no difference between the normal and chronic spinal rat, in regard to the action of capsaicin.

Marsden: The previous discussion also drew attention to the fact that the selectivity of capsaicin for C fibres depends upon the dose, and with Dr Tiseo's direct intrathecal administration of capsaicin, he may be hitting the A fibres.

de Groat: I would agree with that interpretation. We have used systemic administration of capsaicin and Dr Tiseo has used intraspinal administration; those may be two entirely different experiments.

Marsden: Your point is worth emphasizing, in that the interneuronal machinery on which the C fibre or Aδ afferents are acting to control the bladder is poorly understood. The site at which these pharmacological agents delivered into the subarachnoid space are acting on the intraneuronal machinery is still purely speculative.

de Groat: We have studied intrathecal peptide administration in chronic spinal cats where we know more about the organization of the system then in the rat. In cats, VIP is present only in C fibres at sacral levels of the spinal cord. It is present in 25–30% of bladder afferents. Administration of VIP to normal cats inhibits micturition when injected intrathecally, but in chronic spinal cats it stimulates micturition. This fits with our concept that in cats C fibres become important in triggering micturition in spinal animals. VIP administered intrathecally mimics the effect of C fibre afferent stimulation. Therefore we think that VIPergic afferent pathways may be important in inducing automatic micturition in the paraplegic cat.

Marsden: I would add that not only is the intraneuronal machinery of bladder control not understood, but the distribution of the descending fibres from the pontine brainstem micturition centre on that interneuronal machinery in any species is not understood either. For limb movements, the complexity of the interneuronal machinery, and of the distribution of descending inputs to it, is so great that any result could be obtained using pharmacological agents.

de Groat: Something that can explain some of the clonic activity that you have seen, Dr Tiseo, is that visceral afferents in the bladder, in animals and probably in humans as well, can trigger somatic reflexes. We described this initially in chronic spinal cats. In those animals, bladder distension induces hindlimb movement and walking behaviour, prior to urination. Other investigators also observed this when trying to train chronic spinal cats to walk a treadmill. When the bladder was full they walked very well. This is an interaction between visceral and somatic afferents. Some of the movements you see may be due to distension of the bladder, and activation of the afferents. Also in the intact, awake animal, some of the spikes on the baseline may come not from the bladder but from the limbs.

Marsden: In human beings, if muscle spindles in human limbs are vibrated and the bladder is full, there is a different reflex somatic motor response.

Blaivas: Conversely, spasm of the limbs in patients with myelitis often elicits detrusor contraction.

Maggi: May I comment on the problem of the experimental administration of peptides into the spinal cord? We have separated the urethra from the bladder surgically, in rats, and have given capsaicin, either into the bladder or into the urethra, against a background of volume-evoked bladder contractions. If we apply capsaicin to the bladder, there is bladder excitation. But if we administer capsaicin into the urethra, bladder activity is inhibited (Coute et al 1989). This means that we are activating the urethral receptive field of capsaicin-sensitive neurons, and that bladder afferents have an effect which is excitatory, whereas urethral afferents have an inhibitory effect. These sets of nerves probably release the same neurotransmitter centrally, which then acts on distinct second-order neurons that are engaged in different pathways. I think that when you give substance P or VIP or other peptides, which are putatively released from sensory nerves, the lack of an effect, as you have shown, Dr Tiseo, cannot allow any definitive conclusion, because you may be equally stimulating second-order sensory neurons which have opposite effects on what you are measuring.

A second point is that there is considerable enzymic activity in the spinal cord which degrades peptides physiologically, so you cannot exclude the possibility that the infused peptide was broken down in a few seconds. In my view, this type of experiment would be more meaningful using antagonists, rather than agonists.

Tiseo: I agree with both points. There is always a danger of enzymic degradation when working with peptides. This was part of our reason for trying to get the catheter as close to the point of action as possible. We plan to look at antagonists to several of these neurotransmitters in spinally transected rats. We have only done this in the intact animal so far.

Marsden: This would be more meaningful for physiological analysis, but not necessarily so for devising therapeutic strategies!

de Groat: There are many different afferent inputs to any segment of the spinal cord, and the same transmitter may be used in a variety of afferent pathways. Thus if a transmitter substance is applied to the spinal cord it could mimic a massive afferent input from many pathways. For example, VIP is interesting because it is contained in 70% of the afferents from the uterine cervix of the cat, and in a high percentage of bladder (25%) and colon afferents (15%). VIP is also a marker in the cat of sacral C fibre afferents. In our normal animals, when we inject VIP onto the surface of the spinal cord, it inhibits micturition, similarly to stimulation of the uterine cervix. So it is possible to mimic the response of various inputs by the administration of exogenous substances. I agree that using antagonists is a more effective way of looking at the function of putative transmitters, but in many cases effective antagonists are not available.

The efferent pathways to the bladder could be influenced by tonic somatic inputs generated by motor activity in the unanaesthetized animals. Thus when you inject an excitatory amino acid antagonist like MK-801 and observe a facilitation of bladder activity, it is possible that the drug is blocking an afferent pathway that is tonically inhibiting the bladder. This could facilitate the bladder reflex.

Burnstock: The advantage of this experimental model is the absence of anaesthetics, which are supposed to interfere with bladder function. Did you have a chance to look systematically at the effects of different anaesthetics on micturition?

Tiseo: We looked at a variety of anaesthetics, including α-chloralose, ketamine, pentobarbitone, halothane (2% in air), and bupivicaine + 2-chloroprocaine, which are local anaesthetics. They all produced a block of the micturition reflex and overflow incontinence in the rat.

Brading: We obtain micturition reflexes in guinea pigs anaesthetized with urethane and also with ketamine and xylocaine.

Andersson: If we have two ways of emptying the rat bladder, one for territorial marking and one for pure bladder emptying, is there any difference in afferent input in the two types of emptying? Is there any information on that?

de Groat: Territorial marking is said to be triggered by olfactory stimuli; dogs smell a patch of urine from another dog and may respond to that. I don't think it's therefore necessarily an afferent from the bladder that is involved in territorial marking; it is an afferent from some other part of the nervous system. This is similar to penile erection, which can be erotically induced, induced by tactile stimuli, or visually induced. I would imagine that this kind of 'marking' micturition is mediated by input from higher centres in the brain. Just as humans urinate at various bladder volumes, I presume animals can also urinate at various volumes, and probably below the micturition volume threshold at which a normal house-trained animal would attempt to urinate.

Blaivas: Are those reflexes, or is that just a form of heightening voluntary micturition? Do the animals smell something and immediately urinate?

Swash: Animals can be trained to micturate; a house-broken dog can be trained to go outside and micturate, for example.

Blaivas: Dr Tiseo, do you know how rats ordinarily void? Do they do so in spurts, and how often do they void?

Tiseo: It appears to be generally in spurts; but they empty the bladder all at once, not gradually. We infuse at 200 μl a minute, and micturition occurs roughly every five minutes. I don't know what their voiding schedule is when they are just in their cages.

References

Coute B, Maggi CA, Meli A 1989 Vesico-inhibitory responses and capsaicin-sensitive afferents in rats. Naunyn-Schmiedeberg's Arch Pharmacol 339:178–183

Mallory B, Steers WD, de Groat WC 1989 Electrophysiological study of micturition reflexes in rats. Am J Physiol 257:R410–R421

General discussion I

Functional and anatomical correlates

Swash: I would like to hear more about the specificity of the distribution of the innervation of the bladder, in relation to the physiological observations. Geoffrey Burnstock spoke about differences between the dome and lower wall of the bladder. How relevant is the geography of the distribution of the nerves, receptors and neuropeptides to the kinds of physiological data we are hearing about?

Burnstock: We have mainly looked at human preparations, and I am sure that the regional distribution and immunochemistry of the innervation will be critical for our understanding of this system. For example, many pharmacological studies of human bladder have been carried out on the tip of the dome, because that is what is easily available, but I don't think that is typical of the rest of the bladder. One has to be careful about jumping to conclusions on the basis of a limited regional preparation.

Andersson: In bladders removed at cystourethrectomy it is possible to examine the cholinergic and adrenergic innervation, and to correlate it with receptor numbers. We haven't seen any clear difference in the cholinergic innervation within the human bladder. The cholinergic innervation of the urethra was also uniform, but less dense than that in the bladder (Ek et al 1977). The role of the cholinergic inervation in human urethral function is not known. In general it is difficult to correlate the density of nerves and of receptors with contractile responses. For example, there is a sparse adrenergic innervation of the dome of the human bladder but a good response to β-adrenergic agonists, and radioligand experiments have confirmed the existence of β-adrenoreceptors (Andersson 1986). We can also modulate the number of muscarinic receptors; by treating female rabbits with oestrogens we reduced the muscarinic receptors in bladder dome tissue to 10% of the original number, but the response to carbachol didn't change (Batra & Andersson 1989).

Staskin: Do we feel that the presence of receptors implies innervation?

Burnstock: I think the body does not go in for features like receptors unless they play some role. For instance, there are muscarinic cholinergic receptors on vascular endothelial cells. As it turns out, they are *not* related to cholinergic innervation; they are related to another source for acetylcholine, namely the vascular endothelial cells themselves.

Brindley: On this question of local variations in innervation, Dr B. Birch of the Institute of Urology in London has been able to pass a small bipolar electrode through a cystoscope, touch it against the bladder in conscious patients, and stimulate. He has measured thresholds for sensation high in the bladder and lower down, and finds a three-fold variation in threshold from one part of the bladder to the other. By measuring strength–duration curves he has shown that the fibres being stimulated are myelinated. He finds that patients are not good at localizing the stimulus in terms of upper and lower parts of the bladder but they consistently know whether it's on the right or left side. The differences from top to bottom in threshold correlated with the observed density of myelinated fibres in the bladder wall.

Staskin: Is there a consensus that there is true denervation supersensitivity, at least on a pharmacological basis, in the bladder?

Burnstock: A related issue is the concept of plasticity, not only of nerves, but also of receptors. We have worked on many different organs, and the bladder is one of the most remarkable organs for the degree of plasticity that can occur even in the adult animal. If you remove one set of nerves, hyperinnervation by another type occurs and there are concomitant changes in receptor expression too. We have heard from Dr de Groat about entire reflexes emerging under certain conditions, but not in others. The whole question of what controls receptor expression, as well as the expression of nerves and transmitters, remains to be determined.

Marsden: That doesn't answer the specific question about denervation supersensitivity at the functional level; behavioural supersensitivity may not be expressed by changes in receptor numbers.

Brading: Dave Westfall's group find that denervation supersensitivity in smooth muscle is not well correlated with any change in the receptors, in contrast to striated muscle (Westfall 1981). We have looked at the binding of muscarinic antagonists to bladder smooth muscle in various animal models where we see a clear structural reduction in nerve numbers and apparent functional denervation supersensitivity, but we cannot correlate the increased sensitivity with a change in the numbers of muscarinic receptors (unpublished observation). We believe it's more likely to be due to changes in the excitability of smooth muscle. In large mammals, such as man and pig, we do find supersensitivity to acetylcholine with denervation, but in smaller mmmals such as the guinea pig we do not, even when we get denervation and evidence of bladder instability that is very similar to that in the larger species. Dr K. Fujii in my laboratory finds in the guinea pig that acetylcholine does not cause a marked depolarization of the membrane; it is working more through a pharmaco-mechanical coupling, bypassing the excitability of the membrane (Fujii 1988). This may be why we don't see supersensitivity in the muscle. It may be supersensitive to agents which depolarize the membrane, although we have no evidence for this.

Maggi: In relation to the density of innervation, receptor density and functional response, there is one additional possibility to consider, namely a difference in coupling between the receptors and the second messenger systems.

If you take the dome and the neck of the guinea pig bladder and give isoprenaline to relax the muscle and measure cyclic AMP formation, similar amounts are produced in the dome and the neck. Whereas calcitonin gene-related peptide (CGRP), which relaxes the bladder muscle through the same pathway, is much more efficient in stimulating cyclic AMP production in the neck than in the dome. So even in normal (physiological) conditions there may be a regional difference in the coupling between receptors and the second messenger.

Kirby: Supersensitivity dates back to Cannon's law—the concept that if you denervate a smooth muscle the receptor numbers will increase. Patients with distal autonomic neuropathies, who are some of the most profoundly denervated patients seen, don't have much increase in receptor density. In fact there seem to be relatively fewer receptors. I would agree with Alison Brading that if there is denervation supersensitivity it's probably on the basis of an increased excitability in smooth muscle membranes, more than on an increase in receptor numbers.

Burnstock: But you are just talking about adrenoreceptors—what about others?

Kirby: Yes. I cannot give you any information about purinergic receptors.

Marsden: Supersensitivity is a pharmacological functional phenomenon which *may* have a receptor basis. There are many forms of pharmacological functional supersensitivity which cannot be explained on the basis of simple receptor changes.

Burnstock: On the other hand, the reverse is also found. If tissue is exposed to an excess of the transmitter substance, or if there is hyperinnervation, subsensitivity, probably associated with a decrease in receptor numbers, occurs.

Correlations between urinary and anorectal systems

Swash: Can I ask Nick Read how the work on the bladder makes sense in relation to the anorectum? Is there any correlation? It is important to make the comparison.

Read: It's tempting to say that the two systems are entirely parallel; but clearly there are some differences. Both have a storage organ which shows the phenomenon of accommodation, both have a smooth muscle internal sphincter, both have an external striated muscle sphincter which is linked functionally to the muscles of the pelvic floor, and both are supplied by extrinsic parasympathetic nerves which cause contraction of the rectum and bladder and sympathetic nerves that cause relaxation of both organs. The responses to distension of both organs appear to be similar. If you fill the rectum slowly the internal sphincter remains closed for some time and then relaxes. The responses of both sphincters to increases in intra-abdominal pressure appear similar.

The differences between the two systems lie in the fact that there is a very well-developed intrinsic nervous system in the wall of the rectum. This system presumably is there to coordinate the different contractile patterns in the rectum, because the rectum, unlike the bladder, does not contract as a syncytium but shows various patterns. Also the rectum is a secretory organ and an absorptive organ and these functions may well be related and coordinated with functions of motility.

Marsden: One considerable difference is that the bladder is a storage organ and the rectum isn't, in normal circumstances.

Read: In fact the rectum *is* a storage organ, but the entry of material into the rectum is very different from the entry of material into the bladder. There is pulsatile entry into the rectum, and slow entry into the bladder. That is a big difference in behaviour.

Another point concerns the concept of a vascular plexus in the bladder neck and its possible contribution to urinary continence. We have evidence to support the idea that anal cushions may have an important role in maintaining faecal continence. After a radical haemorrhoidectomy, some people become quite incontinent.

Marsden: The emphasis on local reflex circuits within the rectum itself, not involving the spinal cord, was noted earlier. This is a major difference.

Burnstock: The control is very different; there is a dominance of central control mechanisms in the bladder, whereas there is the possibility of a much greater component of local control in the bowel, although probably not the sphincters.

Read: I am not sure about that. We think of the anorectal area as having a local control system that is heavily modulated by the central nervous system. The enteric nervous system controls the complex motor activity of the rectum and coordination with secretion, but stimulation of the extrinsic parasympathetic nerves contracts both bladder and rectum and causes evacuation. Also when we stimulate anterior spinal roots in paraplegic patients, we get a contraction in the descending sigmoid colon and rectum and a complete relaxation of the sphincter, both internal and external components. A similar phenomenon is seen in the bladder.

Brindley: I have also looked at bladder responses, and rectal and anal sphincter responses, to sacral root stimulation. The striated anal sphincter behaves just like the striated urethral sphincter, but the smooth muscle responses of bladder and rectum are not the same. For one thing, rectal responses are about 2.5 times slower than bladder responses. For another, after a long period of spinal root stimulation, bladder pressure goes up, and then slowly decays, but remains elevated for minutes; rectal pressure gives a slow wave, comes right down to baseline and remains there, and then gives a series of little waves that are absent in the unstimulated paraplegic empty rectum. So the patterns of response to spinal stimulation are different in rectal and bladder smooth muscle.

Swash: Defaecation can be induced with an intravenous infusion of neurotensin, indicating that the central or peripheral mechanisms subserving defaecation are susceptible to pharmacological effects (Calam et al 1983).

Burnstock: There are 20 or so transmitters in the intrinsic gut neurons, combined in different ways, whereas in the bladder we have only seen three or four transmitter substances in the intrinsic neurons. That again shows that the bladder has a much more limited repertoire in terms of its intrinsic machinery than the gut.

Read: We have heard that the myenteric plexus in the rectum becomes sparse as you proceed distally. Does it therefore become a bit more like the bladder?

Burnstock: How sparse is it?

Christensen: This gradient in nerve cell density in the rectum is not true in rodents but it is true in cats and other large mammals (Christensen et al 1983, 1984). The density of ganglion cells in the myenteric plexus in such species falls to about 100–150 cells per cm^2 surface area at the lower end of the rectum, whereas at the top, in the area corresponding to the sigmoid colon, it's about 1000–1500 ganglion cells/cm^2.

Burnstock: A lot of these ganglion cells will be sending processes further down, so it doesn't mean, because you have relatively few ganglion cells at the far end of the rectum, that the muscle is not heavily innervated.

Christensen: I agree. We have no idea about the projections. In the rectal plexus, however, there are many large nerve bundles which are really intramural extensions of the extramural nerves, because they have a perineurial sheath and a dedicated blood supply. These are extrinsic neurons projecting down towards the anus. In that connection, is it clear that the innervation of the bladder neck sphincter is by the pudendal nerve?

DeLancey: Huisman et al (1978) put electrodes directly into the striated sphincter of the urethra, going through the lumen and moving towards to the pubic bone, so the only thing they could have entered was in the striated sphincter. They gave those individuals pudendal nerve blocks, and electrical activity increased. The difficulty with trying to look at the nerves to decide about urethral innervation is that you can't easily dissect through the dense tissue in that area to see what innervates it. From all the literature I was unclear about whether there was only one innervation, or were there two, or whether in fact anybody knew. To say that the striated urogenital sphincter is innervated only by the pudendal nerve is an oversimplification, in my view.

Swash: We thought that the intramural component of the striated urethral sphincter muscle was probably innervated by direct somatic efferent branches from the pelvic nerves entering the muscle from its peritoneal surface. Latency studies from spinal stimulation suggested this (Snooks & Swash 1986). So there are two innervations; the periurethral component of the striated urethral sphincter muscles is innervated by the perineal branch of the pudendal nerve, and the intramural component is innervated by direct somatic efferent branches derived from the pelvic plexus.

Blaivas: Retrograde tracer studies have never shown that.

Swash: Those are animal studies; I am talking about human studies, where you cannot do tracer studies. This is the crux of the problem.

de Groat: It seems that the rectum communicates with the internal anal sphincter through the myenteric plexus; it is possible to eliminate the extrinsic nerves and still obtain a sphincter response to rectal distension. I don't know of any evidence for intrinsic nerves in the urinary tract which could mediate a change in the bladder neck and proximal urethra in response to distension of the detrusor. As Geoff Burnstock mentioned earlier, there are peripheral neurons that can mediate interactions in the gut which are apparently not present in the bladder.

Blaivas: Unless you consider the fact that transmission along the smooth muscles themselves can take place?

de Groat: That may occur, but it's not a neural mechanism. I see a difference in the neural connections; however, whether there is transmission through the smooth muscle, from one part of the bladder to the bladder neck and proximal urethra, should be discussed.

Then there is the question of the intrinsic neurons that Geoff Burnstock described in his paper (p 2). An important issue is whether these neurons resemble the myenteric plexus neurons. Geoff said that the myenteric plexus looks like the brain, but what does this plexus in the bladder look like? I suspect it will turn out to resemble the peripheral nervous system, like the shunt fascicles that Jim Christensen has described in the colon.

Another issue is whether neurons in the bladder wall have migrated into the bladder from the pelvic plexus. We know that many species have neurons in the pelvic plexus near the neck of the bladder or on the serosal surface of the bladder, and that some of those neurons move along the nerves into the bladder smooth muscle. This situation is less interesting than one where the intramural neurons represent a different population with unusual properties.

Burnstock: The critical experiment, which has only partially been explored, concerns the embryonic origin of these two groups of neurons. It's clear that in the myenteric plexus, the enteric neurons have a totally different embryonic origin from neural crest tissue from the sympathetic and parasympathetic neurons (Le Douarin 1982, 1984). This is why Langley in 1921 called the enteric nervous system the third component of the autonomic system. And the extrinsic nerves join the gut during development by migration of neurons down the pelvic nerves and then join the plexus. As far I know for the bladder, the neurons largely migrate down into it, rather than having a separate embryonic origin like those in the gut. That supports your view, Dr de Groat.

On your second point, on the morphology of the intrinsic ganglia in the bladder and whether they look like those in the gut or brain, or rather like sympathetic or parasympathetic ganglia, in fact their ultrastructure falls somewhere between enteric and sympathetic ganglia, but marginally perhaps more like sympathetic ganglia, without an extensive neuropil as occurs in enteric ganglia. However, it is still possible that some nerve cells have a separate embryonic origin.

de Groat: I would just like to add a possible modification to the pathways that you described in your talk. This is the parasympathetic sacral innervation to the distal bowel, in the cat and rat. It's possible that there is more than just a two-neuron arc (that is, where the preganglionic neurons in the spinal cord project into the myenteric plexus). In the rat, neurons in the major pelvic ganglion receive input from the spinal cord and then project to the colon and rectum; so there may be a three-neuron arc, consisting of a preganglionic neuron, a plexus ganglion cell, and then neurons in the plexus. We have studied the ganglion cells which lie on the surface of the colon in the cat (de Groat & Krier 1976), and Jim Christensen studied their morphology. These cells receive inputs from the spinal cord and presumably they project into the myenteric plexus along shunt fascicles described by Christensen. Therefore there may be an entirely different organization for the sacral parasympathetic pathways to the gut and to the urinary bladder.

Burnstock: This seems entirely possible. Even in the gut itself we don't know exactly how many relays there are, once fibres penetrate into the plexus.

Brading: There is an interesting similarity in the sympathetic system, in that the ganglia in the bladder wall are the main targets of the sympathetic nerves, in the same way that they are in the myenteric plexus in the gut, and the sympathetic control of these neurons is probably by α-receptor stimulation of this type of neuron, which might otherwise be thought of as the parasympathetic postjunctional neuron.

de Groat: What species are you referring to?

Brading: This is in humans, because John Gosling (Gosling et al 1983) finds that the predominant innervation by the sympathetic nerves in the dome of the bladder is going to these neurons, if it's not going to blood vessels.

Burnstock: A much closer parallel occurs between the lung and stomach. The lung is an embryological offshoot from the stomach, and is much closer to the gut in its organization, in some ways, than the parallel between rectum and bladder.

de Groat: In the cat the adrenergic input to parasympathetic ganglion cells is mediated by local adrenergic neurons that lie within the pelvic plexus, and not by neurons in the sympathetic ganglia (the inferior mesenteric ganglia or sympathetic chain). This input remains after all extrinsic nerves are cut.

Brindley: Very little has been said about sympathetic actions on the bladder. There are patients in whom we can investigate this. There are nine male patients with spinal injuries into whom we have implanted electrodes on the hypogastric plexus in front of the bifurcation of the aorta for the purpose of getting semen. In some of these patients I looked at sympathetic actions on the bladder. I failed to see any systematic effect of stimulating the plexus on the bladder pressure; we know from other evidence that such stimulation makes the bladder neck contract, but it doesn't seem to affect the detrusor.

Blaivas: Did they have reflex bladder contractions, at the same volume?

Brindley: Some of these patients had areflexic bladders because we had cut the posterior roots. Others had reflex bladders. In neither group did hypogastric plexus stimulation cause contraction.

Blaivas: You would expect, from Dr de Groat's work, that it would have the opposite effect, and promote storage?

Brindley: Yes. But I am asking what experiments we should do. One of them is to fill the bladder up, until by natural, pathological non-compliance there is a significant pressure due to filling, and then see whether that pressure is lowered by hypogastric plexus stimulation. It might be!

Blaivas: You would have to know that the pressure rise was due to muscle contraction and not a visco-elastic response to stretch.

Brindley: This would not be impossible to determine, because you could give an anticholinergic drug. If this improved the compliance you would know that the defect in compliance was reflex, not due to fibrosis. This is just one thing we could look at. We could also look at interaction between sacral anterior root stimulation and hypogastric plexus stimulation. If the sympathetic is inhibitory on the detrusor, then perhaps it diminishes the response to sacral anterior root stimulation.

References

Andersson K-E 1986 Clinical relevance of some findings in neuro-anatomy and neurophysiology of the lower urinary tract. Clin Sci 70 (Suppl 14):21s–32s

Batra S, Andersson K-E 1989 Oestrogen-induced changes in muscarinic receptor density and contractile responses in the female rabbit urinary bladder. Acta Physiol Scand 137:135–141

Calam J, Unwin R, Peart WS 1983 Neurotensin stimulates defaecation. Lancet 1:737–738

Christensen J, Rick GA, Robison BA, Stiles MJ, Wix MA 1983 The arrangement of the myenteric plexus throughout the gastrointestinal tract of the opossum. Gastroenterology 85:890–899

Christensen J, Stiles MJ, Rick GA, Sutherland J 1984 Comparative anatomy of the myenteric plexus of the distal colon in eight mammals. Gastroenterology 86:706–713

de Groat WC, Krier J 1976 An electrophysiological study of the sacral parasympathetic pathway to the colon of the cat. J Physiol (Lond) 260:425–445

Ek A, Alm P, Andersson K-E, Persson CGA 1977 Adrenergic and cholinergic nerves of the human urethra and urinary bladder. A histochemical study. Acta Physiol Scand 99:345–352

Fujii K 1988 Evidence for adenosine triphosphate as an excitatory transmitter in guinea-pig, rabbit and pig urinary bladder. J Physiol (Lond) 404:39–52

Gosling JA, Dixon JS, Humpherson JR 1983 Functional anatomy of the urinary tract. Churchill Livingstone, Edinburgh

Huisman AB, Dantuma R, Salome AJ, Jonge MC de 1978 An unexpected effect of pudendal nerve blockade on the urethral EMG. Proceedings of 8th International Continence Society meeting, Manchester

Langley JN 1921 The autonomic nervous system. W. Heffer, Cambridge

Le Douarin NM 1982 The neural crest. Developmental and cell biology 12. Cambridge University Press, Cambridge

Le Douarin NM 1984 A model for cell line divergence in the ontogeny of the peripheral nervous system. In: Black IB (ed) Cellular and molecular biology of neuronal development. Plenum Press, New York, p 3–28

Snooks SJ, Swash M 1986 The innervation of the muscles of continence. Ann R Coll Surg Engl 68:45–49

Westfall DP 1981 Supersensitivity of smooth muscle. In: Bülbring E et al (eds) Smooth muscle: an assessment of current knowledge. Edward Arnold, London, p 285–309

Functional assessment of the anorectum in faecal incontinence

N. W. Read

Sub-Department of Gastrointestinal Physiology & Nutrition, Floor K, Royal Hallamshire Hospital, Glossop Road, Sheffield S10 2JF

Abstract. The functional ability of the anorectum to maintain continence is best assessed by a provocative assessment of continence to a standard load of rectally infused saline. Faecal incontinence is not caused by one condition. The combination of multiport anorectal manometry, electrophysiology and rectal sensory testing can identify several causes, which logically require different treatments. Only time and carefully conducted trials will establish whether such functional testing will be useful.

1990 Neurobiology of Incontinence. Wiley, Chichester (Ciba Foundation Symposium 151) p 119–138

How do we assess the functional of the anorectum as a mechanism for preserving continence? This question really encompasses two different questions. The first is: how do we assess the functional ability of the anorectum to preserve continence? The second: can we devise tests that allow us to identify the component of the mechanism that is at fault and discriminate between different causes of incontinence?

How effective is the continence mechanism?

Patients are often referred for anorectal tests by surgeons who want to know if their patients are likely to suffer with incontinence after an operation, such as colectomy, ileal resection or vagotomy, which gives their patients diarrhoea. Alternatively, they may wish to know the effect of haemorrhoidectomy or sphincterotomy or ileo-anal pouch on the functional ability of the sphincter to maintain continence.

These surgeons are the more enlightened of their profession. Many other surgeons assert that the application of the educated index finger into the anal canal provides them with the most useful assessment of the function of the sphincter. While index fingers may vary in their degree of sensitivity and erudition, we were unable to find any relationship between anal tone assessed with digital examination and either the basal sphincter pressure or the degree of incontinence (Read et al 1979). Similarly, the measurement of resting and squeeze sphincter pressures has failed to discriminate between patients with diarrhoea who complained of incontinence and those with diarrhoea who did not complain of incontinence (Read et al 1979). This is perhaps not surprising, because the continence mechanism is not just a simple muscular resistance and other factors contribute to the maintenance of continence. The best method of discriminating between patients who were incontinent and those who were not was a simple test of the continence to saline (Read et al 1979). In this test, saline warmed to 37 °C was infused into the rectum at a rate of 60 ml/min and the volume infused when the subject first leaked was recorded, as well as the total volume held. Most normal subjects could retain 1500 ml of saline without leakage, whereas all of the incontinence patients tested leaked the fluid and most leaked before 500 ml had been infused. This test, therefore, supports the general principle that in order to get the most accurate functional assessment of the sphincter mechanism, it is necessary to mimic the situation the sphincter may have to cope with. If a patient who claims to be incontinent manages to retain 1500 ml of rectally infused saline, one might suspect that he/she does not have true incontinence but may instead have mucous seepage from a local anal lesion, such as haemorrhoids. Alternatively, he/she may have bile acid malabsorption. We have recently shown that the incorporation of only very small amounts of bile acid into the rectal solution can severely impair continence (Edwards et al 1989).

Normal maintenance of continence

The anorectal mechanism for preserving continence is complicated. It consists of two sphincters, one (internal) composed of visceral smooth muscle, the other (external) of striated muscle and under conscious control; sensors in the rectum and the pelvic floor; and nervous reflexes which control the sphincters.

Under resting conditions and during gradual (approximately 10 ml/min) distension of the rectum (W. M. Sun & N. W. Read, unpublished observations), continence to rectal mucus and faeces is maintained by the tonic contraction of the internal anal sphincter (IAS). The circular fibres of the IAS, however are unable to shorten sufficiently to seal off the anal canal unless they are contracting around an anal lining that is sufficiently bulky to plug the orifice. The bulk of the anal lining is increased by infolding when the sphincter is contracted, and also by the presence of expansile vascular cushions, which act to hermetically seal the sphincter, at the same time stretching the muscle so that the circular muscle fibres can contract at a greater mechanical advantage (Gibbons et al 1986, 1988). A radical haemorrhoidectomy is associated with a high incidence of anal seepage (Read et al 1982). Tonic contraction of the external anal sphincter (EAS) can augment the resting tone of the IAS, but this muscle is almost completely relaxed when the subject is asleep (Whitehead et al 1982).

The tonic contraction of the internal sphincter is unable to maintain continence when this is threatened by rectal contraction, rapid rectal distension and increases in intra-abdominal pressure. This is because rapid rectal distension and contraction causes a reflex relaxation of the IAS, mediated by intrinsic nerves; while rises in intra-abdominal pressure are usually of sufficient magnitude to overwhelm the resting sphincter pressure and may also induce sphincter relaxation. Continence can only be maintained under these conditions by a compensatory contraction of the EAS. Although the EAS responses are present in paraplegic patients and are therefore spinal reflexes, the response to rectal distension is heavily modulated by conscious mechanisms and is very closely linked with rectal sensation (Sun et al 1990). Contraction of EAS during relaxation of the IAS increases the resistance of the sphincter, particularly in its outermost aspect, while allowing the composition of the rectal contents to be sampled by the sensitive anal lining (Duthie & Bennett 1963). The sampling of the rectal contents by the anal sensors has been proposed as the mechanism whereby people can discriminate between solid stool, liquid faeces and flatus. It is possible, however, that solid and fluid (gas or liquid) rectal contents may be identified by their ability to stimulate rapidly adapting rectal stretch receptors in the rectal wall. Most people report that they can perceive gaseous distension as a rectal sensation, and otherwise normal people can find it difficult to distinguish between gas and liquid when they have diarrhoea.

Simultaneous contraction of the puborectalis assists the EAS in maintaining continence by making the anorectal angle more acute. It is easy to see how a more acute anorectal angle will impede the entry of a solid cylindrical stool into the anal canal, but it would be unlikely to aid continence to liquids, unless the upper anal canal was being compressed against a relatively fixed object, such as the cervix uteri or the prostate gland.

The relationship between contraction of the EAS and of the IAS is poorly understood, because of the difficulty in recording the function of both muscles simultaneously in human subjects. Although both muscles relax during defaecation, they contract in a reciprocal manner during attempts to maintain continence. For example, rectal distension and contraction relax the IAS, but contract the EAS, while micturition is associated with relaxation of the EAS and contraction of the IAS (Salducci et al 1982). This reciprocal activity may explain why patients who have weakness of both the IAS and the EAS tend to be more incontinent than patients who have EAS weakness alone.

Investigation of patients with faecal incontinence

Faecal incontinence can result from impairment of any of several components of the continence mechanism. Clinical assessment of the function of the continence mechanism must (a) provide dynamic information about the integrated function of each component, (b) mimic situations where continence is threatened, (c) discriminate between different treatment options, (d) be comfortable for the patient and (e) not interfere unduly with the normal physiological function of the organ.

In our laboratory we use a multi-channel recording technique (Fig. 1) to measure pressures at multiple sites in the anus and the rectum and the electrical activity of the external and internal anal sphincter under resting conditions, during conscious contraction of the external sphincter, and during threats to continence induced by rapid rectal distension and increases in intra-abdominal

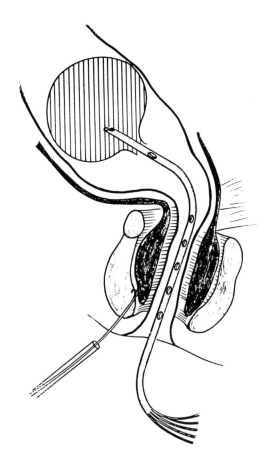

FIG. 1.   A diagram of the anal canal, showing the different muscle components and the probes used to measure pressure in multiple sites in the anal canal and the electrical activity of the internal and sphincter (shaded) and external anal sphincter. (From Read & Sun 1989 with permission.)

pressure (Fig. 2). Rectal sensations during rectal distension are recorded on the chart and any leakage of perfusion fluid is noted.

The recording of anorectal pressures from multiple closely spaced sites facilitates the identification of abnormalities of internal or external sphincter function. The two muscles often exhibit reciprocal activity; hence the EAS contraction that occurs, for example, during rectal distension can mask IAS relaxation in the outermost anal channels, but not in the inner channels. Interpretation of the manometric profiles is greatly facilitated by simultaneous recording of the electrical activities of the EAS and the IAS, allowing changes in pressure caused by the activity of those muscles to be identified.

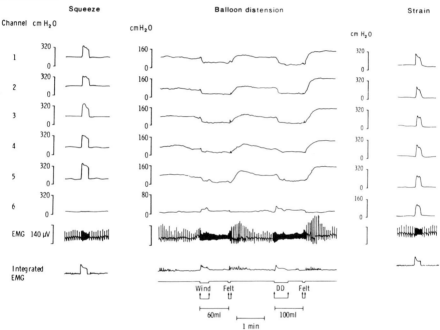

FIG. 2.   Recordings of anorectal pressure and the electrical activity of the external and internal anal sphincter (EAS and IAS) in the typical normal subject before and during conscious contraction of the EAS, during inflation of a rectal balloon with 60 and 100 ml of air, and during increased intra-abdominal pressure induced by the subject blowing up a balloon. Channels 1–6 represent ports situated 0.5, 1.0, 1.5, 2.0, 2.5 and 4.5 cm from the anal verge. Note that the EAS contraction was associated with an increase in EAS electrical activity and anal pressures; rectal distension induced a relaxation in sphincter pressure associated with abolition of the electrical oscillations produced by IAS activity, and an increase in the electrical activity of the EAS, whereas deflation produces a rebound increase in pressure which is associated with marked increase in the slow wave oscillations; and straining to blow up a balloon was associated with increases in rectal pressure, anal pressure and EAS electrical activity. The bar (Felt) indicates when the subject experienced rectal sensations. DD, desire to defaecate.

This test can be used with other clinical information to identify different causes of faecal incontinence, each of which would logically require a different treatment (Table 1).

Tests of anorectal function complement neurophysiological tests, because they test many different components of the continence mechanism and it is often the disturbance of function rather than any underlying neural mechanism that the surgeon is called upon to treat. Pudendal neuropathy is a normal accompaniment of ageing, particularly in women, and its demonstration does not exclude the greater importance of other factors, such as loss of rectal sensation or impaired internal sphincter function. Measurement of external sphincter responses to cerebral or spinal stimulation or the recording of cerebral potentials evoked by rectal stimulation may help to diagnose a lesion in the

TABLE 1   Causes of obstructed defaecation that can be identified by physiological testing

Causes	Features	Possible treatment
Anismus	Paradoxical EAS contraction during defaecation	? Retraining
Short segment Hirschsprung's disease	High anal pressures; failure of IAS to relax on rectal distension	Sphincterotomy
Megarectum	Increased rectal compliance and capacity Reduced rectal sensation	Defaecation retraining
Low spinal lesion	Impaired rectal sensation; reduced rectal tone Absent EAS response to rectal distension and increases in intra-abdominal pressure	Training
Irritable bowel syndrome	Enhanced rectal sensitivity Reduced rectal compliance Increased rectal contractility, and anal relaxation in response to rectal distension	{ Drugs Diet Psychotherapy
Non-prolapsing haemorrhoids	Ultraslow waves High resting pressures Failure of outermost anal canal to relax during rectal distension	Banding Electrocoagulation Haemorrhoidectomy
Partial rectal prolapse	Very low resting pressures Failure of anal pressure to increase above rectal pressure during increases in intra-abdominal pressure	Banding ? Post-anal repair

EAS, external anal sphincter; IAS, internal anal sphincter.

central nervous system, but such lesions are rare and may be suggested on the basis of combined manometric, electrophysiological and sensory testing. Thus CNS stimulation is only indicated if other anorectal function tests and neurological assessment provide a high degree of suspicion.

Pudendal neuropathy

This is perhaps the commonest cause of faecal incontinence. These patients have weak conscious and reflex contraction of the external anal sphincter. The electrical response of the EAS to conscious contraction, rectal distension and increases in intra-abdominal pressure are appropriate, but the mechanical effort is weak. The sphincter pressure often fails to increase above the rectal pressure during rectal distension and increases in intra-abdominal pressure and leakage of perfusion fluid occurs at these times. The weakness of the EAS is thought to occur because the distal segment of the pudendal nerve becomes stretched and compressed against the ischial spine. This situation may arise as a consequence of weakness of the pelvic floor, caused either during childbirth or as a result of prolonged straining. A post-anal repair is often successful, providing the pelvic floor and sphincter are not too weak.

Obstetric trauma

It is not uncommon for patients to be referred many years after their last delivery for investigation of faecal incontinence due to anal tears. The manometric features of a mechanically weak sphincter with normal electromyographic responses cannot be distinguished from pudendal neuropathy. Mapping out the site of the defect by recording EAS activity around the circumference of the sphincter can facilitate diagnosis and guide the surgeon. Sphincter repair is unsuccessful in patients with no EAS electrical activity.

Impaired internal anal sphincter

Twenty-five per cent of the patients referred to us for investigations of faecal incontinence had absent or impaired IAS tone (Sun et al 1989a). The manometric features were very low resting pressures and absent IAS relaxation when the rectum was distended (Fig. 3) and the electrical record showed attenuated or absent IAS electrical oscillations. The abnormally low pressures rule out Hirschsprung's disease (Aaronson & Nixon 1972, Faverdin et al 1981, Meunier et al 1979).

The absent or delayed IAS relaxation in these patients was not associated with an insensitive and hypercompliant rectum (Baldi et al 1982, Lennard-Jones 1985). The maximum squeeze pressures and the EAS pressure responses to rectal distension and to increases in intra-abdominal pressure were lower in patients

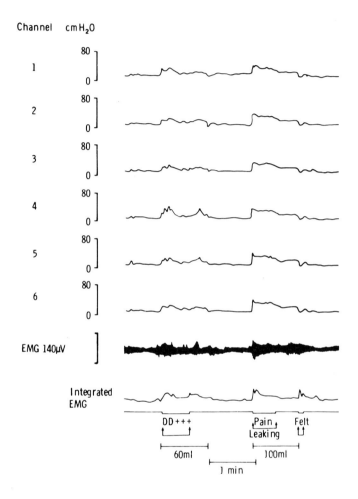

FIG. 3.   Recordings of anorectal pressure and the electrical activity of the sphincter in a female patient with impaired internal anal sphincter (IAS) function before, during and after inflation of a rectal balloon with 60 and 100 ml of air. Channels 1 to 6 represent ports situated 0.5, 1.0, 1.5, 2.0, 2.5 and 4.5 cm from the anal verge. Note the absence of IAS electrical activity and the abnormally low basal anal pressures, and the absence of anal relaxation during rectal distension. This increase is associated with an increase in the electrical activity of the external and sphincter. No rebound pressures were observed when the rectal balloon was deflated. The bars (↑__↑) indicate when the subject experienced rectal sensation. DD, desire to defaecate; +++ indicates the severity of the sensation. (From Sun et al 1989b, with permission from the publishers.)

with IAS dysfunction than in any other group of incontinent patients, and these patients were more severely incontinent than patients who just had weakness of the EAS. Nearly all of these patients also had an abnormal degree of pelvic floor descent. Perhaps the extremely weak striated muscle exposes the IAS to traction by the tissues of the pelvic floor. Alternatively, the abnormal descent of the pelvic floor may damage the delicate sympathetic nerves, that are thought to enhance the tone of the IAS. Unfortunately, our experience suggests that these patients do not do well after post-anal repair. The use of pharmacological agents to increase IAS tone needs to be explored.

Spontaneous transient anal relaxation

Approximately 20% of patients referred for investigation of faecal incontinence showed episodes of spontaneous IAS relaxation at rest lasting at least 15 s and reducing the pressure in the outermost anal channels by at least 20 cm of water (Sun et al 1988) (Fig. 4). The same phenomenon was seen in a similar percentage of normal subjects, but is probably of little significance, because simultaneous contraction of the EAS maintains the anal pressure barrier and guards against incontinence. The relaxations are of a longer duration in incontinent patients and the anal pressure falls to lower values. Fewer than a quarter of the incontinent patients with transient IAS relaxation showed compensatory increases in EAS activity. Some patients, particularly those with diabetes mellitus and other causes of autonomic neuropathy, only have incontinent episodes at night while they are asleep. Since the external sphincter is unable to compensate for a relaxation of the IAS while the subject is asleep (Whitehead et al 1982), transient relaxations of the sphincter may be responsible for nocturnal incontinence.

IAS relaxations are normally evoked by rectal distension, such as might be caused by the entry of faeces into the rectum, or by rectal contraction (Denny-Brown & Robertson 1935, Monges et al 1980, Callaghan & Nixon 1984). The majority of episodes of transient IAS relaxation recorded in these patients, however, appeared to be due either to autonomous losses of internal sphincter tone or to reductions in tone provoked by events that did not increase pressure in the rectum (Meunier & Millard 1977). In 50% of these patients, transient IAS relaxations were also evoked immediately after a conscious contraction or increase in intra-abdominal pressure. Post-squeeze or post-strain relaxation were rare in normal subjects.

Patients with transient relaxations exhibited many of the features of the 'irritable rectum' (see below), but transient relaxations were not a common feature of patients with the irritable bowel syndrome. Surgery is not indicated in patients with transient IAS relaxations unless there is another cause for incontinence, but perhaps the use of drugs to stabilize IAS contractions needs to be explored.

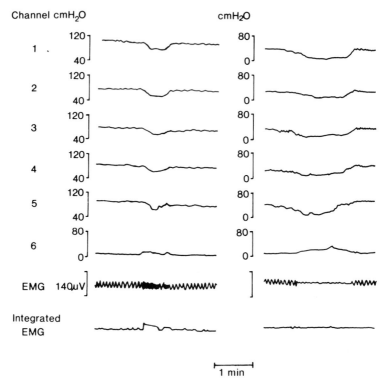

FIG. 4.   Multiport recordings of anal pressure and the electrical activities of the external and internal anal sphincter during and after an episode of spontaneous anal relaxation in a normal subject (*left*) and an incontinent patient (*right*). Channels 1 to 6 represent ports situated 0.5, 1.0, 1.5, 2.0, 2.5 and 4.5 cm from the anal verge. The relaxation lasted longer in the patient and was not associated with a compensatory increase in external sphincter activity. (From Read & Sun 1989, with permission from the publishers.)

Impaired rectal sensation

The ability of the patient to perceive the distension of the rectum caused by, for example, the arrival of faeces, appears to be necessary for the prompt and appropriate contractile response of the EAS (Sun et al 1990). EAS responses occur as soon as a rectal sensation is perceived and last for the same period of time. Conscious perception of rectal distension is not necessary for relaxation of the IAS. Thus patients with impaired rectal sensation may fail to contract the EAS in time to compensate for a relaxation of the IAS, induced by rectal distension or contraction. Two abnormalities can be seen during manometric and electrophysiological tests. In the first, the rectal volume that induces IAS relaxation is lower than that which induces rectal sensation and an increase in EAS activity (Fig. 5) (Wald & Tunuguntla 1984, Sun et al 1990). This abnormality

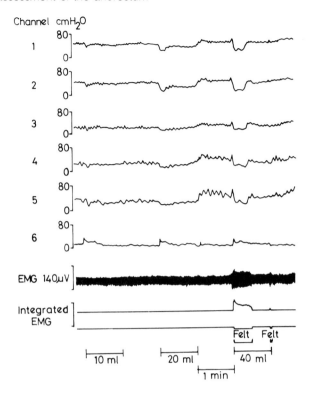

FIG. 5. Recordings of anal pressures at ports situated 0.5, 1.0, 1.5, 2.0, 2.5 and 4.5 cm from the anal margin (channels 1 to 6) and the electrical activity of the external anal sphincter (EAS) during distension of a rectal balloon with 10, 20, and 40 ml of air in a patient. Note that rectal distension of 10 and 20 ml induced internal anal sphincter relaxation and increased rectal pressure but did not elicit rectal sensation, and hence any electrical activity of the EAS. Distension with 40 ml caused rectal sensation which induced increased electrical activity of the EAS.

probably accounts for the incontinence in patients with megarectum and faecal impaction (Read & Abouzekry 1986). In the second, the EAS response is present, but delayed (Fig. 6) (Buser & Miner 1986, Sun et al 1990). Surgery and drugs are ineffective in such patients, but success can be achieved by techniques of sensory and anal coordination retraining.

Spinal lesions

About 10% of patients referred with problems of faecal incontinence exhibit manometric and electrophysiological features which resemble those from patients with lesions in the spinal cord. In most cases, conventional neurological

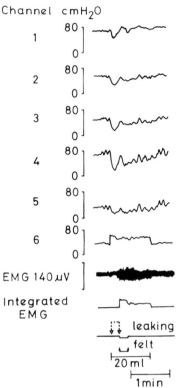

FIG. 6.   Recordings of anorectal pressures at ports situated 0.5, 1.0, 1.5, 2.0, 2.5 and 4.5 cm from the anal margin (channels 1 to 6) and the electrical activity of the external sphincter (EAS) during distension of a rectal balloon with 20 ml of air in a patient. Note that the rectal distension elicits a phasic rectal contraction and internal anal sphincter relaxation. The rectal pressure is higher than the residual anal pressure at the beginning of the distension and leakage occurs. This ceases once the subjects feel the rectal sensation, which triggers the EAS activity, increasing the anal pressure to a value higher than the rectal pressure.

examination and investigation fails to reveal a lesion. Thus occult spinal lesions may be a significant and important cause of faecal incontinence. The features of patients with low spinal lesions, revealed on anorectal testing, are low basal pressures, low squeeze increments, blunted rectal sensation and absent EAS responses to either rectal distension or increases in intra-abdominal pressure or both (Fig. 7). The combination of intact sensation and conscious control of the EAS suggests a lesion in the conus medullaris.

Patients with lesions in the cauda equina have a fairly uniform impairment of conscious and reflex EAS activity with impaired rectal sensation, and neurophysiological tests may be required to distinguish these patients from those with severe pudendal neuropathy.

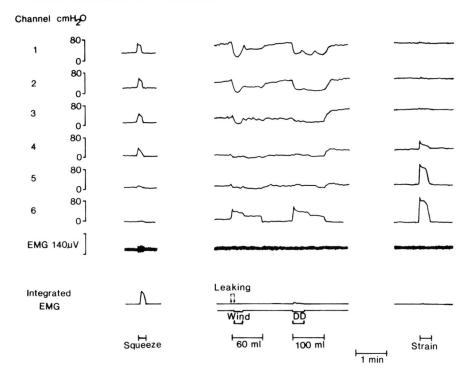

FIG. 7. Multiport recordings of anal pressure and the electrical activity of the external anal sphincter (EAS) during maximum conscious contraction of the EAS, during rectal distension and during straining (as if to defaecate) in a typical patient with a low spinal lesion. Channels 1 to 6 represent ports situated 0.5, 1.0, 2.0, 2.5 and 4.5 cm from the anal verge and in the balloon 5–11 cm from the anal margin. Note that there is appropriate conscious contraction of the sphincter but no increase in activity generated by rectal distension and increase in intra-abdominal pressure. (From Read & Sun 1989, with permission from the publishers.)

Patients with high spinal lesions also have weak sphincter pressures. They often have no conscious contraction of the sphincter and have blunted or often absent rectal sensation, but, unlike the patients with low spinal lesions, reflex activity of the sphincter is often exaggerated when the patient moves and during increases in intra-abdominal pressure and rectal distension (Fig. 8). Thus, the residual pressure during rectal distension is significantly higher in patients with high spinal lesions than in those with low spinal lesions, and a lower percentage of these patients leaked during the manometric test.

Patients with spinal lesions do not respond to anal surgery or drugs. Some success, however, may be achieved by retraining techniques, though patients who are profoundly disabled may require a colostomy.

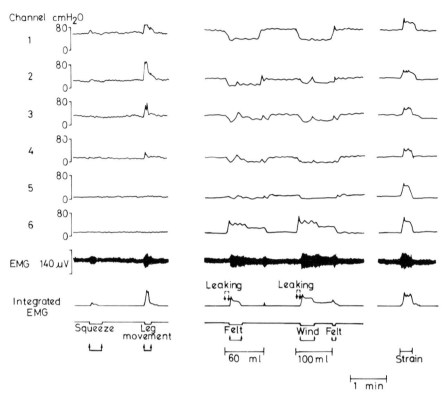

FIG. 8. Recording of anorectal pressures at ports situated 0.5, 1.0, 2.0, 2.5 and 4.5 cm from the anal margin and in the balloon 5–11 cm from anal verge (channels 1 to 6) and the electrical activity of the sphincter complex in a patient with a high spinal lesion during attempts at conscious contraction during rectal balloon distension with 60 and 100 ml of air and during increases in intra-abdominal pressure (strain). There was no conscious contraction of the sphincter but the reflex responses to rectal distension and increase in intra-abdominal pressure were much increased. The pressure and external anal sphincter activity were greatly increased during leg movement. (From Read & Sun 1989, with permission from the publishers.)

The irritable rectum

The rectum in a large cohort of patients with irritable bowel syndrome was much more sensitive to distension than that of normal subjects (Sun & Read 1988, Whitehead et al 1980). Patients feel a desire to defaecate, and experience an urgent desire to defaecate and pain at much lower rectal volumes than normal subjects. The rectal compliance is usually abnormally low (Sun & Read 1988) and sustained relaxation of the IAS and repetitive rectal contractions are induced at abnormally low rectal volumes (Fig. 9).

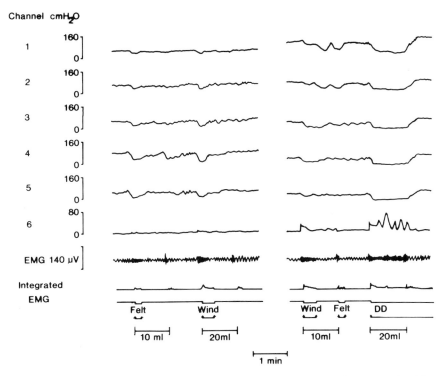

FIG. 9. The anorectal pressure recorded during rectal distension in a normal subject (*left*) and in a typical patient with irritable bowel syndrome (*right*). Channels 1 to 6 represent ports situated 0.5, 1.0, 1.5, 2.0, 2.5 and 4.5 cm from the anal verge. Note that rectal distension induces repetitive rectal contractions, sustained internal anal sphincter relaxations and a desire to defaecate at lower volumes in the patient than in the normal subject. (From Read & Sun 1989, with permission from the publishers.)

Although these physiological features are typical of the irritable bowel syndrome, they can also be found in inflammatory conditions such as ulcerative colitis (Rao et al 1987), and solitary rectal ulcer syndrome (Sun et al 1989b), and they can be induced by rectal infusion of low concentrations (2 mM) of bile acid (Edwards et al 1989). Presumably the inflammatory changes sensitize the rectum. Patients with ulcerative colitis and solitary rectal ulcer syndrome also complain of typical irritable bowel syndrome symptoms.

About 25% of patients with the irritable bowel syndrome complain of episodes of incontinence (Cann et al 1984), but these patients often have an additional weakness of the EAS as a result of obstetric trauma or perineal descent. The combination of large rectal contractions, rectal mucus, and precipitate IAS relaxations with a weak external sphincter is particularly difficult to treat. Pelvic floor surgery is often ineffective unless the irritable rectum is brought under control with drugs or diet or psychotherapy.

References

Aaronson I, Nixon HH 1972 A clinical evaluation of anorectal pressure studies in the diagnosis of Hirschsprung's disease. Gut 13:138–146

Baldi F, Ferrarini F, Corinaldesi R et al 1982 Function of the internal anal sphincter and rectal sensitivity in idiopathic constipation. Digestion 24:14–22

Buser WD, Miner PB Jr 1986 Delayed rectal sensation with faecal incontinence. Successful treatment using anorectal manometry. Gastroenterology 91:1186–1191

Callaghan RP, Nixon HH 1984 Megarectum physiology observation. Arch Dis Child 39:153–157

Cann PA, Read NW, Holdsworth CD, Barends D 1984 The role of loperamide and placebo in the management of the irritable bowel syndrome (IBS). Dig Dis Sci 29:239–247

Denny-Brown D, Robertson EG 1935 An investigation of the nervous control of defaecation. Brain 58:256–310

Duthie HL, Bennett RC 1963 The relations of sensation in the anal canal to the functional anal sphincter; a possible factor in anal continence. Gut 4:179–182

Edwards CA, Brown S, Baxter AJ, Bannister JJ, Read NW 1989 Effect of bile acid on anorectal function in man. Gut 30:383–386

Faverdin C, Dornic C, Ahran P 1981 Quantitative analysis of anorectal pressures in Hirschsprung's disease. Dis Colon Rectum 24:422–427

Gibbons CP, Bannister JJ, Trowbridge GA, Read NW 1986 An analysis of anal sphincter pressure and anal compliance in normal subjects. Int J Colorect Dis 1:231–237

Gibbons CP, Trowbridge GA, Bannister JJ, Read NW 1988 The mechanics of the anal sphincter complex. J Biomechanics 21:601–604

Lennard-Jones JE 1985 Constipation: pathophysiology, clinical features and treatment. In: Henry MM, Swash M (eds) Coloproctology and the pelvic floor: pathophysiology and management. Butterworths, London, p 350–375

Meunier P, Mollard P 1977 Control of the internal anal sphincter (manometric study with human subjects). Pfluegers Arch Eur J Physiol 370:233–239

Meunier P, Marechal JM, Jaubert de Beaujeu M 1979 Recto-anal pressures and rectal sensitivity in child constipation. Gastroenterology 77:330–336

Monges HO, Salducci J, Nandy B, Ranieri F, Gonella J, Bouvier M 1980 The electrical activity of the internal anal sphincter: a comparative study in man and in cats. In: Christensen J (ed) Gastrointestinal motility. Raven Press, New York, p 495–501

Rao SSC, Holdsworth CD, Read NW 1987 Anorectal sensitivity and reactivity in patients with ulcerative colitis. Gastroenterology 93:1270–1275

Read MG, Read NW, Haynes WG, Donnelly TC, Johnson AG 1982 A prospective study of the effect of haemorrhoids on sphincter function and faecal continence. Br J Surg 69:396–398

Read NW, Abouzekry L 1986 Why do patients with faecal impaction have faecal incontinence? Gut 27:283–287

Read NW, Sun WM 1989 Disorders of the anal sphincter In: Snape WJ (ed) Pathogenesis of functional bowel disease. Plenum Medical Book Company, London, p 289–313

Read NW, Harford WV, Schmulen AC et al 1979 A clinical study of patients with fecal incontinence and diarrhea. Gastroenterology 76:747–756

Salducci J, Planche D, Nandz B 1982 Physiological role of the internal anal sphincter and the external anal sphincter during micturition. In: Weinbeck M (ed) Motility of the digestive tract. Raven Press, New York, p 513–520

Sun WM, Read NW 1988 Anorectal manometry and rectal sensation in patients with irritable bowel syndrome. Gastroenterology 94:A450

Sun WM, Read NW 1989 Anorectal function in normal subjects: the effect of gender. Int J Colorect Dis 4:188–196

Sun WM, Kerrigan DD, Donnelly TC, Read NW 1988 Spontaneous anal relaxation—a new mechanism of faecal incontinence. Hepato-Gastroenterology 35:210

Sun WM, Donnelly TC, Read NW 1989a Impaired internal anal sphincter in a sub-group of patients with idiopathic fecal incontinence. Gastroenterology 97:130–135

Sun WM, Read NW, Donnelly TC, Bannister JJ, Shorthouse AJ 1989b A common pathophysiology for full thickness rectal prolapse, anterior mucosa prolapse and solitary ulcer. Br J Surg 76:290–295

Sun WM, Read NW, Miner PB 1990 The relationship between rectal sensation and anal function in normal subjects and patients with faecal incontinence. Gut, in press

Wald A, Tunuguntla AK 1984 Anorectal sensation dysfunction in faecal incontinence in diabetes mellitus. N Engl J Med 310:1282–1287

Whitehead WE, Engel BT, Schuster MM 1980 Irritable bowel syndrome. Dig Dis Sci 25:404–413

Whitehead WE, Orr WC, Engel BT, Schuster MM 1982 External anal sphincter response to rectal distension: learned response or reflex? Psychophysiology 19:57–72

DISCUSSION

Burnstock: This meeting aims to bridge the gap between basic science studies and the clinical picture. One of the words you use frequently as a clinician, Professor Read, is 'lesion'. You seem often to think that the cause of an abnormal condition should be explicable in terms of a lesion in a particular place. Do you really have to think in terms of visible lesions? Could there not be something more subtle, like a change in receptor expression or in transmitter expression, or even a change in the number of gap junctions in the smooth muscle?

Read: That is an appropriate comment. 'Lesion' is actually a bad term because a lesion is a cut, and it is perhaps the wrong word, but it has slipped into common usage. We should also talk about functional as well as structural abnormalities. Many of the changes that I described are functional changes which may not have obvious structural components.

Swash: There is a problem of primary and secondary causation which is intertwined with use of the word 'lesion'. When you talk about 'lesions', you really mean 'causes'. For example, in obstetric trauma, in which there is direct injury to the external anal sphincter muscle, this is easily recognizable because the muscle feels floppy or has a hole in it. But those patients later develop other features; for example, the internal anal sphincter becomes damaged as well, and there is often associated damage to the pelvic floor higher up, because trauma sufficient to damage the anal sphincter muscle directly usually means that the delivery was difficult and that there has also been damage to other pelvic floor muscles and, more importantly, damage to their innervation. The resultant altered behaviour of the pelvic floor causes additional disturbances, especially pelvic floor descent during straining, with recurrent stretch injury to the pelvic innervation leading to progressive weakness of the pelvic floor striated sphincter muscles. In this way a functional disturbance results progressively from the primary 'lesion', or causation. One must separate that aspect that is primary and causes the whole problem, from the cascade of secondary events that may occur over a period of years.

Burnstock: This is fine if you know what comes first. It could be that the first event is a change in the expression of transmitters or receptors that cannot be easily detected, and then there are trophic changes over time to muscle structure and function which are more easily measured.

de Groat: Earlier we discussed the overlap in the central control of the external anal sphincter, other pelvic floor muscles, and the external urethral sphincter. In view of that overlap, one would expect that there are central 'lesions' that might produce a defect in urethral sphincter function. Do your patients also have problems with the urinary tract, and does that help you to define whether there is a specific lesion of the gut, or a general lesion of all the pelvic muscles?

Read: Yes, it does help us. We have now started recording from both anorectum and bladder simultaneously. When we see a defect in one system we also see a similar defect in the other system, in some but by no means all our patients. That is interesting and should tell us something about where the site of the 'lesion' might be. In the patients with high or low spinal lesions that I discussed (p 129–132) we often see comparable abnormalities in the urinary tract as well. We haven't tested enough patients to make that statement very confidently, but it is helpful to be able to look at both systems at once.

de Groat: I think it would be instructive. I suspect that some of these incontinent patients will be shown to have a central lesion, and will exhibit similar changes in several sphincter muscles. On the other hand, some patients may have a problem directly in the gut itself, and will show an internal sphincter problem but not necessarily an external sphincter problem; so by subtraction you may be able to identify the site of the lesion.

Marsden: Have you any hard evidence for an isolated defect in anal performance, due to a central nervous system lesion which spares urinary function? It's remarkable in clinical practice that you never see an isolated anal deficit due to a CNS lesion.

Read: No.

Marsden: Has anybody?

Swash: No. The corollary is also true, that patients with CNS disease who appear to have urinary incontinence only, usually also have faecal incontinence, if you can get them to admit it.

Brindley: Professor Read used the word 'lesion', and then almost retracted it under criticism! I think he should have stuck to his guns. Neurologists have long been familiar with neurological conditions where the abnormality is caused by an anatomically localized lesion, and other conditions, mostly hereditary, which are biochemically determined and the abnormality is present all over the central nervous system. It is therefore not a new idea to think in terms of widespread abnormalities rather than anatomical lesions, but you, Professor Read, were arguing for anatomical localization by analogy. I have doubts about whether you are right, but the argument was clear and it was about anatomical localization: you were saying that in certain patients with no known lesion the picture from your investigations is similar to those with known lesions localized to the lower or upper spinal cord. I am a little sceptical about the conclusion, however. I see many patients with severe spinal cord lesions, often complete or nearly complete. It is striking how rarely they have faecal incontinence, though most have severe bladder problems.

Read: We are seeing an increasing number of patients with urinary problems who have spinal lesions, and it is surprising how many have anorectal problems. They may not all have incontinence; many have a big hard stool in the rectum and are very constipated, which may be one reason that they don't get incontinent. But a lot of them, especially if their motions are liquid, are faecally incontinent.

Brindley: Secondly, on your EMG records, what you showed from the external anal sphincter was clearly a real EMG, but I wonder whether what you recorded from the internal sphincter was in fact electrical activity of smooth muscle, or movement artifact. It showed rather large regular waves. In the bladder, when we see that sort of activity, it is demonstrably artifactual. I know gut smooth muscle is different from bladder smooth muscle and perhaps it does produce bigger electrical activity, but there is a theoretical argument against that. A smooth muscle cell is tiny compared with the electrodes, whereas a motor unit in a skeletal muscle is not so small by comparison. I think smooth muscle could only produce such waves as a real manifestation of a membrane phenomenon in the smooth muscle cells if gap junctions were causing simultaneous activity in a very large region of the smooth muscle. In the bladder it seems that they don't. The piece of smooth muscle analogous to a motor unit in skeletal muscle is very small in the bladder, and therefore the electrical signals picked up by large electrodes are tiny.

Read: It is a very regular phenomenon, that occurs at the known range of the slow wave of the internal sphincter, recorded using intracellular electrodes which are put into that muscle. There is often a mechanical component at the same sort of frequency, which might support your argument, but could support the view that slow wave represents an oscillation in membrane potential.

Christensen: On the EMG question, I don't think you can distinguish a movement artifact from a true action potential in such a study. Movement artifacts often appear as rapid electrical transients, looking just like action potentials.

Stanton: I was fascinated by the earlier discussion of comparisons that can be made between investigations of the urinary system and the bowel, and by the results you have obtained. You mentioned that some of your control subjects were also found to be incontinent. How much of a problem is this? We face exactly the same problem with our controls. How does one overcome this? Do they say that their bowel never becomes so full anyway, and that they are being 'over-filled' with the saline infusion, much as a woman with a normal bladder would say, when she acts as a control?

Read: What really is 'normal', and what is 'abnormal'? Our saline continence test is a provocative manoeuvre. The normal subjects who leaked during that test may perhaps have had a degree of pudendal neuropathy; many had had children previously. If they had severe diarrhoea, they may well have complained of incontinence and been 'patients', but as they passed solid stools, their weak sphincters did not worry them.

Stanton: Do you use biofeedback therapy in the management of any incontinent patients? Can they recognize a signal that you feed to them and modify their bowel control?

Read: Biofeedback is useful, but I wonder what the mechanism is. We did a controlled study during which patients also underwent the manoeuvres without receiving any feedback or instructions. Some patients (not as many as when we gave feedback) actually got better without any feedback. When we measured to see what was happening to the sphincter at the end of the trial, we found that the biofeedback had done nothing to anal pressures or to recto-anal coordination or anorectal angle, but had improved rectal sensation. So there were no objective changes, but there were subjective changes in sensation. Patients also felt more confident, having been under the care of a doctor for a period of time. I do therefore wonder what biofeedback does, but it is an effective treatment for about 70% of incontinent patients.

Stanton: On a more philosophical point, one begins to wonder whether we shouldn't re-think our teaching, or our practice of medicine, and have unified departments of 'excretion', where there is one person who is trained in physiology and in the management of both bowel and bladder, because they are so closely linked, as you have emphasized.

Read: That would be a good idea.

Functional assessment of the bladder

Jørgen Nordling

Department of Urology, Herlev Hospital, University of Copenhagen, DK-2730 Herlev, Denmark

Abstract. The urinary bladder has two functions: to store and to empty. A frequency–volume chart completed by the patient provides useful information about voiding intervals, possible factors provocative for incontinence, functional bladder capacity and daily urine volume. Filling cystometry is used primarily to evaluate reflex function in the storage phase, giving information about the presence or absence of detrusor instability and (in combination with urethral EMG) about detrusor–sphincter coordination. Information is also obtained about bladder sensation, bladder capacity and bladder compliance. Detrusor function during emptying is closely related to outflow conditions and therefore demands simultaneous registration of detrusor pressure and urinary flow rate. An inverse relation exists between detrusor pressure and flow rate, which means that reduced flow rate causes increased detrusor pressure for the same detrusor power. Underactive detrusor function will result in low detrusor pressure and low flow rate. The finding of a non-contractile detrusor may indicate psychogenic inhibition or a neurogenic lesion. Sacral evoked potentials and denervation supersensitivity tests may help to distinguish between these conditions.

1990 Neurobiology of Incontinence. Wiley, Chichester (Ciba Foundation Symposium 151) p 139–155

The urinary bladder has two functions: to store and to empty. The assessment of bladder function includes an evaluation of both.

Frequency–volume chart

A frequency–volume chart should provide information about the number of and time intervals between voidings during 24 hours. The volume of each voiding and total urine volume during 24 hours should also be measured. According to Klevmark (1987), four diagnostic prototypes of frequency–volume charts are often found:

Type 1 with normal single volumes and normal 24 hours volume denotes normal bladder function.

Type 2 with normal single volumes and increased 24 hours volume denotes normal bladder function, but polyuria as the cause of frequency. Polyuria can be either habitual or secondary to diabetes or renal insufficiency.

Type 3 with small single volumes day and night is usually found in cases of motor or sensory urgency.

Type 4 with large morning volume and variable small volumes during the daytime is usually seen in psychosomatic conditions.

A parameter such as functional bladder capacity should be determined from a patient's normal voiding and must be distinguished from the cystometric bladder capacity measured during artificial bladder filling at cystometry.

Cystometry

Cystometry records the pressure–volume relationship of the urinary bladder. The method yields information on the elastic properties of the bladder wall, the sensory qualities of the bladder, and the central control of the detrusor muscle.

In 1927, Rose reported on the clinical applications of cystometry. Since then cystometry has become a routine investigation in the urological clinic and the technical equipment has undergone several modifications. The first cystometries were done with water as the filling medium. The filling was incremental and the intravesical pressure was recorded between each increment. Later investigators preferred continuous inflow and continuous pressure recording.

The bladder can be filled at different rates and with water or CO_2 as the filling medium (Nordling et al 1978). A normal cystometrogram is shown in Fig. 1. It is characteristic that under normal circumstances the bladder can be filled to cystometric capacity (the volume at which the patient has a normal strong desire to void) with only a small rise in intravesical pressure and without the occurrence of detrusor contractions. Bladder compliance is defined as Δ volume divided by Δ pressure and under normal circumstances is high. Low bladder compliance is seen in conditions where the bladder has lost its normal elasticity as a result of fibrosis, as for example after X-ray treatment or in combination with bladder hypertrophy in cases of neuromuscular bladder dysfunction.

During bladder filling the volume at first sensation to void is registered. A normal voiding sensation confirms intact sensory pathways from the bladder to the cerebral cortex.

The main reason for doing filling cystometry is however to evaluate the voluntary control of the micturition reflex. Over-active detrusor function is defined by the International Continence Society (Abrams et al 1988) as involuntary detrusor contractions during the filling phase, which may be spontaneous or provoked and which the patient cannot completely suppress. Involuntary detrusor contractions may be provoked by rapid filling, alterations in posture, coughing, walking, jumping and other triggering procedures. The presence of involuntary detrusor contractions is termed 'detrusor hyperreflexia' if over-activity is due to a disturbance of the nervous control mechanism. If

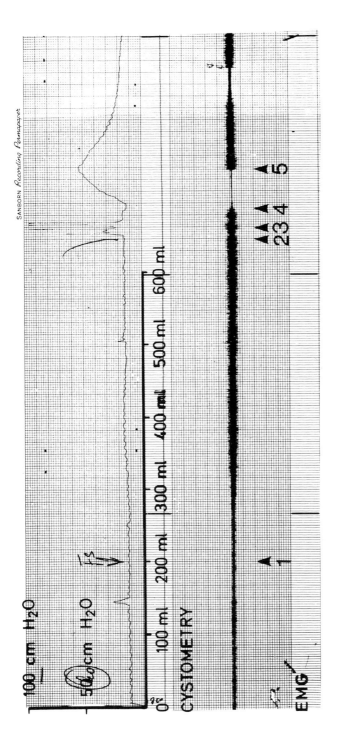

FIG. 1. Normal CO_2 cystometrogram and urethral electromyogram. 1: First sensation to void. 2: Cystometric bladder capacity. 3: Patient asked to cough. 4: Patient asked to void. Complete relaxation of the sphincter is seen followed by a detrusor contraction. 5: Patient asked to stop voiding. The patient is squeezing followed by complete suppression of the detrusor contraction within 50 seconds.

there is no evidence of relevant neurological disorder, detrusor over-activity is referred to as 'unstable detrusor'.

Hodgkinson et al (1963) were the first to describe the condition in which neurologically normal women were incontinent in association with uninhibited detrusor contractions. The pathophysiology of this condition is still obscure. In detrusor hyperreflexia the cause is a neurological lesion which compromises normal cerebral inhibition of the micturition reflex. In detrusor instability there is also a failure of central control and there might be an unrecognized underlying neurological abnormality. Even local factors in the detrusor muscle itself might be responsible. It has for example been postulated that vasoactive intestinal polypeptide (VIP) may play a role (Kinder & Mundy 1985).

The aetiology of detrusor instability is idiopathic. It may be psychosomatic, neuropathological or myogenic. In men with infravesical obstruction the preoperative incidence of detrusor instability may be as high as 80% (Meyhoff et al 1984). After relief of the obstruction, detrusor instability disappears in a little under half of the patients, indicating that bladder outflow obstruction might be an aetiological factor.

Detrusor instability is probably rather common and may occur in 10% of

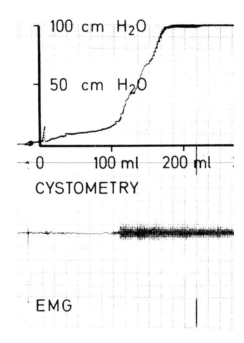

FIG. 2. CO_2 cystometry and urethral electromyography in a patient with a spinal cord lesion at T2. At a bladder volume of 100 ml a detrusor contraction is elicited, accompanied by increased sphincter activity.

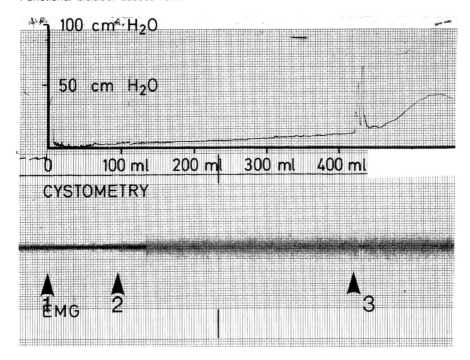

FIG. 3. CO_2 cystometry and urethral electromyography in a patient with urge incontinence. 1: start of bladder filling. 2: first sensation to void at a bladder volume of 100 ml. 3: cystometric bladder capacity. Bladder filling is stopped and the patient is asked to cough. This elicits an involuntary detrusor contraction. That the patient is not voiding is confirmed by the continuous high activity in the electromyogram.

the population. The incidence increases with age (Abrams 1985), independent of the presence of obstruction.

In females with urinary incontinence the incidence of unstable bladder varies from 10 to 55% (Hodgkinson et al 1963, Arnold et al 1973, Arnold 1974, Walter 1978, Nordling et al 1979a). The actual incidence depends on whether provocative procedures are used. In the supine position, about 15–20% will demonstrate bladder instability (Fig. 2); provocation by coughing and filling in the standing position will add another 20% (Fig. 3).

In the standardization report from the International Continence Society (Abrams et al 1988) it is stated that involuntary detrusor contractions may be provoked by rapid filling. This is not our experience. In a comparative study of water and CO_2 cystometry with filling rates of 50 ml/min and 200 ml/min respectively, we found that some patients were able to suppress the micturition reflex for the relatively short time that a rapid-filling cystometry lasted (Nordling et al 1978). If pressure monitoring continued after filling, an uninhibited contraction occurred within one to two minutes. We therefore started to ask all patients with normal inhibition during filling voluntarily to elicit a detrusor contraction after cystometric capacity was reached and bladder filling had stopped. We then further tested the voluntary control over the micturition reflex by asking the patient to hold the water and suppress the micturition reflex. In normal individuals this was possible within half a minute or so, but some patients could not do this. From our experience we therefore more or less arbitrarily selected a limit of 50 seconds, within which time bladder pressure should be back to premicturition pressure. If suppression of the reflex lasted longer, or the reflex could not be suppressed at all (Fig. 4), the patient was classified as having abnormal voluntary control of the micturition reflex.

This procedure also has the advantage of giving several important pieces of information about detrusor innervation. The occurrence of a detrusor contraction gives information about an intact motor innervation from the cerebral cortex via the brainstem, the spinal cord and the peripheral parasympathetic nervous system. As we routinely do urethral electromyography with a surface electrode mounted on the urethral catheter, we also get information about voluntary sphincter control and about patient cooperation.

A pattern like that seen in Fig. 2, with an uninhibited detrusor contraction accompanied by increased sphincter activity, might be due to detrusor–sphincter

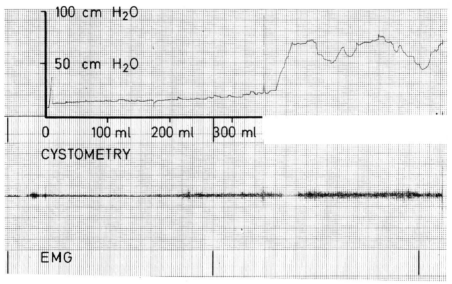

FIG. 4. CO_2 cystometrogram and urethral electromyogram from a patient with stress and urge incontinence. After bladder filling is stopped at a bladder volume of 350 ml, the patient voluntarily elicits a detrusor contraction. She is however not able to suppress this, which indicates abnormal cerebral control of the micturition reflex.

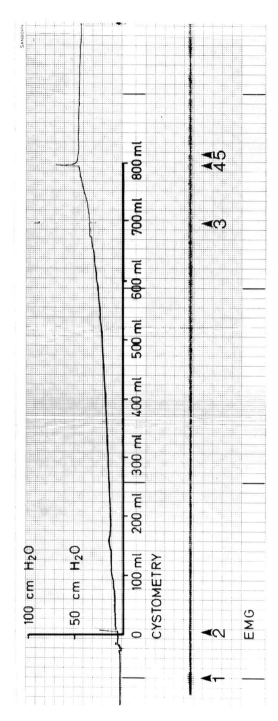

FIG. 5. CO_2 cystometry and urethral electromyography in a patient with voiding difficulties after radical hysterectomy. 1: Squeezing before start of bladder filling. 2: Start of bladder filling. 3: 'First sensation to void' at a bladder volume of 700 ml. 4: Cystometric bladder capacity of 800 ml. The patient is asked to cough and bladder filling is stopped. 5: The patient is asked to void without straining. She can only briefly relax the sphincter and no detrusor contraction is elicited.

dyssynergia, but will also be seen if the patient tries to inhibit the detrusor contraction by squeezing. To distinguish these it is necessary to ask the patient to relax and void instead of squeezing. The actual patient could not do that because of a spinal cord lesion.

If a detrusor contraction cannot be demonstrated during cystometry, this might be due to either psychogenic inhibition or a lesion of the peripheral motor innervation of the bladder (Fig. 5). To distinguish between these conditions, sacral evoked potentials (Nordling et al 1979b) and denervation supersensitivity tests (Glahn 1970) may be helpful.

The function of the detrusor muscle during voiding is to act as a pump to expel urine through the urethra. Assessment of the detrusor is almost exclusively done by measuring intravesical pressure during voiding (Schäfer 1983). This pressure is dependent on both detrusor power and urinary flow rate. To diagnose whether poor bladder emptying and/or a weak urinary stream is due to detrusor weakness or infravesical obstruction, it is therefore necessary to measure detrusor pressure and urinary flow rate simultaneously (Abrams & Griffiths 1979). These considerations are however more relevant in the evaluation of infravesical obstruction, and therefore of minor importance in this symposium, which deals with urinary incontinence.

References

Abrams P 1985 Detrusor instability and bladder outlet obstruction. Neurourol Urodyn 4:317–328

Abrams P, Griffiths D 1979 The assessment of prostatic obstruction from urodynamic measurements and from residual urine. Br J Urol 51:129–134

Abrams P, Blaivas JG, Stanton SL, Andersen JT 1988 The standardisation of terminology of lower urinary tract function. Scand J Urol Nephrol Suppl 114:5–19

Arnold EP 1974 Cystometry-postural effects in incontinent women. Urol Int 29: 185–186

Arnold EP, Webster JR, Loose H et al 1973 Urodynamics of female incontinence. Factors influencing the results of surgery. Am J Obstet Gynecol 117:805–813

Glahn BE 1970 Neurogenic bladder diagnosed pharmacologically on the basis of denervation supersensitivity. Scand J Urol Nephrol 4:13–24

Hodgkinson CP, Ayers MA, Drukker BH 1963 Dyssynergic detrusor dysfunction in the apparently normal female. Am J Obstet Gynecol 87:717–730

Kinder RB, Mundy AR 1985 The inhibition of spontaneous contractile activity in isolated human detrusor muscle strips by vasoactive intestinal polypeptide. Br J Urol 57:20–23

Klevmark B 1987 The frequency–volume chart in diagnosis and for control of treatment. Nord Med 102:340–342

Meyhoff HH, Nordling J, Hald T 1984 Urodynamic evaluation of transurethral versus transvesical prostatectomy. Scand J Urol Nephrol 18:27–35

Nordling J, Hebjørn S, Walter S, Hald T, Christiansen HD 1978 A comparative study of water cystometry and CO$_2$ cystometry. Urol Int 33:60–67

Nordling J, Meyhoff HH, Andersen JT, Walter S 1979a Urinary incontinence in the female. The value of detrusor reflex activation procedures. Br J Urol 51:110–113

Nordling J, Andersen JT, Walter S, Meyhoff HH, Hald T, Gammelgaard PA 1979b
Evoked response of the bulbocavernosus reflex. Eur Urol 5:36–38
Rose DK 1927 Cystometric bladder pressure determinations: their clinical importance.
J Urol 17:487–502
Schäfer W 1983 The detrusor as the energy source of micturition. In: Hinman F, Boyarsky
S (eds) Benign prostatic hypertrophy. Springer-Verlag, New York, p 450–469
Walter S 1978 Detrusor hyperreflexia in female urinary incontinence treated
pharmacologically. Urol Int 33:316–321

DISCUSSION

Brading: Dr Nordling, if you were recording from the bladder without knowledge of the history of the patient, I assume you would be unable to distinguish between what you would call detrusor hyperreflexia and what you call unstable bladder?

Nordling: That is correct; the cystometrogram is just the same.

Brading: Is there any real evidence in the two cases that hyperreflexia is caused by increased motor activity, leading to the unstable contractions of the detrusor? From our work on pigs with detrusor instability, my feeling is that in both conditions in the human the behaviour of the smooth muscle, and its pathology, will be very similar. But have you any real evidence here?

Nordling: We have no evidence allowing us to determine that. We don't know where the unstable detrusor contraction is generated; it might be in the muscle or in the central nervous system, or in both.

de Groat: I presume that the test of whether instability is neurally mediated or due to intrinsic smooth muscle contractions is to remove the neural input and see if the contractions change. In animals you can cut nerves, or transect the spinal cord, or give ganglionic blocking agents or postganglionic receptor blocking drugs like atropine, and see if the response changes. I presume that some of this work has been done in humans as well. What are the effects of drugs on these patients?

Nordling: If the bladder nerves are cut in a patient you won't see any detrusor contraction because the micturition reflex is abolished, but that doesn't mean that the cause can't lie in the detrusor muscle in patients with detrusor instability. The micturition reflex nervous pathways are needed for a coordinated contraction to occur, but the defect might be in the muscle.

de Groat: My suspicion is that both contribute, and that part of these unstable contractions may be intrinsic but the contraction itself is amplified by reflexes through the central nervous system. If one could do the appropriate tests in humans for example, and block ganglionic transmission, the amplitude of those contractions might be altered. In some patients they may disappear completely, and in others they may be reduced. Dr Blaivas has some data on this, I think?

Blaivas: Yes. Both the unstable contractions and the hyperreflexic contractions are always basically a micturition reflex, which means that they are preceded by electrical silence and sphincter relaxation continues throughout voiding. We have reported on 550 consecutive patients (Blaivas 1982), but we have observations on many thousands. In virtually all patients who appear to have an intact neuroaxis, when the bladder contracts involuntarily it is preceded by a period of electrical silence in the EMG, which implies that it's a micturition reflex and not a local response of the muscle.

Conversely, the patients who have neurological lesions which are in a location where they interfere with the connections to the pontine micturition centre (i.e., spinal lesions) usually do not have a period of silence preceding the detrusor contraction, implying that there is a local spinal reflex, or possibly some event in the muscle. But I think there is good evidence that hyperreflexic and unstable contractions, in the absence of a specific neurological lesion in the spinal cord, are simply uninhibited micturition reflexes, which are neurological events and not local events in the muscle.

Marsden: Could you clarify the difference between an unstable and a hyperreflexic contraction?

Blaivas: They look the same physiologically. The only difference is in the presumed aetiology. We think that the aetiology of a hyperreflexic contraction is a neurological process, namely the removal of an inhibitory neural impulse that would prevent the bladder from contracting involuntarily. An unstable contraction is an involuntary detrusor contraction in a neurologically normal person. But they look the same and the difference may be a semantic one.

de Groat: The fact that a change in the external urethral sphincter precedes the large unstable contraction of the bladder implies that the unstable contraction is a centrally generated event, rather than a peripheral, smooth muscle event.

Brading: How separate are these events in time? Could one have a small rise in detrusor pressure which is triggering the urethral relaxation?

Blaivas: The events are crystal clear. Normally there is a sudden electrical silence which precedes the detrusor contraction. The problem is that in some people there may be volitional sphincteric activity. Most normal people can voluntarily contract the striated sphincter at any time, so a person who is about to have an involuntary bladder contraction can contract the sphincter momentarily in an attempt to inhibit the onset of the detrusor contractions. But in all the people we have seen, even those who voluntarily contract the sphincter prior to voiding, there is a period of electrical silence just before the bladder actually contracts. The only way that the electrical silence can be overridden is if someone has a strong voluntary contraction and is trying to stop at the same time that the bladder is trying to start.

Nordling: We don't see that silence in the electrical signal in our patients with bladder instability. Probably this is because we are doing the cystometry in a different way. We ask the patient to hold water during bladder filling, while

Dr Blaivas instructs them to do nothing. Then we will see a voluntary sphincter contraction when the patient tries to abolish the uninhibited detrusor contraction.

Blaivas: I think you would if you used needle electrodes and oscilloscopic monitering; I noticed on your tracings that the increased EMG activity in the hyperreflexic and normal bladders was obtained with surface electrodes. I would submit that the apparent increased activity is more likely to be either an artifact of the recording, or recordings from muscles distant to the urethral sphincter.

Nordling: Most certainly the latter.

Fowler: To what extent do you feel that needle electromyography interferes with normal voiding patterns, Dr Blaivas?

Blaivas: Needle EMG will interfere with normal micturition patterns in many people, particularly if insertion is painful or if the person is nervous or inhibited. It should not be used routinely for these reasons. Our data are from selected patients who are willing to participate, knowing what is about to happen. Most of these people are able to void and relax. However, if I think they will not be able to cooperate during the examination, we don't use the needle. So there is a considerable selection process.

Fowler: Would you say that if you had EMG sphincter activity simultaneously with a detrusor contraction, it had a neurological cause—an upper motor neuron lesion?

Blaivas: If the bladder contracts involuntarily, it is by definition detrusor instability. The International Continence Society subdivides this according to the presumed aetiology of the unstable bladder, into hyperreflexia or no hyperreflexia, in which case it is still called instability. The hyperreflexia can be part of a normal micturition reflex which loses its inhibition, in which case the sphincter relaxes first and the spinal cord pathways are intact; or the sphincter can contract simultaneously with or just before the detrusor contraction, which we call detrusor–external sphincter dyssynergia. I did not say that we can distinguish unstable contractions from hyperreflexia. I said we could distinguish detrusor–external sphincter dyssynergia from a normal micturition reflex. Detrusor–external sphincter dyssynergia is, in our opinion, due to a spinal neurological lesion. A patient with a suprabulbar neurological lesion usually has an uninhibited micturition reflex, but never dyssynergia.

Brading: Has anybody looked at the detrusor smooth muscle and its innervation in these hyperreflexic patients?

Blaivas: We don't have the technology with which to evaluate the innervation of smooth muscle, unfortunately!

Brading: Can one get samples of the bladder smooth muscle from these patients?

Blaivas: Yes, but we wouldn't really know what to do with them.

Brading: We could suggest something! I was interested in your patients who start a contraction and can't stop, Dr Nordling, because that would suggest an alteration in the smooth muscle allowing increased spread of activity. Once you began such a contraction it would spread throughout the bladder. Because bladder smooth muscle doesn't have an inhibitory innervation, there is no way to stop it.

Nordling: Many normal subjects can stop a detrusor contraction.

Brading: If they can, that would suggest that they are stopping the excitatory innervation. I am suggesting that there may be two ways of increasing intravesical pressure. In the normal bladder, activity is entirely correlated with nerve activity, but in the unstable bladder, activity starts in the smooth muscle and is a property of that muscle. It cannot be stopped because there is no inhibitory innervation. It looked to me as if those patients who cannot inhibit a contraction once it has started fall into the latter category.

Nordling: But if you block the micturition reflex with anticholinergic drugs, you won't see the unstable contractions.

Brading: That is presumably because it hasn't started; you haven't triggered the initial contraction. In normal bladder you will only get contraction if you trigger all the smooth muscles with the nerves; as soon as you stop activity in the nerves, the smooth muscle contractions are no longer synchronized, and the pressure will drop. Whereas, in the unstable bladder, the initial contraction may be triggered by some nerve activity, but will then spread myogenically to involve all the detrusor.

Marsden: Does the entity of myotonia of the bladder exist?

Brading: It certainly happens in the outflow obstruction type of instability, where the smooth muscle properties are different and there is marked denervation of the bladder.

Blaivas: Is there an electrical spread through the muscle itself or is it nerve mediated?

Brading: We think the former happens.

Andersson: Dr Nordling, what is the importance of the Lapides and Glahn tests for diagnosing neuronal damage?

Nordling: We still use them a lot. It is impossible to tell whether an areflexia seen during cystometry is neurogenic because of neurological damage or because of psychogenic inhibition. The Lapides test gives a measure of bladder compliance during the first 100 ml of filling, before and after the administration of carbachol, while the Glahn test measures pressure during a period of 20 minutes with 100 ml in the bladder. So you would expect to see many more false positive and negative results from the Lapides test, because compliance during cystometry is such an inconsistent thing.

Maggi: Has there been any systematic study on the influence of filling rate on the behaviour of the bladder in disease states and in normal subjects? From the animal data, one would expect this parameter to be important, both for the response of nerves and for the response of muscle. The nerves may be influenced by different filling rates, because there are probably several sets of sensory nerves with different thresholds. Also, the occurrence of inhibitory reflexes to the bladder may be influenced by the degree of distension. The muscle can be influenced by very rapid distension of the bladder, because we know that stretch of the muscle can produce a myogenic reaction. It is important to try to understand the origin of these uninhibited contractions, whether they are myogenic in part, neurogenic in part, or only myogenic or only neurogenic. Has there been any systematic study on the effect of filling rate on cystometry in humans?

Nordling: There have not been many studies in the human on this matter. Dr Klevmark did studies in the cat demonstrating that physiological filling rates during cystometry give very different results from rapid filling rates (Klevmark 1974). In humans, we used different filling rates with water and carbon dioxide, 50 ml/min and 200 ml/min respectively. The rate has no great impact on reflex activity, but it affects the volume at first sensation and cystometric bladder capacity. I found some differences, but they were the opposite of what you might expect, namely that unstable detrusor contractions were a little more frequent with slow filling rates.

Brindley: There is a straightforward test which would decide whether, in a given patient, detrusor instability involves the central nervous system, or only structures within the bladder. This is to do a sacral epidural block. I don't know of anybody having done it, probably because it is assumed that detrusor instability is always neurogenic and would be abolished by sacral epidural block. Dr Brading's observations on pigs with artificial outflow obstruction tell us that someone should do this test, in man.

Kirby: It would just block the micturition reflex completely, wouldn't it?

Brindley: It doesn't in Dr Brading's pigs, so it might not in man.

Blaivas: Although there are no formal studies on this, we do give epidural and spinal anaesthesia frequently; it is the method of choice for quadriplegic and paraplegic patients. They almost never have involuntary contractions during the surgical procedure. So it is clinically evident that in the majority of patients the involuntary contractions are neurologically mediated.

Brindley: Of course, these are the neurologically caused instabilities; they are not the instabilities that are due to outflow obstruction. The possible human analogues of Dr Brading's pigs are men with prostatic hypertrophy.

Blaivas: There too, probably 90% of operations for prostatic obstruction are done under spinal anaesthesia.

Brading: The problem is that this is largely anecdotal evidence and one doesn't know the degree of anaesthesia. Anaesthetics of any sort can affect smooth muscles as well as nerves. In our animal models, although the unstable contractions are myogenic and persist under anaesthesia, increasing the depth of anaesthesia can block them. I would very much like to see a good study on the effect of anaesthesia on urodynamics in humans with unstable bladders; presumably this could be done quite easily.

Blaivas: I thought your hypothesis was that even if the detrusor contraction is mediated neurologically, once it has started, in the experimental preparation, it would continue unabated, so this experiment wouldn't answer the question. I think we agree clinically that you could abolish the onset of almost all these detrusor contractions by spinal or epidural anaesthesia; the real question is why they persist once they start and cannot be controlled, whether or not there is an electrical spread of the contraction to start with. You would need a preparation in which you could allow the detrusor contraction to start, and then try to abolish it with some kind of intervention aimed at blocking the excitatory neural input.

Stanton: Ted Arnold has done that study, looking at different filling rates, and this is why the Middlesex Hospital adopted the idea of 100 ml/min as a rate which would initiate detrusor contractions, or provoke them, and in a normal subject it would function as a physiological test; but that is open to dispute.

On the effect of anaesthesia, I recall that Pat Doyle showed that urethral pressure was profoundly affected by anaesthesia, but I don't know if he looked at cystometry.

Brading: Mr D.E. Neal's group in Newcastle is doing ambulatory monitoring of 'natural fill' cystometry. They find significant differences between that and conventional 'medium fill' cystometry on the same patients. They are finding far more 'unstable contractions' occurring with 'natural fill' cystometry.

Read: We have not studied filling rates in the bladder, but we have done it in the rectum, and there is a tremendous difference in responses and sensations according to the rate of filling.

If you fill a rectal balloon intermittently and rapidly there is a much steeper pressure–volume relationship, and you see rectal contractions, and prompt internal sphincter relaxation at low volumes. If you fill the rectum by ramp inflation, the result depends on the rate. The faster you fill the rectum, the less it accommodates to the distension, and sensations are delayed. This tells us something about the sensory mechanisms. I imagine that there are populations of rapidly adapting and slowly adapting receptors in the rectum, and you get different results if you alter the conditions of the experiment.

Staskin: Are there accepted classification systems now for rectal monitoring? There are several different methods used to classify bladder incontinence, including a temporal system of acute versus persistent incontinence, and a neurogenic system, of areflexic, normoreflexic and hyperreflexic bladders, with or without sphincter coordination. We also use a functional classification which says that incontinence occurs when intravesical pressure overcomes outlet resistance, and therefore leakage must be either an abnormal elevation of pressure or a decrease in resistance. Is there a classification for rectal monitoring that helps to group various diseases into the type of abnormality which you would expect, or, if you saw an abnormality and didn't know what was wrong, would you be able to use the classification system in your investigation to look for the aetiology?

Read: There isn't a classification system in the way you described. This probably reflects the different systems we are dealing with, and the fact that you are dealing with something which is liquid, and in faecal incontinence we deal with something which is solid sometimes and liquid at other times. There perhaps needs to be a classification but we are still talking about it and we haven't reached any general agreement. I presented a scheme which might provide a way of dividing patients up, but I don't think everybody is going to agree with that. We need a lot more experience.

Staskin: Does anyone in your field use a semi-solid or solid provocative test? Your provocative tests seem to use liquid and not solid material.

Read: That is because most patients leak, when they have liquid or gas in the rectum. We have used different sized spheres for testing the ability to defaecate; we haven't used a solid to test incontinence.

Swash: One method of radiological assessment is to use an intrarectal, radio-opaque paste, of the consistency of normal faeces. This test, defaecating procto-graphy, has proved valuable in coloproctological practice. Other laboratories use balloons for anorectal manometry rather than a perfusion method.

Read: But not necessarily to test continence.

Swash: No, to test the equivalent of stress incontinence in the anorectal system, where the anal sphincter system is overcome by the presence of the material in the anorectum; or where there is 'urge' faecal incontinence, when there is a CNS lesion but a normal sphincter system, and the patient is unable to inhibit the onset of the defaecation response. Defaecation occurs, like micturition, either voluntarily, or in response to the arrival of an overwhelming amount of material in the anorectum which indicates the necessity to defaecate. It also occurs as a regular time-locked phenomenon, just as micturition does on waking in the morning, for example.

Stanton: Sometimes in the bladder there can be a sensation of urgency which is totally sensory, and not motor. Can the same occur in the rectum?

Read: Yes, the sensation of urgency can occur with no motor correlates.

Marsden: You can also get an irritable rectum, like an irritable bladder. It fascinates me that you don't impugn the central nervous system as a cause of irritable rectum, due to uninhibited contractions of the rectum.

Read: A high spinal lesion could lead to an irritable rectum, but enhanced rectal contractility is probably more frequently related to local irritation or to modulation from the brain.

Marsden: In the group of patients that Dr Nordling and Dr Blaivas deduce to have an uninhibited bladder of central nervous system origin, what proportion have an identified neurological cause? When you follow such patients for a long period of time, in what proportion does a neurological cause emerge, bearing in mind that neurology tends to be progressive?

Blaivas: Unfortunately, we do not routinely evaluate patients in that way. We don't look for central nervous system causes if the only presumed neurological abnormality is detrusor instability. There are many clinical data on detrusor instability, however. For example, approximately 30% of stress incontinent women have detrusor instability on a cystometrogram or by history. In a group of unselected patients who are evaluated because of bladder symptoms of any cause, who do not complain of urge incontinence, we find 10–20% have detrusor instability in the absence of a clinical reason to suspect a neurological aetiology. In unselected, normal controls, cystometrograms reveal 5–10% with unstable detrusor contractions. But if you see detrusor–sphincter dyssynergia, almost 100% will either have an identifiable neurological lesion or will go on to show one within a year or so.

Nordling: In the material of Steen Walter, which was unselected patients referred for urinary incontinence, about 1% of the total had neurological disease. This was three or four out of 300 patients, and they all had multiple sclerosis (Walter & Olesen 1982).

Marsden: I raised this point because so often, in my experience, neurologists, presented with a report of detrusor hyperreflexia due to some neurological cause, are unable to identify it!

Swash: You have to be sure you are talking about the same thing. Dr Blaivas's paper will make clear the definition of detrusor–sphincter dyssynergia. The term is often used relatively loosely, and this leads to confusion over its clinical significance. I must admit that I am relieved to hear the controversy about hyperreflexia versus the unstable bladder, because the literature is not easy to follow. I still have difficulty in understanding how it can be thought that the unstable contractions can originate in the bladder muscle. We have discussed the control of bladder muscle by the nervous system and noted that the bladder musculature does not initiate spontaneous contractions, because it has no pacemaker, and, unlike the gut, no intrinsic nervous system from which spontaneous contractions could be initiated. This suggests that the unstable contraction is a primary response of the muscle fibre syncytium itself— perhaps like myotonia in striated muscle? Surely it is more likely that it originates in the central nervous system, unless a specific change occurs in that hypertrophied bladder smooth muscle that changes its physiology. This seems unlikely.

Brading: It does occur! It is well established experimentally in many systems that if you make an obstruction which gives rise to hypertrophy, you get significant changes in smooth muscle behaviour and in cell–cell connections. This happens in the gut (Bortoff & Sillin 1986, Gabella 1987). By putting rings of cellulose around the gut in various animal species one can produce a type of obstruction and obtain extensive hypertrophy of the smooth muscle which alters its properties. In the uterus there is a marvellous example of hypertrophy in pregnancy, with large changes in both smooth muscle behaviour and cell–cell connections.

Swash: But do the cells now fire spontaneously?

Brading: Any cell on its own will fire spontaneously, but it's when they all fire together that you get pressure changes. Spread of electrical activity from cell to cell, or some other chemical or mechanical factor, achieves this synchrony. It is normally the nerves that synchronize activity in an organ like the bladder, where cell electrical coupling is less developed than in other smooth muscles; but if there is a change in the smooth muscle cells which increases cell coupling, any focus that increases activity (such as stretch or local nerve activity) can spread, and will produce synchronized contraction which will put the pressure up.

References

Blaivas JG 1982 The neurophysiology of micturition: a clinical study of 550 patients. J Urol 127:958–963

Bortoff A, Sillin LF 1986 Changes in intracellular electrical coupling of smooth muscle accompanying atrophy and hypertrophy. Am J Physiol 250:C292–C298

Gabella G 1987 Dynamic aspects of the morphology of the intestinal muscle coat. In: Szurszewski J (ed) Cellular physiology and clinical studies of gastrointestinal smooth muscle. Elsevier Science Publishers, Amsterdam

Klevmark B 1974 Motility of the urinary bladder in cats during filling at physiological rates. I. Intravesical pressure patterns studied by a new method of cystometry. Acta Physiol Scand 90:565–577

Walter S, Olesen KP 1982 Urinary incontinence and genital prolapse in the female: clinical, urodynamic and radiological examinations. Br J Obstet Gynaecol 89:393–401

The neurogenic hypothesis of stress incontinence

Michael Swash

Department of Neurology, The London Hospital, London E1 1BB and Anorectal Physiology Laboratory, St Mark's Hospital, City Road, London EC1V 2PS, UK

Abstract. There are a number of causes of incontinence. The common forms of urinary incontinence, faecal incontinence or double incontinence, are stress related, in that voiding of urine or faeces occurs in response to a sudden increase in pressure in the bladder or anorectum that is not opposed by an adequate pressure increase in the sphincteric region. This weakness of the sphincter mechanism is due to chronic partial denervation of the striated sphincter muscles of the pelvic floor, comprising the external anal sphincter muscle and puborectalis (puboanalis) components of the voluntary anal sphincter musculature, and the periurethral and intramural components of the urinary striated sphincter musculature. Denervation of these muscles occurs progressively following injury initiated during childbirth and then sustained by repeated stretch-induced injury during straining behaviour at stool. Age-related changes to this innervation may also be important. Weakness of the pelvic floor, and perineal descent during straining, lead to secondary changes in the anatomy of the bladder neck, of the anorectal angle, and of the smooth muscle of the internal urinary and anal sphincters. The cystometric and anal manometric changes found in patients with stress incontinence are secondary to this neurogenic weakness of the pelvic floor.

1990 Neurobiology of Incontinence. Wiley, Chichester (Ciba Foundation Symposium 151) p 156–175

The maintenance of urinary and faecal continence is fundamental to ordinary life. Continence implies the ability to micturate and defaecate at will, in response to appropriate signals arising in the vesico-urethral and anorectal tracts, and in relation to internal stimuli, particularly time-locked habits. Both the urinary bladder and the colo-rectum function as storage organs pending evacuation at some suitable time. Incontinence is a term that is generally understood to mean inappropriate evacuation of urine or faeces. Thus incontinence can result from involuntary, accidental or inadvertent evacuation, due to lesions in the central or peripheral control systems in the nervous system or due to local dysfunction in the sphincter mechanism itself. These differing functional disorders are summarized in Table 1. In the attempt to understand a functional disorder of a complex control system, progress is usually most easily achieved by studying

156

TABLE 1   Classification of incontinence

1. Local sphincter pathology
Congenital perineal anomalies
Obstetric anal sphincter tears
Trauma
Perineal suppuration
Perineal and pelvic neoplasms

2. Lower motor neuron pathway lesions

Peripheral (intrapelvic) nerve lesions
Pudendal, perineal and intrapelvic nerve stretch lesions
Obstetric nerve injuries
Intrapelvic tumour and endometriosis
Diabetic neuropathy
Cauda equina lesions
Lumbosacral spinal trauma
Lumbosacral disc prolapse
Lumbar canal stenosis
Ankylosing spondylosis
Idiopathic arachnoiditis of cauda equina
Cauda equina tumours
Conus medullaris and sacral cord lesions
Ischaemia
Multiple sclerosis
Multiple system atrophy
Parkinson's disease?

3. Upper motor neuron lesions

Spinal cord lesions
Trauma
Cord compression
Ischaemia
Tumour
Multiple sclerosis
Syringomyelia
Cerebral
Dementia
Cerebrovascular disease
Hydrocephalus
Multiple sclerosis
Tumours (especially of frontal lobe)

4. Multifactorial

5. Enteric and bladder

Sphincter overwhelmed by diarrhoea
Irritable bowel syndrome
Acute cystitis
Urge incontinence due to unstable bladder

the effector mechanism itself. In the context of incontinence, therefore, dysfunction due to damage to the sphincter mechanism ought to offer a naturally occurring disorder that could provide the basis for a pathophysiological description of disturbances of the storage and evacuation of urine and faeces.

Stress incontinence

The commonest type of incontinence, *stress incontinence*, is due to weakness of the pelvic floor sphincter muscles. In this form of incontinence loss of urine or faeces occurs when the pressure in the bladder or rectum exceeds that generated by the urinary or anal sphincter musculature respectively. Stress incontinence is thus associated with incompetence of the sphincter mechanism itself. The structural abnormality in stress urinary incontinence consists essentially of loss of support of the bladder neck (Tanagho 1974), and there is a similar loss of support of the anorectum in stress faecal incontinence, resulting in straightening of the normal anorectal angulation, and descent of the anorectum in relation to the plane of the pelvic floor (Parks 1975, Henry & Swash 1985).

Neurogenic aetiology of stress faecal incontinence

The neurogenic hypothesis of stress incontinence arose from studies of idiopathic anorectal incontinence carried out at St Mark's Hospital and The London Hospital (Parks 1975, Swash et al 1985). In this functional disorder of the anorectum faecal incontinence occurs inadvertently, often without the patient's awareness of incontinence until it is discovered that the underclothes are soiled. This form of faecal incontinence is predominantly a disorder of women, occurring especially after the menopause. It is particularly associated with a history of difficult childbirth some years previously, but some cases occur in women who have never experienced childbirth. The latter usually give a history of constipation with prolonged straining at stool during many years. In a few patients there is a history of previous persistent backache and sciatica, or of laminectomy for lumbosacral disc prolapse (Henry & Swash 1985). In this form of faecal incontinence both the resting pressure and the maximum squeeze pressure in the sphincteric region of the anal canal are reduced. Indeed, in severe cases there may be almost no recordable increase in anal canal pressure during a maximal voluntary squeeze contraction or during a sudden cough (Neill et al 1981, Henry et al 1985). During coughing or straining as though defaecating there is usually marked descent of the posterior part of the perineum towards the examiner; this, and the weakness of the external anal sphincter, can often best be appreciated by asking the patient to cough during digital examination of the rectum (Henry et al 1982). The anal canal is usually patulous, and there may be a slight diminution in sensory acuity in the anal canal and at the anal margins (Roe et al 1986, Rogers et al 1986). Often the patient is unable to distinguish between the presence of flatus or faeces in the anorectum. The disorder progresses inexorably from minor degrees of dysfunction, e.g. incontinence of liquid motions, to frequent incontinence of formed stools (Parks 1975).

Histopathological evidence

Repair of the pelvic floor has been attempted by a number of related surgical techniques. During repair by the posterior approach the external anal sphincter and the associated voluntary sphincter muscles, especially the puborectalis and the lowermost fibres of the levator ani, together with the internal anal sphincter muscle, are exposed and available for biopsy. In a study of these muscles, histological features of chronic partial denervation were recognized, especially in the puborectalis and external anal sphincter muscles (Parks et al 1977, Beersiek et al 1979). In addition, the internal anal sphincter muscle showed loss of smooth muscle fibres, with disruption of the normal architecture of the muscle, and fibrosis (Lubowski et al 1988a). The elastic tissue component that provides a non-muscular closing force in this circular muscle was strikingly stretched and disrupted. A few extrinsic autonomic nerve fibres were present in relation to the remaining muscle fibres. Studies of small somatic afferent and efferent nerve fibre bundles innervating the external anal sphincter muscle showed marked loss of myelinated and unmyelinated nerve fibres, with collagenous replacement. These features were consistent with denervation of the voluntary striated muscles that form the voluntary anal sphincter, due to damage to the innervation of these muscles at a distal site. The changes in the internal anal sphincter are thought to be secondary to weakness of the striated muscle of the pelvic floor (Swash et al 1988).

The external anal sphincter is innervated by inferior rectal and inferior haemorrhoidal branches of the pudendal nerves that reach this muscle by traversing Alcock's canal after passing out of the pelvis beneath the sacrospinous ligament. The pudendal nerves also give rise to perineal branches which pass anteriorly on either side of the vagina to innervate the two sides of the peri-urethral striated sphincter muscle (Fig. 1). The puborectalis muscle, however, although equally severely affected by the denervating process that damages the external anal sphincter muscle, receives its innervation not from the pudendal nerves, but from direct motor branches derived from the same S2–S4 roots, that project to its peritoneal surface from the lumbosacral plexus (Percy et al 1981). The differences between the innervations of these two muscles suggest that they have different embryological origins, the external anal sphincter being derived from the sphincter cloacae and the puborectalis from the pelvi-caudal muscle group (Snooks & Swash 1986).

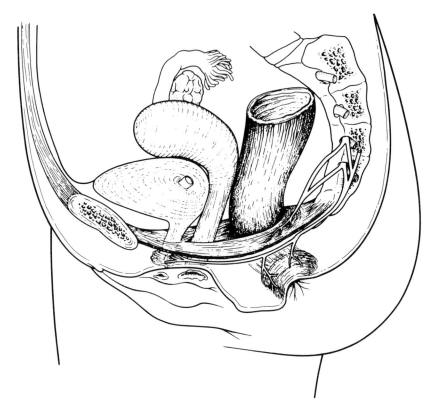

FIG. 1.   Sagittal section of female pelvis, to show pudendal and perineal nerves, and the direct motor branches that innervate the puborectalis from the sacral plexus.

Electrophysiological evidence

Damage to the innervation of the external anal sphincter and puborectalis muscles in idiopathic stress anorectal incontinence can be directly assessed by concentric needle or single-fibre EMG techniques (Neill & Swash 1980, Bartolo et al 1983). These studies (Fig. 2) show a gradually increasing degree of abnormality, representing compensatory reinnervation rather than denervation, with increasing degrees of functional abnormality in pelvic floor disorders (Table 2), ranging to incontinence at the end of the scale (Swash et al 1985). The innervation of the external anal sphincter muscle can be studied directly by measuring the terminal motor latency in the pudendal nerves (PNTML) utilizing an intra-anal electrode array with a fixed inter-electrode distance (Kiff & Swash 1984). In pelvic floor disorders, and especially in idiopathic neurogenic anorectal incontinence (Fig. 3), the PNTML is increased (Snooks et al 1984a, 1985a).

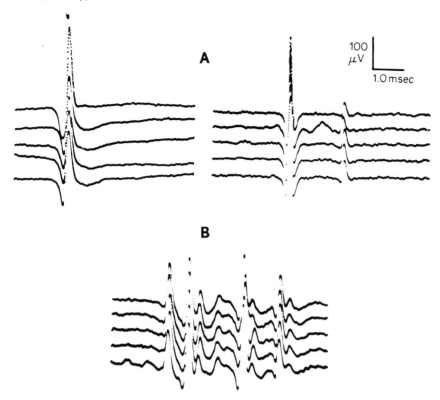

FIG. 2.   Single-fibre EMG of external anal sphincter muscle. A: normal units consisting of one or two spike components. B: polyphasic units of increased duration from a patient with neurogenic stress faecal incontinence.

TABLE 2   Pelvic floor disorders

Neurogenic faecal incontinence
Stress urinary incontinence
Double incontinence
Anismus-type constipation
Solitary rectal ulcer syndrome
Anterior rectal prolapse
Complete rectal prolapse
Genito-urinary prolapse
Haemorrhoids
Idiopathic anal, perineal and rectal pain syndromes
Secondary pelvic floor disorders
   e.g. Denervation from cauda equina disease
    Parkinson's disease etc. (see Table 1)

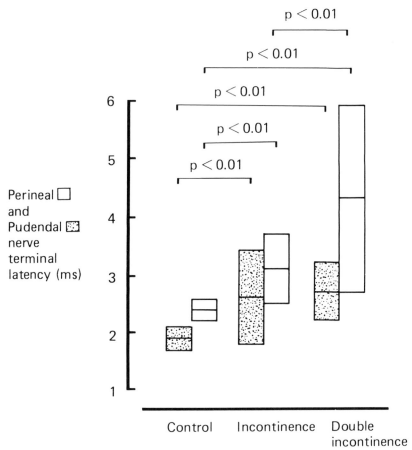

FIG. 3. Increased pudendal nerve terminal motor latency in patients with faecal incontinence (Incontinence) and double incontinence (means ± 2 SD).

In a few patients the primary neural abnormality is found in the cauda equina rather than distally in the innervation of these muscles within the pelvis. This can be investigated by utilizing direct transcutaneous stimulation of the cauda equina, and recording the evoked muscle response in the external anal sphincter or puborectalis muscle with surface recording electrodes placed in the anal canal. An electrical stimulator developed for transcranial stimulation of the motor cortex is used to deliver sufficient current to the cauda equina by the transcutaneous route (Fig. 4). An increased motor latency is found in patients with cauda equina disease and, in some of these patients, the latency from the T12/L1 stimulation site is found to be increased while that from the L4/L5 level is normal, indicating a lesion localized within the cauda equina nerve roots between these two spinal levels (Swash & Snooks 1986).

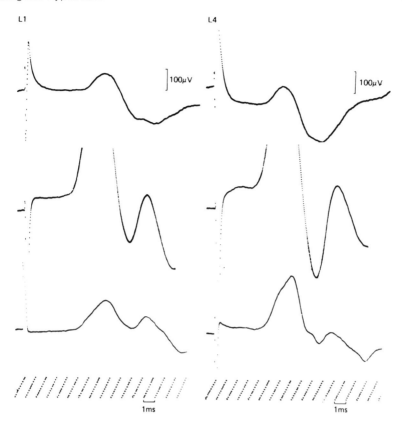

FIG. 4. Motor latencies to external anal sphincter, puborectalis and external urethral sphincter muscles (top to bottom) after transcutaneous electrical stimulation of cauda equina nerve roots at the L1 and L4 levels respectively. Note that the latencies after the more caudal stimulation are shorter than those after more rostral stimulation.

Effect of childbirth

The effect of pregnancy and childbirth on the innervation of the striated pelvic sphincter musculature has been investigated in a prospective study by Snooks et al (1984b). This study showed that the PNTML was more increased in multipara than in primipara, and that prolonged labour, the application of forceps, and delivery of a large baby were all factors that resulted in more pudendal nerve damage. Women delivered by Caesarean section show no evidence of damage to the innervation of their pelvic floor muscles. In multipara the PNTML was more likely still to be abnormal two months after delivery, indicating the development of cumulative and irreversible damage to the innervation of the pelvic floor muscles with increasing numbers of vaginal

deliveries. Pudendal and spinal anaesthesia during childbirth had neither deleteri-
ous nor beneficial effects on the pelvic floor innervation (Snooks et al 1984b, 1985c).

Stress urinary incontinence and genital prolapse

The striated urinary sphincter musculature is as vulnerable to denervation from
damage to its innervation during childbirth as are the pudendal and intrapelvic
innervations of the external anal sphincter and puborectalis muscles (Anderson
1983, Fowler et al 1984). Studies of the innervation of the striated peri-urethral
sphincter muscle, achieved by recording the terminal motor latency in the

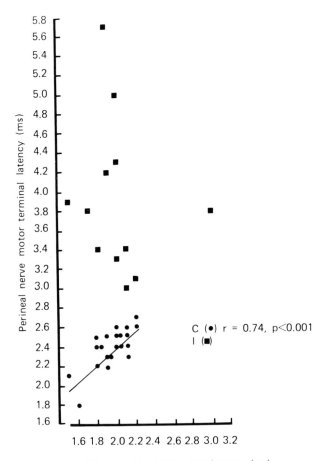

FIG. 5. Perineal and pudendal nerve terminal latencies in genuine stress urinary
incontinence. Note that there is selective increase in the perineal latency in all but one
of the patients examined. I, incontinent subjects; C, controls.

perineal component of its pudendal innervation (PerNTML), have shown that the PerNTML is selectively increased in women with genuine stress urinary incontinence (Fig. 5) (Snooks & Swash 1984). In a few women with stress urinary incontinence the PerNTML is only relatively slightly increased, and in these women there is electrophysiological evidence of denervation of the peri-urethral striated sphincter musculature as a consequence of disease in the cauda equina rather than from neuropathy in the pelvic floor itself (Snooks et al 1985b).

There is a close relationship between stress urinary incontinence and idiopathic (stress) neurogenic faecal incontinence (Parks et al 1977). About 15% of women presenting with anorectal incontinence also have stress urinary incontinence (double incontinence), and in women in whom neurogenic faecal incontinence is the only symptom the PerNTML is abnormal, although not so increased as in those who also have stress urinary incontinence (Snooks et al 1984a). The clinical features in the pelvic floor of women with stress urinary incontinence are similar to those of women with neurogenic (stress) faecal incontinence, especially in relation to the presence of perineal descent on straining. In stress urinary incontinence perineal descent is more marked anteriorly than posteriorly, reflecting the greater degree of damage to the anorectal components of the pelvic floor musculature in faecal incontinence. Similarly, in genital prolapse it has been shown that there is weakness of the pelvic floor due to denervation of the affected muscles, and accompanied by an increase in the PNTML, implying that there is damage to the pudendal innervation distally in the pelvic floor itself (Smith et al 1989). Direct measurement of the integrity of the motor innervation of the puborectalis in these conditions shows that there is similar damage to the innervation of the pelvi-caudal component of the pelvic floor musculature, in addition to that of the external anal sphincter and of the peri-urethral sphincter musculature (Swash et al 1985). When this is directly due to childbirth it is probable that it is the result of stretching of the birth canal during delivery, and of direct pressure or injury to the innervation of these muscles at the level of the lumbo-sacral plexus (Snooks et al 1984b). Clearly, this is especially likely to occur during a difficult childbirth, as was commonly experienced in developed countries before the advent of modern obstetric techniques.

Perineal descent and stretch-induced nerve injury

When the pelvic floor is weakened by damage to its innervation, the normal diaphragmatic function of this muscular sheet is compromised, so that caudally directed forces caused by abdominal straining during defaecation, laughing, or coughing are not fully withstood. The pelvic floor then bulges downward during such strains, causing repeated and sometimes sustained stretching of the pudendal nerves and of the intrapelvic nerves (Henry et al 1982). These nerves are short and are thus liable to damage, as are all peripheral nerves, when stretched by more than about 10% of their length. Repeated stretch-induced injuries of this type may therefore lead to progressive denervation, with compensatory reinnervation of the pelvic floor muscles. The distribution of these abnormalities will depend on the individual vulnerability of the nerves in the pelvis, and to the distribution of any pre-existing damage sustained during childbirth.

The effect of straining on the pelvic floor innervation has been tested directly by measuring the PNTML before, and at intervals after, a 60-second maximal defaecation strain in patients with abnormal perineal descent. In these experiments the PNTML increased after the strain and then gradually returned to its former value. In patients without abnormal perineal descent this manoeuvre resulted in much less change in the PNTML (Lubowski et al 1988b). Further evidence supporting a direct role of perineal descent in leading to progressive denervation of the pelvic floor and its striated sphincter muscles is obtained from the linear relationship found between the amount of perineal descent on straining and the PNTML measured in the resting position. The slope of the regression line is greater in women with increased perineal descent than in those without this clinical abnormality. A similar relationship was found between the PerNTML and perineal descent, confirming the close similarity between the clinical and electrophysiological abnormalities in stress faecal and stress urinary incontinence (Jones et al 1987).

Effect of age of the pelvic floor

Age effects on the pelvic floor are also important. It is a common clinical feature of these two types of incontinence, and of the development of pelvic floor disorders as a whole, that they are commoner with increasing age, and that they are especially a feature of postmenopausal women. The factors leading to the relatively selective involvement of the perineal and pudendal components of the innervation of the sphincter-cloacae muscles of the pelvic floor are, as yet, uncertain. However, age effects are well documented in cystometric studies of bladder and urinary sphincter function, and in manometric investigations of anorectal function. Studies of normal women show marked changes in the anal maximal squeeze pressure, the single-fibre EMG fibre density in the external anal sphincter muscle, the pudendal nerve terminal motor latency, and in the amount of perineal descent with straining, all occurring at about the time of the menopause. The change in PNTML precedes that in fibre density. These changes suggest that the changing hormonal environment at this time may be a relevant contributory factor leading to susceptibility to stress incontinence at this time of life, given the other contributory and initiating factors discussed above (Laurberg & Swash 1989). Anal function in geriatric patients with faecal incontinence shows abnormalities consistent with multifactorial causes for the incontinence, including pelvic floor denervation and other anorectal disorders (Percy et al 1982, Barrett et al 1989).

Smooth muscle and continence

The role of the smooth muscle of the internal urethral and internal anal sphincters in the maintenance of continence has been much discussed in the past. It is evident that continence, micturition and defaecation are under volitional control, and the functional and electrophysiological data suggest that the striated sphincter components are the major factors in the maintenance of continence. The internal anal sphincter is probably important in sensory sampling of intra-anal contents, and in the maintenance of continence when the contents of the rectum are fluid rather than solid. It may also take on an important compensatory role in some patients with denervation or damage to the striated sphincter mechanism sustained in infancy or childhood, for example through poliomyelitis or meningomyelocele. Occasionally an adult presents with faecal incontinence after haemorrhoidectomy as a consequence of inadvertent damage to this compensatory mechanism. In the urinary system there is doubt that the non-striated internal urinary sphincter is ever capable of maintaining urinary continence in the absence of a competent striated urinary sphincter.

Implications of the neurogenic hypothesis of incontinence

The neurogenic hypothesis of the pathogenesis of stress urinary and faecal incontinence (Fig. 6) has particular importance when the treatment and

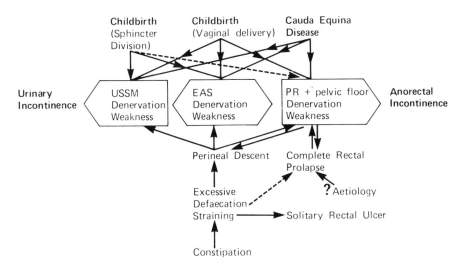

FIG. 6.   Algorithm of the neurogenic hypothesis of stress urinary and faecal incontinence, illustrating its dependence on denervation of the pelvic floor striated sphincter muscles following obstetric injury, straining at stool and cauda equina disease, and the role of perineal descent in leading to stretch injury to the pelvic innervation. USSM, periurethral striated sphincter muscle; EAS, external anal sphincter muscle; PR, puborectalis muscle.

prevention of these types of incontinence is being considered. Reparative procedures are essentially plastic repair procedures, and these can only be expected to be successful when there is sufficient innervated muscle remaining in the pelvic floor to enable the surgeon to re-fashion a striated sphincter system. Similarly, biofeedback, and physiotherapy (including pelvic floor exercises), will not be effective if there is severe pelvic floor denervation. Unfortunately, there is no method of repairing nerves damaged by this process. Treatments involving the construction of innervated sphincters are perhaps more likely to be successful. Prevention of stress incontinence will depend on close attention to the development of obstetric techniques that monitor the risk factors during childbirth for pelvic floor injury, and allow their correction. The lesson from Caesarean section that the damage to the innervation occurs during vaginal delivery is clear, and it is possible that the contemporary trend toward 'natural childbirth' may have hitherto unrecognized consequences for the pelvic floor that will become evident in the future. The underlying disease process in the relatively smaller group of women in whom neurogenic stress incontinence develops as a consequence of cauda equina disease requires further assessment. In some of these women there is no immediately apparent cause.

Finally, it is important to recognize that the neurogenic theory of the origin of stress urinary and faecal incontinence does not necessarily exclude other contributory factors, including damage to ligamentous suspensory mechanisms for pelvic floor support. Indeed damage to such factors may be important in explaining the clinical differences between stress incontinence arising in the context of childbirth from that arising from pure denervation of the pelvic floor, for example with cauda equina disease.

Acknowledgements

These ideas on incontinence have developed in studies with Research Fellows from many countries, whose work is accessible through their publications from the Sir Alan Parks Physiology Laboratory at St Mark's Hospital, and from The London Hospital. I am grateful for the generous financial support of a number of research trusts, charities, and individuals without whom this work would not have been carried out.

References

Anderson RS 1983 Increased motor unit fibre density in the external anal sphincter in genuine stress incontinence; a single fibre EMG study. Neurourol Urodyn 2:45–50
Barrett JA, Broddehurst JC, Kiff ES, Ferguson G, Faragher EB 1989 Anal function in geriatric patients with faecal incontinence. Gut 30:1244–1251
Bartolo DCC, Jarratt JA, Read NW 1983 The use of conventional EMG to assess external sphincter neuropathy in man. J Neurol Neurosurg Psychiatry 46:1115–1118
Beersiek F, Parks AG, Swash M 1979 Pathogenesis of idiopathic anorectal incontinence. J Neurol Sci 42:111–117
Fowler CJ, Kirkby RS, Harrison MJG, Milroy EJG, Turner-Warwick R 1984 Individual motor unit analysis in the diagnosis of disorders of urethral sphincter innervation. J Neurol Neurosurg Psychiatry 47:637–641

Henry MM, Swash M 1985 Coloproctology and the pelvic floor. Butterworths, London, p 407

Henry MM, Parks AG, Swash M 1982 The pelvic floor musculature in the descending perineum syndrome. Br J Surg 69:470–472

Henry MM, Snooks SJ, Barnes PRH, Swash M 1985 Investigation of disorders of anorectum and colon. Ann Coll Surg Engl 67:355–360

Jones PN, Lubowski DZ, Swash M, Henry M 1987 Relation between perineal descent and pudendal nerve damage in idiopathic faecal incontinence. Int J Colorect Dis 2:93–95

Kiff ES, Swash M 1984 Normal proximal and delayed distal conduction in the pudendal nerves of patients with idiopathic (neurogenic) anorectal incontinence. J Neurol Neurosurg Psychiatry 47:820–823

Laurberg S, Swash M 1989 Effects of aging on the anorectal sphincters and their innervation. Dis Colon Rectum 32:737–742

Lubowski DZ, Nicholls RJ, Burleigh DE, Swash M 1988a The internal anal sphincter in anorectal incontinence. Gastroenterology 95:997–1102

Lubowski DZ, Swash M, Nicholls RJ, Henry MM 1988b Increase in pudendal nerve terminal motor latency with defaecation straining. Br J Surg 75:1095–1097

Neill ME, Swash M 1980 Increased motor unit fibre density in the external anal sphincter muscle in anorectal incontinence; a single fibre EMG study. J Neurol Neurosurg Psychiatry 43:343–347

Neill ME, Parks AG, Swash M 1981 Physiological studies of the pelvic floor musculature in idiopathic faecal incontinence and rectal prolapse. Br J Surg 68:531–536

Parks AG 1975 Anorectal incontinence. Proc R Soc Med 68:681–690

Parks AG, Swash M, Urich H 1977 Sphincter denervation in anorectal incontinence. Gut 18:656–667

Percy JP, Neill ME, Swash M, Parks AG 1981 Electrophysiological study of motor nerve supply of pelvic floor. Lancet 1:16–17

Percy JP, Neill ME, Kandiah TK, Swash M 1982 A neurogenic factor in faecal incontinence in the elderly. Age Ageing 11:175–179

Roe AM, Bartolo DCC, Mortensen McNJ 1986 New method of assessment of anal sensation in various anorectal disorders. Br J Surg 73:310–312

Rogers J, Henry MM, Misiewicz JJ 1986 Combined sensory and motor deficit in primary neuropathic faecal incontinence. Gut 29:5–9

Smith ARB, Hosker GL, Warrell DW 1988 The role of partial denervation of the pelvic floor in the aetiology of genitourinary prolapse and stress incontinence of urine: a neurophysiological study. Br J Obstet Gynaecol 96:24–28

Snooks SJ, Swash M 1984 Abnormalities of the innervation of the urethral striated sphincter musculature in incontinence. Br J Urol 56:401–405

Snooks SJ, Swash M 1986 The innervation of the muscles of continence. Ann R Coll Surg Engl 68:45–49

Snooks SJ, Barnes PRH, Swash M 1984a Damage to the innervation of the voluntary anal and periurethral striated sphincter musculature in incontinence; an electrophysiological study. J Neurol Neurosurg Psychiatry 47:1269–1273

Snooks SJ, Swash M, Setchell M, Henry MM 1984b Injury to innervation of pelvic sphincter musculature in childbirth. Lancet 2:546–550

Snooks SJ, Badenoch D, Tiptaft R, Swash M 1985a Perineal nerve damage in genuine stress urinary incontinence; an electrophysiological study. Br J Urol 57:422–426

Snooks SJ, Swash M, Henry MM 1985b Abnormalities in peripheral and central nerve conduction in anorectal incontinence. J R Soc Med 78:294–300

Snooks SJ, Swash M, Henry MM, Setchell M 1985c Risk factors in childbirth causing damage to the pelvic floor innervation. Br J Surg 72:S15–S17

Swash M, Snooks SJ 1986 Slowed motor conduction in lumbosacral nerve roots in cauda
    equina lesions; a new diagnostic technique. J Neurol Neurosurg Psychiatry 49:808–816
Swash M, Snooks SJ, Henry MM 1985 A unifying concept of pelvic floor disorders and
    incontinence. J R Soc Med 78:906–911
Swash M, Gray A, Lubowski DZ, Nicholls RJ 1988 Ultrastructural changes in internal
    anal sphincter in neurogenic anorectal incontinence. Gut 29:1692–1698
Tanagho EA 1974 Simplified cystometry in stress urinary incontinence. Br J Urol 46:295–302

DISCUSSION

Bourcier: We use physiotherapy with biofeedback or electrostimulation in incontinent patients referred to our clinic from the urology or gastroenterology departments. Generally, we have patients with urinary incontinence, and only a few of these patients complain of faecal incontinence. However, patients treated for faecal incontinence usually also suffer from urinary incontinence.

In 1977 I became involved in a physiotherapy programme for incontinent menopausal women. This treatment has a high cure rate. In addition, since 1986, nulliparous or multiparous sportswomen have been referred to me for conservative mangement of stress (urinary) incontinence; however, these patients responded less well to physiotherapy.

Electrophysiological studies in this group of patients have shown abnormalities in the innervation of the pelvic floor musculature. I am interested to know whether this poor response to physiotherapy relates to the neurogenic causation of pelvic floor dysfunction in these patients.

Swash: Not all patients with idiopathic neurogenic faecal incontinence are also incontinent of urine; only 10–15% show this relationship. Furthermore, there are electrophysiological differences between patients with isolated faecal incontinence, isolated stress urinary incontinence, and double incontinence (Snooks et al 1984a, 1985).

As regards incontinence in sportswomen, I have had similar experience with female ballet dancers; urinary incontinence is an occasional hazard.

Stanton: With the very young nulliparous incontinent female patient, for example a 14-year-old girl trampolining, we must remember that there are many other causes of stress incontinence apart from denervation of the pelvic floor. Sometimes just a subtle change in the position of the bladder neck can tip the balance between continence and incontinence. It may not be a denervation process; it may be either something hereditary, a change in collagen for example, or weakness of the pelvic fascia in that age group of women who are not used to exercise and suddenly start jogging or taking up exercise. We can expect more such problems now that jogging and similar exercise have become popular.

Marsden: In the hypothesis of a peripheral neurogenic cause for idiopathic anal or urinary incontinence related to childbirth, is the mechanism in the majority of women stretch, rather than cut or tear?

Swash: Damage occurs during the second stage of labour when the head and shoulders are pushing down onto the perineum through the elongated birth canal. There is a combination of stretching and direct injury to the innervation of the stretched pelvic floor sphincter musculature.

Marsden: The nervous system at that age is remarkably good at regeneration. Why do you not see effective regeneration of damaged nerves which are still in continuity?

Swash: In our follow-up studies we did find an improvement in pudendal latency two months after delivery, so there was partial recovery. But at a subsequent delivery, there was a greater risk, in that multiparous women showed more marked abnormalities in fibre density in the external anal sphincter muscle, and in the pudendal nerve terminal motor latency (Snooks et al 1984b). There is probably a crucial point at which sufficient nerve fibres have been damaged during the birth process, especially during repeated childbirth or during even a single forceps delivery, to cause loss of sufficient motor units to produce significant weakness in the pelvic floor. When that has occurred, the patient is not protected against straining efforts in defaecation, which leads to further stretch-induced damage to the pelvic innervation.

Christensen: When a somatic nerve regenerates, does it build a whole new myelin sheath and everything else as it grows, or is the nerve more likely to sprout and form an unmyelinated fibre? In other words, are you measuring myelination, rather than nerve regeneration?

Swash: If the nerve fibre is stretched or torn a little, it will retract slightly and then regeneration occurs in the zone of Wallerian change, distal to the damage in the nerve. The axon grows down as a sprout. If the basic epineurial and endoneurial structure of the nerve is preserved, including the basal lamina tubes, regenerating axons grow through that system and reinnervate the partially denervated muscle, more or less accurately. The myelin is re-formed, but the myelinated segments are usually slightly shorter than normal and there is some slowing of conduction for some time afterwards.

Christensen: That might account for the persistent delay in conduction that you see. If the striated muscle has atrophied as a result of the loss of innervation, that might mean that the nerves will not regenerate so readily.

Swash: Totally denervated muscle is very unlikely to recover fully.

Christensen: This could explain the discordance between the concepts of nerve regeneration and the persistence of the abnormalities.

Swash: Yes, and it is consistent with the idea that biofeedback might help patients with partially denervated sphincter muscles, giving them an increased sensory awareness, rather than by improving muscular strength.

Marsden: The two components of the hypothesis are complementary, with an original neural insult from which you would expect recovery, and, as a consequence of that neural insult, you get pelvic floor descent as a second factor that perpetuates the neural insult.

Fowler: I am doubtful of the significance of a prolongation of distal motor latency as an indicator of denervation. These patients have weakness of the pelvic floor; in other words, they have lost motor units. We agree that prolongation of distal motor latency is a poor indication of denervation, but it seems even more unlikely that this prolongation would correlate with any functional deficit. The prolongation of any distal motor latency reflects the degree of demyelination in that nerve, and I don't understand how that could be reflected as impaired function. In carpal tunnel syndrome, for instance, the weakness of the abductor pollicis brevis is not claimed to be related to latency.

Swash: I agree entirely, but we were looking for a simple test that would directly assess some functional aspect of the nerve itself, when we already knew that there was a chronic partial reinnervation of the sphincter musculature, from the EMG studies. We chose this method because it is used routinely for other peripheral nerves. If nerve damage is due, as we suggest, to an acquired disturbance—that is, stretch-induced damage to axons—there will be some immediate recovery, and some axons will presumably recover by regeneration. Probably the length of these new Schwann internodes will be decreased so that conduction will be slightly impaired. There has been no study, for example, in carpal tunnel syndrome correlating the EMG change with the motor latency change.

Kirby: I agree about the limitations of pudendal latency as a measure of denervation. You could look for weakness of the striated muscle or the external urethral sphincter, to see whether stress urinary incontinence is related to denervation, by looking at individual motor units. This is something that Clare Fowler and I have been intending to do for some time. David Warrell has some evidence to support your denervation theory, but Barnick & Cardozo (1989) have claimed that individual motor units from the external urethral sphincter in stress incontinent patients were normal. What puzzles me is that the patients I see with partial cauda equina lesions, who probably have the most profound denervation of all in the pelvic floor, do not seem to be particularly troubled by stress incontinence, although they may have some. Nor do they have an excessive amount of pelvic floor descent. According to your theory, those people should be completely incontinent.

Swash: One major difference between patients with incontinence due to cauda equina disease and patients with the common syndrome of stress urinary incontinence is that the former is unrelated to pregnancy. One musn't discount the simple mechanical effect of the childbirth experience on the pelvic floor itself. After all, there are patients with stress urinary incontinence who have *no* denervation of the pelvic floor, so this is not the only explanation, although it seems to be the most common. There must also be direct hormonal effects of pregnancy on the pelvic floor itself, on the urethra and its supporting tissues, and on the perineal muscles themselves, as well as on the nerve supply to these structures.

Stanton: Could the actual pelvic mass, whether of the pregnant uterus or even fibroids, initiate the denervation process? Mark Krieger's work seemed to indicate that some of the women he studied who had large pelvic masses but were not pregnant had evidence of denervation. Could this denervation in fact start before the second stage, namely during pregnancy itself?

Swash: I agree that the pelvic mass of pregnancy could be important. The older literature suggests that stress urinary incontinence can occur during pregnancy, prior to delivery, and this has been confirmed.

DeLancey: Incontinence during pregnancy is associated with the subsequent development of stress incontinence. In fact, Diokno et al (1990) have found that this is a predictor of stress incontinence.

Bartolo: We did some work which to some extent answers the earlier question about reinnervation, and also confirms what Michael Swash has been saying. We looked at patients who are continent and had obstructed defaecation. We took a group of men and a group of women; the men by definition could not have had children, so the effects of pregnancy were removed. They had all strained at stool over many years. The women were all parous. We measured reinnervation by motor unit potential duration rather than fibre density. In the external anal sphincter the reinnervation changes were similar to those in other patients who were incontinent, despite the fact that the incontinent patients had very low sphincter pressures, and these patients with obstructed defaecation had normal pressures. But the obstructed male patients had no changes indicating reinnervation in the puborectalis at all; so the puborectalis was entirely normal in this respect, in males. But in the women, although the external anal sphincter changes were the same as in the men, there were profound changes in the puborectalis. So presumably all these people were damaging their sphincters by chronic straining at stool, they were reinnervating and so maintaining their normal anal pressures, but we inferred that the puborectal changes were the result of previous childbirth, and, once they failed to keep up with the injury, they became incontinent.

Swash: That is interesting. Age-related effects in relation to the pathogenesis of stress incontinence should also be discussed. The combination of childbirth-induced injury to the pelvic innervation plus age-related effects on the perineum, urethra, bladder and anorectum may account for the frequent late presentation of genuine stress incontinence of urine or of faeces.

DeLancey: If you had asked a group of gynaeologists ten years ago what was involved in genital prolapse and urinary incontinence (they didn't talk about anal incontinence except for external sphincter division), most would have said that it had to do with connective tissue and had nothing to do with muscle. However, looking at the interplay of connective tissue and muscle may become more important, because causation may not be as simple as a single insult to a nerve, and evidently regeneration will play some role.

An analogy from the biomechanical system of the musculoskeletal system may help, namely that muscle has a capacity for maintaining stability over a dynamic range and that the fibrous ligamentous tissues are responsible for keeping a joint stable once it exceeds that range. We may be seeing that damage to the muscular system of the pelvic floor happens at childbirth, so that it is not as capable of holding things up. The connective tissue must then take over, and, over many years of needing to do that, it stretches. This might explain why women may have children at age 25 but develop genital prolapse and urinary incontinence at a much later age; we may be seeing part of an initiation of a series of events that occur later in life because the muscle no longer plays its role and fibrous connective tissues must take over. This muscular damage is something that people had talked about in gynaecology in genital prolapse for many decades but had not put into perspective with the other 'fascias and ligaments'.

Stanton: I would disagree slightly in terms of the presentation of symptoms. Frequently when one questions a woman patient one finds that incontinence is linked very directly to her first, second, third or fourth child, without any gap in time, and if there is a gap it is because the woman hasn't come forward; but she is almost always able to associate it with one particular childbirth. I think women are conditioned not to complain!

DeLancey: Or it is because the severity of her symptoms increases with age.

Stanton: Yes. And also prolapse is a gradual process. It has a fairly subtle onset, whereas incontinence is a more dramatic symptom.

Burnstock: It seems curious to me that for anorectal incontinence you talk about the pelvic floor and also the external anal sphincter, which are all striated muscles, without mentioning the very complicated autonomic neuromuscular machinery in the rectum itself and the internal anal sphincter, which must also go wrong sometimes. How many other forms of faecal incontinence are due to the smooth muscle and its innervation, and how much do they contribute to the overall picture of anorectal incontinence?

Swash: Most patients with anorectal incontinence turn out to have pelvic floor denervation, but a small proportion, depending on the kind of hospital in which you are working and the selectivity of the referral pattern, have no evidence of denervation but have some other disturbance. These are the patients with urge incontinence, due either to heightened sensory stimulation from disturbances in the anorectum itself, perhaps an inflammatory disorder or irritable bowel syndrome, or some other unknown primary abnormality in the muscular system of the anorectum.

Burnstock: What is all the complex nervous system in the rectum actually doing?

Swash: The rectum is primarily a storage organ.

Burnstock: Then why isn't it just a sac, like the bladder?

Swash: Because it's part of the gut! The faecal content has to be propelled along through the rectum before and during defaecation.

Burnstock: So you don't think the autonomic neuromuscular system has much to do with incontinence, but just with normal propulsion?

Swash: Yes. There is some peristalsis in the rectum, as well as a massive contraction of the rectum during defaecation itself. One question we should be asking is what happens during normal defaecation, because that's not well understood.

Marsden: The rectum does something that the bladder doesn't do, namely it distinguishes between flatus and faeces. How much of that is sensory?

Swash: It is mostly sensory.

Read: I find it difficult to understand how the internal anal sphincter can become so weak, and I wonder whether the histological picture is compatible with stretching or the lack of support. Should we consider other mechanisms, such as damage to the sympathetic nerves or the blood supply to the internal sphincter?

Swash: One problem is that the nerve supply to the internal anal sphincter is quite sparse. There are noradrenergic sympathetic fibres which traverse through the muscle, but stimulation of these sympathetic nerves seem to result in relaxation of the internal sphincter, so weakness of this muscle in anorectal incontinence cannot be due to 'denervation' of the muscle. Secondly, cutting the autonomic nerves that supply the gut doesn't result in atrophy of enteric smooth muscle, so one wouldn't expect the internal non-striated sphincter to become atrophic after direct damage to its nerve supply. Thirdly, we know that electron and light micrographs reveal the smooth muscle fibres to be stretched and damaged in a way which suggests that this damage must be mechanical (Swash et al 1988).

References

Barnick CF, Cardozo L 1989 Electromyography of the urethral sphincter in genuine stress incontinence: a useless test? Neurourol Urodyn 8:318–319

Diokno AC, Brock BM, Herzog AR, Bromberg J 1990 Medical correlates of urinary incontinence in the elderly. Urology, in press

Snooks SJ, Swash M, Setchell M, Henry MM 1984a Injury to innervation of pelvic sphincter musculature in childbirth. Lancet 2:546–550

Snooks SJ, Barnes PRH, Swash M 1984b Damage to the innervation of the voluntary anal and periurethral striated musculature in incontinence; an electrophysiological study. J Neurol Neurosurg Psychiatry 47:1269–1273

Snooks SJ, Badenoch D, Tiptaft R, Swash M 1985 Perineal nerve damage in genuine stress urinary incontinence; an electrophysiological study. Br J Urol 57:422–426

Swash M, Gray A, Lubowski DZ, Nicholls RJ 1988 Ultrastructural changes in internal anal sphincter in neurogenic anorectal incontinence. Gut 29:1692–1698

General discussion II

Rectal function and parallels with urinary continence

Arhan: Five years ago we studied anorectal motility in 93 children after surgery for myelocele or meningomyelocele (Arhan et al 1984). A previously described method was used (Martelli et al 1978). The rectal, anal and marginal pressures were recorded by a special probe (Arhan & Faverdin 1972). The recto-anal inhibitory reflex was elicited by distending the rectal ampulla with balloons inflated with increasing volumes. Finally, the subjects were asked to contract the perineal muscles. The results were compared with those obtained in 80 normal children.

Statistical analysis of the results showed that motor disorders of the lower limbs were related to faecal incontinence. It was also shown that continent patients had a higher resting pressure in both the upper and lowest part of the anal canal, compared with incontinent patients. However, the rectal pressures were similar in the two groups.

The standard deviation of the pressure around the mean value was called the 'activity index'. This index was only increased in patients in the upper part of the anal canal. When the recto-anal inhibitory reflex was elicited both in the upper anal canal and at the anal margin, faecal incontinence was observed. This phenomenon is also observed in young babies before the usual age of faecal continence. Ninety per cent of patients who had a recto-anal inhibitory reflex recorded up to the anal margin were incontinent and only 47% who did not were incontinent.

A normal resting trace was observed in 61% of the patients. In this first group, 63% of patients were incontinent.

In a second group (13% of patients), spontaneous relaxations of the upper and lower anal canal were recorded simultaneously with contractions of the rectum. In this group, 91% of the patients were incontinent.

A third group was characterized by ultra-slow pressure waves in the anal sphincter. In this group, 92% of the patients were incontinent.

A fourth group of seven children were characterized by a very flat rectal and sphincteric trace at rest and by the absence of any recto-anal inhibitory reflex. All seven children were under two years of age; continence oculd not be appraised in this group.

A comparison of these findings with those obtained by cystometry of neurogenic bladders suggested that the patients in group III had a central neurogenic rectum and that those in group IV had a peripheral neurogenic rectum. On the other hand, in the patients in groups I and II, the motor function of rectal and sphincteric smooth muscle appeared normal but there is a lack of tonicity of the perineal and sphincteric striated muscle, which unmasks the natural contractions and relaxations of the internal anal sphincter. This may explain why in these groups of patients the relaxation of the internal sphincter obtained by rectal distension can be recorded up to the anal margin and that ultra-slow waves are easy to record.

Read: You seem to be seeing much the same things as we have observed in adults with faecal incontinence, and we agree that there are many different causes of faecal incontinence to consider. The interrelationship between what is happening in the rectum and in the sphincter muscles, what pressure excursions are occurring in the rectum, and the importance of relaxations of the internal sphincter that are not covered by an appropriate external sphincter contraction—all those things may become important in certain patients, particularly some of those that you see with meningomyelocele.

Staskin: There are other things to correlate in the urinary tract with the descending colon and sigmoid function. You cannot have a large reservoir in the rectum, or you will form a bolus that can't pass through the anal canal. When you consider the need to use peristalsis to move the bolus along, and the idea that you also need a peristaltic wave to move urine through the ureter, it may be that many of the electrophysiological correlates that you might look for are more similar in the *ureter* than in the bladder.

Read: This bears on what we were saying about the amount of neural machinery in the rectum. It looks more complicated than the bladder; the rectum can exhibit various patterns of motor activity—peristalsis and retrograde repulsion, for example. If you put material into the rectum, relatively small objects can find their way half way back round the colon. Thus the rectum is not the same as the bladder, which is just a simple reservoir; it does other things and therefore its neural machinery is more complicated. When you consider just defaecation and faecal continence, from the viewpoint of its extrinsic control, which is very important, there are great similarities between the bladder and the rectum.

Burnstock: I would stress that in the ureter, peristalsis is myogenic, whereas in the gut it is clearly neurogenic, so you can hardly make that comparison, in my view.

Staskin: But there is also intrinsic bladder activity; and you can stimulate peristalsis in the ureter during surgery. Is there not a myenteric plexus within the ureter?

Brading: There is almost no excitatory innervation in the ureter (there may be some sensory innervation). There are no muscarinic receptors; the isolated ureter doesn't respond to bath-applied agonists. Direct activation of the smooth muscle gives a propagated contraction which is purely myogenic.

Burnstock: The normal ureter has a plateau-like action potential, which has a long refractory period that prevents reflux of urine.

Marsden: So we have a rectum that is packed full of nerves, a bladder which has a few, and a ureter that has none.

Stanton: Some workers have hypothesized the presence of a pacemaker at the vesico-ureteral junction which they suggest may become partly disordered in cases of unstable bladder.

Burnstock: I don't understand that. There undoubtedly are pacemaker cells in the ureter, with characteristic action potentials (see Zawalinski et al 1975), but I don't see how that would have any influence on the bladder itself.

Brading: There is no evidence for a pacemaker in the ureter.

Bartolo: One should not dismiss the importance of the rectum as a storage organ, because although the rectum is not normally full of faeces, the ability to defer defaecation is related to our ability to have a compliant rectum. Although in neurogenic disease, faecal incontinence is primarily a sphincter disorder, in ulcerative colitis, Crohn's disease and radiation injury patients have a non-compliant rectum in which they can't abolish the high pressure wave and become incontinent despite having a normal external anal sphincter. In reconstructive surgery we make reservoirs which are compliant pouches constructed from the ileum. We also now make rectal pouches, because with a straight colo-anal anastomosis the patient is commonly incontinent. So we need to be able to store faeces, and the ability to defer defaecation seems to be the most important function of adequate rectal capacity.

Christensen: Dr Swash speculated about why the internal anal sphincter was weak in patients with pudendal nerve damage. When we were examining the innervation of the colon, we found we could not destroy the myelinated fibres that run in the shunt fascicles in the cat colon simply by pelvic nerve section; we had to cut the pudendal nerves as well (Christensen & Rick 1987). This led me to conclude that there is some parasympathetic pudendal innervation that extends into the smooth muscle of the colon. This would support the observation that patients with what looks like pudendal neuropathy might also have weakness of the internal anal sphincter.

Kirby: It surprises me that there is so much difference between the internal anal sphincter and the bladder neck, in women at least. When I put a pressure transducer at the bladder neck in women and filled up the bladder with saline, there was a steady rise in bladder neck pressure during filling. I attributed that to a reflex arc informing the bladder that it was filling, by sending information up the spinal cord to the thoraco-lumbar outflow and increasing the sympathetic tone of the bladder neck. When we gave an α-adrenergic blocking drug, phentolamine, intravenously, the rise in bladder neck pressure was reduced.

The internal anal sphincter seems to be completely different. As the rectum fills, Dr Swash is saying that it relaxes rather than closes, which is the opposite of what you would expect of a sphincter. Yet it's clearly a sphincter in its structure. How do you explain that?

Swash: There is controversy about this, but the rectum is said to be empty in normal subjects. As it fills it dilates and initiates the recto-anal reflex, an entirely enteric, intramural reflex in which dilatation of the internal anal sphincter occurs when the rectum is distended. This is the beginning of the defaecation response, induced by rectal filling. This filling can occur after a meal, as a post-prandial response to colonic contractions (the gastro-colic reflex). This is not to say that some normal subjects do not have faeces in the rectum, so it's more complicated than that.

Read: As you distend the rectum, the internal sphincter relaxes at times when the subject experiences no sensation. There is no correlation between the sensation of filling and desire to defaecate and internal sphincter relaxation. But there is another correlation: as the rectum is distended by ramp inflation, the rectal pressures rise rapidly to their plateaus; this is followed by a terminal rapid rise in pressure. The point of inflection between the plateau and the second rise is when you get a desire to defaecate, irrespective of the distension rate.

Burnstock: Charles Hoyle and Rahima Crowe in my laboratory have been looking at the human internal anal sphincter, and when you say there are only a few sympathetic nerves, I would tend to agree, since dopamine β-hydroxylase (DBH)-immunoreactive nerve fibres were found in nerve bundles and around blood vessels. Further, it is densely innervated by neuropeptide Y-immunoreactive nerves (many of which may represent sympathetic nerves), and we have found nerves containing CGRP, [Met]enkephalin, substance P, VIP and occasionally 5-HT in nerve bundles in this sphincter. Inhibitory junction potentials have also been recorded, which might account for the strong dilator effect when intramural nerves are stimulated. So probably neural control of the internal anal sphincter is important, involving not just extrinsic nerves, but also intrinsic fibres coming from enteric plexuses.

Swash: I was struck by your comment that the numbers of nerve cells and fibres diminished caudally through the gut, because there is no more gut to which the enteric neurons might project. However, I am sure you are correct that I have underestimated the innervations of the internal anal sphincter.

Read: I always believed that sympathetic nerves were excitatory to the internal anal sphincter. But Lubowski et al (1987) stimulated presacral nerves at operation and found an inhibition of internal sphincter tone. Is it possible that you could be stimulating parasympathetic fibres to the sphincter, as well as sympathetic fibres? I am confused about this area!

Swash: Everybody is confused. We thought we were stimulating sympathetic fibres, but of course we were stimulating a *nerve*, and might therefore have noted effects relating to either the rostral or caudal input direction resulting from our stimulation. For example, rostral effects might induce reflex effects differing from the caudal-going effects. The question is open!

Christensen: In terms of our expectations of what the bladder neck and internal anal sphincter should do, it seems to me that the internal sphincter does exactly what one would expect that a sphincter should do. It works exactly like the lower oesophageal sphincter; that is, it is contracted at rest. A large fraction of that tone is myogenically rather than neurogenically maintained. When the smooth muscle of the oesophagus above the oesophageal sphincter is stretched, the oesophageal sphincter relaxes. The internal anal sphincter is also myogenic and it relaxes on rectal distension. In both cases relaxation is apparently mediated by non-adrenergic inhibitory nerves. These two sphincters are very much alike. But the pylorus and the ileo-colonic sphincter seem to be a little different.

Kirby: Of course the oesophageal sphincter is not designed to hold food in the oesophagus; it is supposed to relax as food comes down. The bladder and the rectum are the opposite; they should not leak.

Christensen: The function of a sphincter is to keep things on both sides where they belong, but at the same time to allow flow when required; the internal anal sphincter may be doing just that. Continence, in my view, is more a function of the external anal sphincter than the internal sphincter.

Marsden: Could someone explain how one can have voluntary incontinence of what one perceives as wind, but voluntary continence of what one perceives as faeces?

Christensen: If the faeces are liquid, patients often can't make this distinction between wind and faeces, and so they have faecal incontinence.

Bartolo: Duthie has explained this most satisfactorily (Duthie & Gairns 1960). The middle part of the anal canal is lined by sensory nerves, and during periods of rectal distension the recto-anal inhibitory reflex causes the anal canal to open, so we can sense whether there is liquid, gas or solid there and take appropriate action. If the rectal pressure wave is high and doesn't relax, we leak; if we sense that it's gas, we can pass it; and if we sense that it's liquid and the pressure wave doesn't relax, we take the necessary action!

Marsden: How is the sensing actually done?

Swash: Besides the sensory receptors in the anorectal mucosa, there are Pacinian corpuscles in mesentery and a few muscle spindles in the striated sphincter muscles.

Marsden: But what is one doing? Is one using sphincter contractions to test whether the rectal contents can be compressed or not?

Read: That wouldn't distinguish between gas and liquid. I do not believe the anal sphincter is a good mechanism for discrimination between liquid and gas, but the rectum probably discriminates between solid and fluid stool. When you feel gas or liquid coming into the rectum, you can compress it and this gives rise to different sensations from the arrival of solid.

Bartolo: I think the anal sphincter is a wonderful mechanism! If you remove the rectum and replace it by an ileal pouch, then with a perfect sphincter, these patients, who always have a liquid stool, can sometimes pass gas.

Read: Not many such patients with an ileal pouch can tell the difference between solid and liquid.

Bartolo: Some can, although many will never pass flatus; they only do so at the end of the defaecation. Certainly some patients with ileal pouches can pass gas, standing up. They have a liquid stool but they can discriminate gas.

Marsden: What part of the anal sphincter has been left in position?

Bartolo: We leave the whole of the internal sphincter, with the transitional zone. Some patients in whom that transitional zone has been removed can still discriminate.

Read: There is a voluntary compressing mechanism, made up of the levator ani and the external sphincter. That may be how it is done, by compressing fluid and detecting the alteration in sensation.

Marsden: Do you see this compression going on in any of the tests? Do you actually see the anal sphincter doing this?

Swash: You can see the external anal sphincter and puborectalis muscles contracting and relaxing during defaecation proctography.

Marsden: Testing it out? This information would reach the brain very quickly.

Swash: Yes. The sensory receptors resemble those in glabrous skin—for example, Meissner-type corpuscles and free endings from unmyelinated C and Aδ nerve fibres.

Kuijpers: We remove the proximal anal mucosa in performing an ileo-anal procedure. In our results, 75% have normal control for gas, liquid and solid stool. This indicates that the proximal anal mucosa is not so important in faecal continence; probably is not important at all.

References

Arhan P, Faverdin Cl 1972 Une sonde à ballonnets pour l'étude de la mécanique rectoanale. Path Biol 20(3,4):191–194

Arhan P, Faverdin C, Devroede G, Pierre-Kahn A, Scott H, Pellerin D 1984 Anorectal motility after surgery for spina bifida. Dis Colon Rectum 27:159–163

Christensen J, Rick GA 1987 The distribution of myelinated nerves in the ascending nerves and myenteric plexus of the cat colon. Am J Anat 178:250–258

Duthie HL, Gairns FW 1960 Sensory nerve-endings and sensation in the anal region of man. Br J Surg 47:585–594

Lubowski DZ, Nicholls RJ, Swash M, Jordan MT 1987 Neural control of external anal sphincter function. Br J Surg 74:668–670

Martelli H, Devroede G, Duguay C, Dornic C, Faverdin C 1978 Some parameters of large bowel motility in normal man. Gastroenterology 75:612–618

Zawalinski V, Constantinou CE, Burnstock G 1975 Ureteral pacemaker potentials recorded with the sucrose gap technique. Experientia 31:931–932

Stress urinary incontinence

Stuart L. Stanton

Urodynamic Unit, Department of Obstetrics and Gynaecology, St George's Hospital Medical School, Lanesborough Wing, Cranmer Terrace, London SW17 0RE, UK

Abstract. Stress urinary incontinence due to urethral sphincter incompetence (genuine stress incontinence) afflicts some 5–15% of women. The mechanism of continence is imperfectly understood, as is the precise mode of its cure, whether conservative or surgical. The pathophysiology is a reduction in urethral resistance in the absence of detrusor activity. Aetiological factors include congenital malformation of the bladder neck, denervation of the pelvic floor and sphincter mechanism following childbirth, trauma causing disruption of the urethral sphincter mechanism, fibrosis associated with bladder neck surgery for prolapse, oestrogen deprivation at the menopause, and urethral relaxation or instability. Conventional investigations include urethral pressure measurement, urethral electric conductance, electrophysiological tests, and cystometry or videocystourethrography (the latter procedures diagnose by exclusion). A more precise evaluation of the role of urethral resistance is hampered by lack of suitable techniques for measuring urethral and sphincteric function. Treatments include pelvic floor exercise, drugs to increase urethral resistance, and surgery, either to evaluate the bladder neck or to increase urethral resistance.

1990 Neurobiology of Incontinence. Wiley, Chichester (Ciba Foundation Symposium 151) p 182–194

Stress incontinence is loss of urine on physical effort. It occurs in many conditions and it is wiser to regard this term as a symptom or a sign and not as a diagnostic label. When stress incontinence occurs secondary to incompetence of the sphincter mechanism, it is termed either urethral sphincter incompetence or genuine stress incontinence (the latter is the preferred term used by the International Continence Society) (Bates et al 1976).

The following questions are posed: their answers are germane to any improvement in management of this condition.

1. What is the mechanism of urethral sphincter incompetence?
2. How do we investigate urethral function?
3. Why are drugs ineffective in controlling this condition?
4. Which operation for continence?

This paper will try to address these questions under the following headings.

1. Pathophysiology

Urethral sphincter incompetence (genuine stress incontinence) is defined as involuntary loss of urine when the intravesical pressure exceeds the maximum urethral pressure in the absence of detrusor activity. The causes of this are:

(a) Loss of urethral resistance due to factors such as epispadias, urethral and periurethral scarring following previous bladder neck surgery, hypo-oestrogenization of the urothelium and underlying submucosa containing vascular plexus, and denervation of smooth and striated muscle within the urethra.

(b) Descent of the bladder neck following childbirth, due to denervation and stretching of the pelvic floor and its fascial supports. Here there is failure of transmission of the intra-abdominal pressure to the proximal urethra, so producing a negative pressure gradient between bladder and urethra leading to incontinence.

(c) Lack of posterior support for the bladder neck and proximal urethra. When this occurs, the cough force transmission is unable to compress the proximal urethra.

(d) Urethral relaxation. The urethra appears to have more tone and resistance but progressively relaxes after a cough force, so that incontinence follows. Hilton (1988) has demonstrated that the mean Δ maximum urethral closure pressure (relative) is a useful discriminant. This is taken as the variation in centimetres of water above and below the mean MUCP as a percentage of the mean MUCP itself. In a group of 145 women with urethral sphincter incompetence, 38% were found to have an unstable urethra.

Denervation of the pelvic floor muscles and the smooth muscle in the pubo-cervical fascia (Sayer et al 1989) is the underlying pathology in many of these causes. There are also congenital or degenerative changes in the collagen in these tissues.

2. Investigation

Whilst the bladder can be reliably investigated using twin-channel subtracted cystometry, and bladder and urethra can be investigated with a combination of cystometry and radiological screening as videocystourethrography (VCU), there is a dearth of reliable methods of urethral investigation.

Urethral pressure measurements have been in vogue for the past 20 years, initially as static pressures derived from a water-filled catheter (Brown & Wickham 1969) and now using twin microtip transducer sensors mounted on a solid catheter, and recording simultaneous dynamic bladder and urethral pressure measurements. Most clinicians find these measurements unreliable and unable to differentiate sphincter incompetence from other forms of incontinence. Versi et al (1986) found that there was significant overlap in maximum urethral closure pressure between normal patients and those with urethral sphincter incompetence, and that this was a valueless parameter for distinguishing between them.

In an effort to simplify the diagnosis of urethral sphincter incompetence and to minimize the invasiveness of these investigations, Peattie et al (1988a) used a technique known as distal urethral electric conductance (DUEC) as a screening test for female urinary incontinence. A DUEC catheter containing two gold brass-plated electrodes 1 mm wide and 1 mm apart was placed in the urethra and fixed 1.5 cm proximal to the external urethral meatus. A non-stimulatory voltage of 20 mV was placed across the electrodes and the current, recorded in microamps, was a measure of impedance. Urine gave a low impedance; three patterns were demonstrated. Two of these showed respectively a conductance rise greater than 8 μA for two seconds or a conductivity rise during intra-abdominal pressure with super-imposed spikes of conductivity of 8 μA, and were found in urethral sphincter incompetence ($\chi^2 = 40.2$, $P > 0.001$). A third pattern showed rises in conductivity greater than 8 μA and lasting for longer than three seconds, which were indicative of detrusor instability. A broader application of the urethral electric conductance principle was to measure UEC at the bladder neck in conjunction with cystometry, to enhance the diagnosis of the unstable urethra.

A further approach to the assessment of urethral function has been the measurement of urethral elastance by Lose et al (1989). Using a probe which simultaneously measured urethral cross-sectional area and urethral and vesical pressures, they studied the ability of the urethra to resist dilatation in the resting state with measurements taken at the bladder neck and mid and distal urethra. Patients with urethral sphincter incompetence had a statistically significant decrease in elastance at the bladder neck compared to normal patients.

Ultrasound is a recent addition to urodynamic investigations. Scanning can be performed using a perineal, transrectal or vaginal probe. At present, the vaginal probe gives the clearest definition. The rectal probe is sometimes uncomfortable. Quinn et al (1989) have extensive experience of this technique applied to urodynamics and suggested its role in the diagnosis of urethral sphincter incompetence. However, because the technique used is unable to detect uninhibited detrusor contractions, its main use so far has been to detect bladder neck opening, station and excursion of the bladder neck (Gordon et al 1989), to detect residual urine, and to detect abnormal urethral, paraurethral and bladder anatomy. I think the approach to bladder neck movement will be the most exciting, with measurement of intra-abdominal force as a prerequisite (A. Clark, M. Pearce, S. Creighton & S. L. Stanton, unpublished paper presented to the American Urogynecological Society, Phoenix, Arizona, 4–7 October 1989).

3. Treatment

The clinical spectrum of dysfunction produced by sphincter incompetence means that a variety of treatments are usually required. Conservative methods are used for temporary alleviation, where incontinence is mild or the patient elects to postpone surgery or where surgery is inappropriate because the patient is physically or mentally frail.

Drug treatment of stress incontinence due to sphincter incompetence is singularly disappointing. α-Adrenergic stimulation (e.g. with phenyl-propanolamine or midrodine) has been used with inconsistent relief and often with the appearance of sympathomimetic side-effects such as tachycardia. Oestrogen has been given to the post-menopausal patient, again with inconsistent results.

Electronic stimulation of the pelvic floor has been attempted, using implanted electrodes at the bladder neck and removable vaginal or anal plug electrodes. In all modes, there has been uncertainty about the route of stimulation and the parameters of stimulation have varied enormously. One of the more useful approaches has come from Vereecken et al (1989) who utilized the moment of detrusor pressure increase to initiate electrical stimulation via anal or vaginal plug electrodes. The stimulus for the control of the sphincter incompetence was a current intensity of 10 mA at a frequency of 250–300 Hz (slower frequencies of 5–50 Hz can be used for detrusor instability). The stimulus intensity is adjusted until minimal pain and maximal effects are found. The short stimulus excludes muscle fatigue and the device can be used by the patient at home.

Simple pelvic floor exercises have been in use for years and wide variations in success are reported. The Kegel perineometer, used to measure pelvic floor tone and demonstrate to the patient a visual display of intravaginal pressure change, has the disadvantage that vaginal pressure can be artifically raised by increasing the intra-abdominal pressure, which would mask any contribution from the pelvic floor muscles. Plevnik (1985) described an innovative approach to determining pelvic floor tone and to augmenting this by pelvic floor exercises, using plastic vaginal cones containing metal of increasing weight, from 20 to 100 g (Figs. 1 and 2). A cone is inserted into the vagina with the tapered end pointing downwards and the patient tries, both passively and actively, to retain this cone, using only her pelvic floor muscles. Any use of the abdominal musculature will cause the cone to be extruded. Peattie et al (1988b) demonstrated the effectiveness of cones in reducing urine loss, measured by a standard urine pad test and by a reduction in the number of women opting for continence surgery. It should be noted that these exercises require 1–3 months before change is evident and have to be continued for life, if improvement or cure is to be maintained.

The urinary catheter completes the list of conservative treatments. It is either a temporary or a permanent method and may be inserted either urethrally or suprapubically. The latter is more comfortable and there is less risk of urinary tract infection, but it does require a doctor to insert it initially. Urethral catheterization is simpler and easily accomplished by a nurse but has the disadvantage of being uncomfortable. A new silicone-coated latex Foley catheter

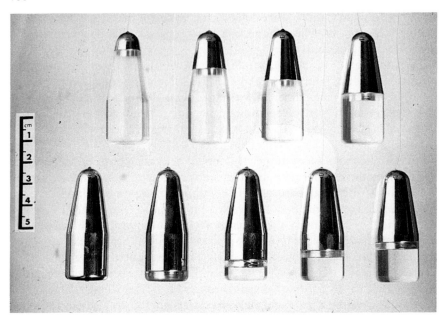

FIG. 1.   Vaginal cones of varying weights, between 20 and 100 g.

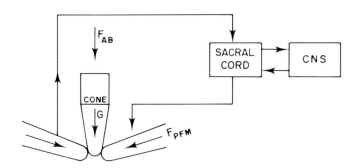

FIG. 2.   Diagram to show biofeedback from the weight (G) of the vaginal cone acting on the pelvic floor muscles and sending impulses back to the sacral spinal cord, central nervous system and then to the pelvic floor muscles again. F_{AB}, force due to abdominal pressure; F_{PFM}, force developed by pelvic floor muscles.

has been devised by Brocklehurst et al (1988) to minimize these disadvantages and to avoid bypassing. The catheter has a soft compliant intra-urethral portion which conforms to the shape of the urethra and has been found to be more acceptable than a standard Foley catheter.

The surgical management of urethral sphincter incompetence remains the mainstay of permanent and effective treatment. Uncertainty about the pathophysiology has led to a variety of procedures, with four or five ultimately being used as the most effective operations. The choice depends on clinical and urodynamic parameters, and again lack of an effective method of investigating the urethra is notable.

The aims of surgery are:

1. To elevate the bladder neck and enhance intra-abdominal pressure transmission to the proximal urethra, to produce a positive closure pressure.

2. To support the proximal urethra so that the cough force effectively compresses this.

3. To increase urethral resistance, so that it exceeds any intravesical pressure increase.

A scheme has been devised by which to select these operations (Stanton 1986) (Fig. 3). Clinical urodynamic assessments detect voiding difficulty and detrusor instability and these are treated appropriately.

The next stage is to decide the elevation of the bladder neck. If it is not elevated, and if the patient is elderly or frail, a Raz procedure (endoscopic bladder neck suspension operation) is recommended. This has a brief operating time and low operative and postoperative morbidities, and minimal postoperative analgesia is required.

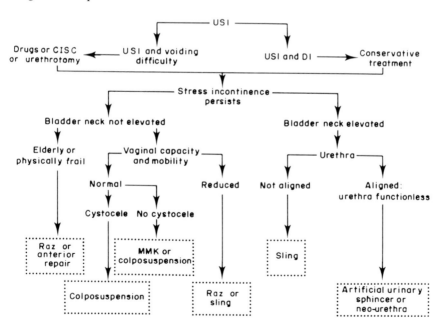

FIG. 3. Schema for the choice of continence surgery. USI, urethral sphincter incompetence; DI, detrusor instability; CISC, clean intermittent self-catheterization; MMK, Marshall–Marchetti–Krantz procedure.

If the patient is fit and healthy a clinical decision is made as to whether the vaginal capacity and mobility have been impaired by previous operative scarring, menopause or nulliparity. If they are impaired, a sling or Raz procedure is technically more satisfactory than a colposuspension or a Marshall–Marchetti–Krantz procedure, which are used when vaginal capacity and mobility are not compromised. The colposuspension is particularly indicated when there is coexistent anterior vaginal wall prolapse.

Finally, when bladder neck elevation has been achieved but the bladder neck and proximal urethra are not supported or aligned to the symphysis pubis, a sling is recommended. If urethral function studies indicate a decrease in urethral resistance, then urethral reconstruction or the insertion of an artificial urinary sphincter, which will increase outflow resistance, should be considered.

The technique of paraurethral injection for minimal incontinence (e.g. improvement of incontinence but not cure after incontinence surgery) using Teflon or Silastic material became less popular when it was found that these substances migrated to the lungs and brain. A new substance—glutaraldehyde cross-linked bovine collagen (GAX collagen)—has been used by Appell et al (1989) and is effective in increasing urethral resistance, without causing local foreign body reaction or migration. It is thin enough to be injected by a fine needle with or without a general anaesthetic and is biodegradable, so that after 24 weeks it is replaced by the host collagen.

Conclusion

This paper has tried to show the state of the art of urethral sphincter incompetence and where gaps in knowledge exist. Enhanced diagnostic techniques are crucial to any improvement in success by conservative and surgical treatments.

References

Appell R, Goodman J, McGuire E et al 1989 Multicenter study of periurethral and transurethral GAX-collagen for urinary incontinence. Proceedings of 19th Annual Meeting of the International Continence Society, Ljubljana. Neurourol Urodyn 8:339–340

Bates P, Bradley W, Glen L et al 1976 First report on standardisation of terminology of lower urinary tract function. Br J Urol 48:39–42

Brocklehurst J, Hickey D, Davies I, Kennedy A, Morris J 1988 A new urethral catheter. Br Med J 291:1691–1693

Brown M, Wickham J 1969 The urethral pressure profile. Br J Urol 41:211–217

Gordon D, Pearce M, Norton P, Stanton SL 1989 Comparison of ultrasound and lateral chain urethrocystography in the determination of bladder neck descent. Am J Obstet Gynecol 160:182–185

Hilton P 1988 Unstable urethral pressure: towards a more relevant definition. Neurourol Urodyn 6:411–418

Lose G, Colstrup H, Thind P 1989 Urethral elastance in healthy and stress incontinent women. Proceedings of 19th Annual Meeting of the International Continence Society, Ljubljana. Neurourol Urodyn 8:370-372

Peattie A, Plevnik S, Stanton SL 1988a DUEC test: a screening test for female stress incontinence. Proceedings of 18th Annual Meeting of the International Continence Society, Oslo. Neurourol Urodyn 7:173-174

Peattie A, Plevnik S, Stanton SL 1988b Vaginal cones: a conservative method of treating genuine stress incontinence. Br J Obstet Gynaecol 93:1049-1053

Plevnik S 1985 New method for testing and strengthening of pelvic floor muscles. Proceedings of 15th Annual Meeting of the International Continence Society, London. p 267-268

Quinn M, Farnsworth B, Pollard W, Smith P, Stott M 1989 Vaginal ultrasound in the diagnosis of stress incontinence: a prospective comparison to urodynamic investigations. Proceedings of 19th Annual Meeting of the International Continence Society, Ljubljana. Neurourol Urodyn 8:302-303

Sayer T, Dixon J, Hosker G, Warrell DW 1989 A histological study of pubocervical fascia in women with stress incontinence of urine. Int Urogynaecol J 1:18

Stanton SL 1986 Choice of surgery. In: Stanton SL, Tanagho E (eds) Surgery of female incontinence, 2nd edn. Springer-Verlag, Heidelberg, p 275-278

Vereecken R, Dhaene P, Van Nuland T, Sansen W, Puers B 1989 A new concept for electrostimulation in incontinence. Proceedings of 19th Annual Meeting of the International Continence Society, Ljubljana. Neurourol Urodyn 8:360-361

Versi E, Cardozo L, Studd J, Cooper D 1986 Evaluation of urethral pressure profilometry for diagnosis of genuine stress incontinence. World J Urol 4:6-9

DISCUSSION

Burnstock: You appear to use a very high frequency of stimulation (250-300 Hz) in your treatment. It is possible that you are directly stimulating the muscle with these stimulation parameters. Sympathetic nerves, which you are most interested in, are usually stimulated at about 10-15 Hz. It has been claimed that very high frequency stimulation favours the release of peptides such as VIP, which is a potent vasodilator. It would be important to think very carefully about what is actually being stimulated with the stimulation parameters selected.

Stanton: This is right. The stimulators are placed in the vagina and anus, which are large areas in relation to specific nerve endings. People have implanted stimulators, as I said, but even then, where are you implanting those stimulators in relationship to nerves? This was never clear. So the actual direction of current flow is very vague. But you are quite right; a lot of different parameters have been used—square waves, sinusoidal waves. Certainly 250-300 Hz is quite a fast frequency, but I made the point that when these devices are used to treat detrusor instability where a different muscle is being stimulated, a slower frequency (5-50 Hz) is used. I am sceptical about the concept of stimulation, but it is a mode of treatment that many clinicians use in Europe, particularly in Scandinavia, and also in parts of the USA.

Bourcier: For many years electrical stimulation has been used as an aid in the control of urinary incontinence. According to several reports of very interesting studies by M. Fall and S. Plevnik, both stress and urge incontinence have been successfully treated in 30% to 80% of cases.

In France since 1981 we have used electrical stimulation for urinary incontinence. According to these previous studies, the different parameters are: alternating pulses at 20 Hz for bladder instability; alternating pulses of 50–100 Hz for urethral closure pressure. Muscle fatigue is less marked. Because of the impedance of the vagina in relation to age (305 ohms for menopausal women and 460 ohms for young women), the current used ranged from 10 mA to 70 mA. To achieve optimal stimulation without causing discomfort to the patient the voltage has to be adjusted to values below the threshold for pain.

Is it possible to go back to the English definition of sphincter incompetence? In France, we have another definition of genuine stress incontinence; it is the association of an open bladder neck and a low pressure with a weak urethral sphincter. As the impact of pelvic floor support is very important and the rate of relapse is high in this group, we prefer, before surgery, to use a combination of stimulation and biofeedback.

I agree with Dr Stanton that the new type of therapy represented by the use of cones is an effective and cost-effective method of physiotherapy. My view is that this method could be adapted as a primary treatment or for prevention in nulliparous women and in sportswomen.

The only problem with the use of cones is that whatever the weight is, in a patient with 'reversed (inverted) perineal command' (see p 48) she can retain the cone through an abdominal contraction and by pushing down. Another problem occurs in sportswomen with a very strong abdominal wall; the cone simply drops out.

A further point is that there is no relationship between a good score with cones (40–50 g) and the strength and endurance of the pelvic floor.

Burnstock: I am surprised by what appears to be the very preliminary use of drugs in the treatment of incontinence. There are many strategies that could be explored, as we begin to understand more about the various neurotransmitters contained in nerves supplying the urethra. For instance, a noradrenaline uptake inhibitor would enormously potentiate the effect of the noradrenaline that would be released by stimulation.

Stanton: For this condition of incompetent sphincter, very few drugs have been explored. For detrusor instability, more have been used.

Burnstock: You appear to be assuming that incontinence is largely a urethral problem, but is it not true that contraction of the bladder is an equally important part of the voiding mechanism and that urethral opening and bladder contraction are normally linked activities?

Stanton: No. I was simply trying to conform to the topic that I was intended to cover, because otherwise the subject is so broad. I therefore didn't want to deal with the combination, which we frequently encounter, of mixed instability and sphincter incompetence, but of course one cannot separate them, and it is fallacious to do so.

Swash: Why is it fallacious to separate the two, if they occur together?

Stanton: Really because of the practical consequences, that in a number of patients the two coexist and you have to think about treating them together, and also because sometimes you can induce instability by the effects of surgery.

Blaivas: In addition to pelvic floor exercises and their biomechanical effects, the patients also gain a heightened awareness of voiding events. All these things together—the strengthening exercises, the possible reciprocal inhibition by contracting the sphincter and avoiding detrusor contractions, and the fact that the patients are now thinking about their voiding habits in a way they never did before—contribute to what I think is a reasonably good success rate for these therapeutic modalities. At present there are a large number of prospective trials of medical treatments for benign prostatic hyperplasia. In these studies, the patients all keep a diary of their voiding habits. The actual keeping of the diary is considered to be part of the placebo effect but, in fact, in some studies 60–70% of the patients get better on placebo. I would suggest that keeping a voiding diary and heightening one's awareness of micturitional events is not a placebo, but part of the treatment.

My second point is a philosophical comment on ways of looking at incontinence. In simplistic terms there are only two possibilities for sphincteric incontinence: (1) the walls of the urethra are not normally coapted (that is what you describe as decreased resistance; the urethra itself somehow doesn't function properly); or (2) there is an abnormality of bladder neck descent such that the pressures are not transmitted equally from the abdominal cavity to the bladder and urethra. Bladder pressure transmission is greater than urethral, and leakage occurs. The thrust of diagnosis used to be: does the patient have stress incontinence or not? But that can usually be answered by a very simple history and examination. I think we can all make this distinction with a great degree of reliability just by standing the patient and having her cough or strain, and observing the pattern of urinary loss. But we want to know more precise details nowadays. We want to know the pathophysiology and which of those two entities (stress or urge), either alone or in combination, is causing the condition. And we want to know more about the bladder and how well it can contract. That is the purpose of the diagnostic process. In that regard, I see ultrasound, urethral conductance and stress urethral pressure profiles as not being very useful in answering those questions. Potentially, urethral elastance, as described by Lose et al (1989), might be a good way of making the diagnosis.

Finally, treatment will depend conceptually on (1) whether you are trying to prevent the descent of the bladder neck and urethra, or (2) whether you are trying to compensate for an urethra whose walls don't stay coapted. These are conceptually very different. In the latter circumstance you want to compress the urethra, and in the former you simply want to prevent the descent. I think that is the direction in which we should be going.

Stanton: I quite agree, and that's why I tried to focus my comments about bladder neck descent on what I think is the best objective method of diagnosis that we have at the moment, namely ultrasound. There isn't anything to compare with ultrasound in terms of safety, absence of irradiation, non-invasiveness, and a technique you can do in your own department and can therefore replicate with your patients.

Blaivas: But compared to a fluoroscopic study, ultrasound *is* more invasive, because you have a large probe in the vagina. It is like putting the cone inside the vagina and asking the patient to cough and relax at the same time!

Stanton: Nevertheless, it is the most accurate method we have for localization of the bladder neck.

Blaivas: X-ray is more accurate.

Stanton: You have then to look at the projection distance; you must ensure that the patient is standing the same way each time, and so on.

Blaivas: I agree that we haven't done these studies with such great precision in the past, but they are quite easy to do, and will allow one to answer the questions.

Stanton: At least we both agree that descent or excursion of the bladder neck is important, whatever the technical details of the diagnostic methods.

de Groat: We have discussed the active properties of the sphincter and the urethra, but John DeLancey earlier brought up collagen and elastic fibres, and that came up again with the mention of elastance by Stuart Stanton. In an animal study Jack Krier examined the length–tension relationships of the striated muscle of the cat external anal sphincter and concluded that the passive length–tension curve is much stiffer for this particular muscle than it is for the typical mammalian skeletal muscle, and that the passive tension is more dependent on elastic and connective tissue in this muscle than in limb muscles (Krier et al 1989). It was very much like the oesophageal sphincter, and also like cardiac muscle. I think this is important.

John DeLancey pointed out that in post-menopausal women, oestrogen levels change, connective tissues also change and that a major part of sphincter weakness is due to an alteration in the passive properties of this muscle. Thus both active and passive properties are important. Krier mentions that 44% of the resting tension of the external anal sphincter muscle is passive, and is due to its elastic properties. Even in the active state, during muscle contraction, almost 13% of the tension results from the passive properties of the muscle. His conclusion was that this may be an adaptive response of this particular muscle to its sphincter function. I wonder whether not only the anal sphincter, but many of the muscles that make up the pelvic floor, may have this kind of property. It would be interesting to look at the length–tension properties of all the pelvic floor muscles. This may be a major property that changes with age.

Stanton: I would agree, and would add to that the contribution of vascular turgor, which is thought to be as high as 30% of the resting tone of the urethra.

Blaivas: The elastance measurement doesn't separate passive from active forces, but it is looking at length and tension in relation to changes in radius and pressure.

Marsden: The force exerted in response to a nervous input depends upon the passive length–tension relationship of a muscle, so what you get out from a nervous input is also determined by the passive properties of the muscle.

de Groat: Krier also said that the external anal sphincter muscle is linked through connective tissue to smooth muscle in the bowel, and thus smooth muscle by pulling on the striated muscle can cause an increase in the passive tension that occurs in it. At this meeting we have been interested in the mechanisms for the coordination of smooth and striated muscle systems, and we have often thought about autonomic nerves affecting striated muscle, but here is an indirect approach where the smooth muscle can increase the tension in the striated muscle.

DeLancey: It is interesting that although we use the term 'ligament' for the supportive tissues of the pelvic viscera, they all contain surprising amounts of smooth muscle. The 'ligament' is not the usual ligament that we think of, which connects bone to bone. There have not been any published studies of the contractile properties of this supposed 'fibrous tissue', where for some reason evolution has put an unusual quantity of smooth muscle into the tissue.

Andersson: To revert to pharmacological treatment, it is true that the success rate so far is very limited, but other agents besides oestrogens and α-adrenergic receptor agonists have been used for treatment. Noradrenaline uptake inhibitors have been tried, including imipramine. Favourable results were reported (Gilja et al 1984), but the study was not controlled. Good results have been reported with β-receptor antagonists (Kaisary 1984), which would be expected to increase intraurethral pressure. Again, studies have not been controlled, so we cannot say if there are effective alternatives to the existing drug treatments.

Stanton: This is why I did not discuss this more, because there isn't anything yet that has been tried and is effective, in controlled studies.

Burnstock: I mentioned noradrenaline uptake inhibitors because if you are thinking about drug development, the nice thing about these inhibitors is that you are not adding something new; you are simply enhancing the endogenous release of noradrenaline and in this way increasing the efficiency of an abnormally diminished physiological event.

Andersson: It's an attractive idea, but you always have to think of the lack of selectivity and the toxic effects of for example tricyclic antidepressant agents. You don't die from stress incontinence, but you may from overdosage with these drugs!

DeLancey: One topic that many of us have been talking about increasingly with stress incontinence is trying to define the problem that each individual has.

We all have experience with an individual patient who improves dramatically with drug therapy. If you use that drug on one hundred people, the other 99 may not respond. One of the new areas that I find interesting is to try to select out the patient who will respond to oestrogen, or who might respond to a noradrenaline uptake inhibitor, or will only respond to surgery. It may not be a uniform condition in all people.

Burnstock: You need more basic studies, to find out for example at what age oestrogen does affect receptor expression. Perhaps beyond a certain age it doesn't work any more, and you are wasting your time. You need many more fundamental studies before being in a position to decide on the best strategy.

Stanton: The short practical answer is that you need a large number of treatments to offer, because you certainly never get, in any age group, a single effective cure for stress urinary incontinence.

Swash: How effective are oestrogens in patients with genuine stress incontinence of urine?

DeLancey: Individual patients do become completely cured, but they are very few.

Swash: Does this improvement persist for a long time?

DeLancey: I don't know that anyone has studied such patients over years; studies are usually fairly short-term. The vast majority of post-menopausal women don't respond at all to oestrogen treatment, however.

References

Gilja I, Radej M, Kovačič M, Parazajder J 1984 Conservative treatment of female stress incontinence with imipramine. J Urol 132:909–911

Kaisary A V 1984 Beta adrenoceptor blockade in the treatment of female urinary stress incontinence. J Urol (Paris) 90:351–353

Krier J, Meyer RA, Percy WH 1989 Length–tension relationships of striated muscle of the cat external anal sphincter. Am J Physiol 256:6773–6778

Lose G, Colstrup H, Thind P 1989 Urethral elastance in healthy and stress incontinent women. Proceedings of 19th Annual Meeting of the International Continence Society, Ljubljana. Neurourol Urodyn 8:370–372

Detrusor-external sphincter dyssnergia

Michael B. Chancellor, Steven A. Kaplan and Jerry G. Blaivas

Departments of Urology, College of Physician and Surgeons, Columbia University, 622 West 168th St, New York, NY 10032 and Helen Haynes Hospital, West Haverstraw, New York, NY 10032, USA

Abstract. Detrusor-external sphincter dyssynergia (DESD) is characterized by involuntary contractions of the external urethral sphincter during an involuntary detrusor contraction. It is caused by neurological lesions between the brainstem (pontine micturition centre) and the sacral spinal cord (sacral micturition centre). These include traumatic spinal cord injury, multiple sclerosis, myelodysplasia and other forms of transverse myelitis. There are three main types of DESD. In Type 1 there is a concomitant increase in both detrusor pressure and sphincter EMG activity. At the peak of the detrusor contraction the sphincter suddenly relaxes and unobstructed voiding occurs. Type 2 DESD is characterized by sporadic contractions of the external urethral sphincter throughout the detrusor contraction. In Type 3 DESD there is a crescendo–decrescendo pattern of sphincter contraction which results in urethral obstruction throughout the entire detrusor contraction. In patients with sufficient manual dexterity the most reasonable treatment option is to abolish the involuntary detrusor contractions (to ensure continence) and then to institute intermittent self-catheterization (in order to empty the bladder). The bladder may be paralysed pharmacologically or may be surgically converted to a low pressure urinary reservoir by the technique of augmentation enterocystoplasty. In quadriplegic men, transurethral external sphincterotomy may be performed and the incontinence managed with an external urinary appliance. Without proper treatment over 50% of men with DESD develop serious urological complications within about five years. In women these complications are much less common.

1990 Neurobiology of Incontinence. Wiley, Chichester (Ciba Foundation Symposium 151) p 195–213

Dyssynergia is a condition in which two muscles contract simultaneously and thereby oppose each other's action. When the external urethral sphincter (EUS) contracts during a detrusor contraction, urinary flow is impeded by the resulting increased urethral resistance—hence the term detrusor–external sphincter dyssynergia (DESD).

Since the external urethral sphincter is a striated muscle it is under voluntary control. During normal micturition the EUS is completely relaxed and open. Contraction of the external sphincter during a detrusor contraction occurs only during voluntary attempts to interrupt the urinary stream. This will usually cause the bladder contraction to abate within several seconds. Previous studies have shown that DESD only occurs in patients with neurological lesions of the spinal cord (Blaivas et al 1981a, Blaivas 1982, Siroky & Krane 1982). Unpublished observations from our urodynamic laboratory in over 10 000 patients confirm the fact that DESD is almost never seen in the absence of a spinal cord lesion. The only possible exception to this is Parkinson's disease. We (Berger et al 1987) and others (Pavlakis et al 1983) demonstrated that patients with Parkinson's disease may also have sporadic increases in sphincter EMG activity during micturition. Unlike the situation in DESD, in these patients the increased EMG activity is not accompanied by demonstrable or clinically relevant urethral contractions. Hence, these patients are not clinically obstructed.

The term 'detrusor–external sphincter dyssynergia' has also been applied to a group of non-neurological clinical syndromes characterized by contractions of the EUS during voluntary micturition (Allen 1977, Kaplan et al 1980, Raz & Smith 1976). It is our belief that these conditions, variously termed 'the non-neurogenic neurogenic bladder', and 'external sphincter spasticity', are nothing more than learned behaviours which are either conscious or subconscious attempts to abort micturition. These syndromes are seen most often in children with recurrent urinary tract infections, in women with 'urethral syndrome', and in men with 'prostatitis syndromes'.

Neurophysiology

Anatomy

Although precise anatomical details remain controversial, the external urethral sphincter is thought to be a condensation of slow- and fast-twitch skeletal muscles about the membranous urethra in the male and the middle half of the urethra in females (Woodburn 1968, Gosling & Dixon 1987). Somatic innervation is classically thought to derive from the second to fourth sacral spinal cord segments via the external pudendal nerve (Kuru 1965, Elbadawi 1982). Gosling & Dixon (1987) have observed that slow-twitch muscle fibres are innervated by somatic fibres within the pelvic nerve. The role of the autonomic innervation of the human urethral external sphincter is controversial (Morita et al 1981, Rossier et al 1982).

Coordination of micturition

Previous data from our laboratory (Blaivas et al 1981a, Blaivas 1982) have demonstrated that in humans micturition is normally initiated by relaxation of the external urethral sphincter followed within seconds by a rise in detrusor pressure as the detrusor contraction begins. This sequence of events remains intact in patients with neurological lesions above the level of the pontine mesencephalic micturition centre. However, in patients with suprasacral spinal cord lesions this orderly sequence is usually lost and detrusor–external sphincter dyssynergia ensues (Blaivas et al 1981a, Blaivas 1982, Yalla et al 1977a, McGuire & Brady 1979).

The classic works of Barrington (1915, 1921, 1925, 1928, 1931, 1933, 1941), Bradley & Teague (1968) and de Groat & Ryall (1969) clearly document the fact that the micturition reflex is a spinobulbospinal reflex which is integrated and coordinated in the pontine micturition centre of the brainstem. Descending inhibitory and excitatory influences acting reciprocally balance and coordinate the potentially antagonistic states of the detrusor and sphincter. Negative and positive feedback both exist (Galeano et al 1986, Kuru 1965, Morrison 1987a,b).

In our series of 550 patients who underwent urodynamic studies (Blaivas 1982), 149 patients had detrusor hyperreflexia and 53 of these (36%) had DESD. All the patients with dyssynergia had a well-defined neurological lesion of the spinal cord, whereas none of 249 patients with supraspinal neurological lesions or neurological integrity had dyssynergia. Moreover, in the patients with DESD we never observed a decrease in EMG activity before the onset of the detrusor contraction. Similarly, in a study of over 200 patients with spinal cord injury a pre-voiding decrease in urethral pressure was never seen in patients with DESD (Yalla et al 1977). These data suggest that when the integrity of the pontine mesencephalic micturition pathway is lost the detrusor contraction itself is a stimulus for sphincter contraction. Rudy et al (1988) also observed a direct correlation between detrusor and sphincter contraction in spinal cord injury patients with DESD.

Urethral reflexes

A number of different reflexes involving the striated urethral musculature have been described. In the cat and human there is increased urethral sphincter activity in response to bladder filling (Barrington 1931, 1941, Blaivas et al 1977, Blaivas 1983, Galeano et al 1986, Kuru 1965), to increased abdominal pressure such as in cough, and Credé and Valsalva manoeuvres (Blaivas et al 1977, Blaivas 1983, de Groat & Ryall 1969, Galeano et al 1986, Siroky & Krane 1982), and to urethral distension (Galeano et al 1986, Garry et al 1959; Kuru 1965).

Galeano et al (1986) described the effects of complete C5–C6 transection on vesico-urethral function in a urodynamic study of 46 unanaesthetized spinally transected cats. In the control animals they described five spinal reflexes: (1) vesico-vesical contraction reflex, (2) vesico-urethral relaxation reflex, (3) urethro-vesical contraction reflex, (4) vesico-urethral contraction reflex and (5) a urethro-urethral contraction reflex. The net result of these reflexes is that in the control animals micturition was always accomplished in a synergistic fashion with urethral relaxation preceding or occurring simultaneously with the detrusor contraction. In contrast, all the spinalized cats developed DESD. This was due in great part to the intense exaggeration of the urethro-urethral contraction reflex whereby flow through the urethra caused a reflex increase in urethral pressure and EMG activity. In addition, in the spinalized cats two important brainstem reflexes, the vesico-vesical contraction reflex and the urethro-vesical contraction reflex, were impaired. The net result of this is impairment of detrusor contraction. Galeano et al (1986) also noted that isolated peripheral manipulations of bladder and urethra do not improve micturition because increased detrusor contractions simply cause a reflex increase in the dyssynergia. This is similar to what Yalla et al (1976) showed in humans, namely that the so-called 'voiding manoeuvres', such as Credé, Valsalva, suprapubic tapping and administration of bethanechol, actually impede micturition by exaggerating the degree of DESD.

de Groat (1975) compared the somato-vesical reflexes of chronic spinal cats with those present during postnatal development in kittens. An excitatory spinal reflex can be elicited from the perineal skin of kittens which results in contraction of the bladder and voiding. The reflex is organized in the lumbosacral cord and utilizes a pelvic nerve efferent pathway. The kittens void and defaecate when the mother licks their perineal region. The reflex disappears at the age of 5–7 weeks, and the latency of response more than doubles by the time the response disappears, presumably due to the development of myelinated bulbospinal pathways. This reflex can be elicited in adult cats only after spinal transection, and its absence in normal adults is presumed to be because of inhibitory descending pathways that suppress it.

Jolesz et al (1982) suggested that the physiology of the external urethral sphincter is similar to that of a flexor muscle. Single-shock stimulation of skin nerves in the hindlimb of a spinal cat, which elicited contraction of ipsilateral flexor muscles in that limb, also evoked distinctive reflex discharges in the ipsilateral pudendal nerve. These discharges had the electrophysiological characteristics of 'flexor' reflexes seen in the nerves to flexor muscles. As with flexor reflexes, the external sphincter was suppressed by input that regularly inhibit flexor muscles.

Diagnosis

The diagnosis of DESD requires that detrusor pressure and sphincter electromyography be performed simultaneously. Ideally, intra-abdominal and intravesical pressure should be monitored and detrusor pressure should be displayed by subtracting the former from the latter. Radiographic contrast may be used as the infusant for bladder filling so that the bladder and urethra can be visualized simultaneously (Blaivas 1988). This provides valuable information on the anatomy of DESD. Sphincter electromyography is most accurately performed with needle electrodes and oscilloscopic and audiographic monitoring.

It is essential to observe the sphincter electromyogram (EMG) pattern on an oscilloscope screen. The EMG display at a speed of 10 ms/cm allows for a detailed evaluation of individual motor units. Conventional paper speeds of 0.5 to 1 mm/s are too insensitive for proper electromyographic evaluation. The slightest increase in electrical activity is grossly exaggerated and may simulate a complete interference pattern. Moreover, distant muscle activity cannot be distinguished from the true external sphincter.

Detrusor–external sphincter dyssynergia is defined as an involuntary detrusor contraction (Blaivas et al 1981a). Since DESD is an involuntary condition, it is impossible to arrive at this diagnosis by examining a paper tracing after the urodynamic evaluation has been completed. The judgement must be made at the time of the study by noting whether the observed bladder and sphincter contractions were voluntary.

DESD must be differentiated from other conditions in which there is increased EMG activity during detrusor contractions. In some instances patients may voluntarily contract the sphincter during involuntary detrusor contractions in an attempt to prevent incontinence. Others may exhibit a 'learned behaviour' of starting and stopping during voiding. Both these conditions can be distinguished from DESD because the sphincter EMG becomes completely silent just before or coincident with the onset of the detrusor contraction. It is only after the detrusor contraction commences that the sphincter contractions occur.

Berger et al (1987) and Pavlakis et al (1983) found that there were often sphincter contractions during involuntary detrusor contractions in patients with Parkinson's disease. According to Pavlakis and coworkers, 7% had pseudo-dyssynergia, which they defined as a voluntary contraction of the pelvic floor in attempts to prevent incontinence. Eleven per cent had sphincter bradykinesia—a failure of the pelvic floor to relax during the detrusor contraction. We have also seen a picture similar to Type 2 DESD (see below) in some patients with Shy–Drager syndrome (Salinas et al 1986).

Classification

On the basis of the temporal relationship between electromyographic activity and detrusor contraction, three types of dyssynergia were described (Blaivas

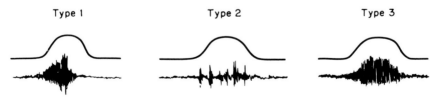

FIG. 1.   Classification of detrusor–external sphincter dyssynergia. (Reproduced with permission from Blaivas et al 1981b.)

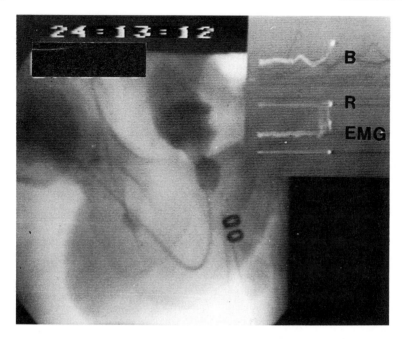

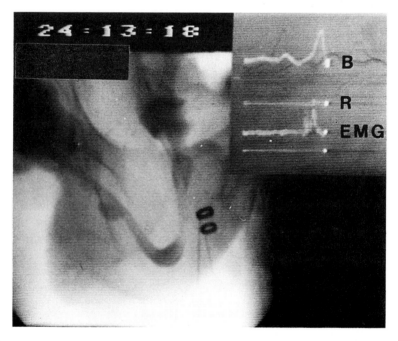

FIG. 2 (*caption opposite*)

et al 1981b) (Fig. 1). In Type 1 dyssynergia there is a simultaneous increase in both detrusor pressure and EMG activity (Fig. 2, upper). At the peak of the detrusor contraction there is sudden and complete relaxation of the external sphincter (Fig. 2, lower). Voiding occurs only during the down-slope of the detrusor pressure curve, during sphincter relaxation. Thirty per cent of our series of 54 patients with DESD had Type 1 dyssynergia (Blaivas et al 1981b).

Type 2 dyssynergia is characterized by clonic contractions of the external urethral sphincter interspersed throughout the detrusor contraction (Fig. 3). These patients usually void with an interrupted spurting stream. Only 15% of our patients had Type 2 dyssynergia.

In Type 3 dyssynergia there is a crescendo–decrescendo increase in both EMG activity and detrusor pressure which persists throughout the detrusor contraction (Fig. 4). These patients are obstructed throughout the entire detrusor contraction. Fifty-five per cent of the patients in our series had Type 3 dyssynergia.

Rudy et al (1988) did serial urodynamic investigations on 14 patients with acute spinal cord injury, at intervals of 2–4 weeks. During the evolution of neurological recovery, Rudy and coworkers observed only one pattern of dyssynergia. They found that 'increased electromyographic activity and resting external urethral sphincter pressure correlated closely with a positive slope of the intravesical pressure trace. With a slope of less than zero the electromyographic activity and resting urethral sphincter pressure always decreased'. They further observed that voiding occurred only during negative slopes—that is, when detrusor pressure was falling. From these results they concluded that the previously described patterns of dyssynergia are variations, largely owing to the techniques used, of the single pattern that they observed. This pattern is the waxing and waning of the elevated intravesical pressure and associated external sphincter activity seen with reflex bladder activity. Furthermore, synergia-like urethral responses were observed in some patients during the negative slope of the intravesical pressure, suggesting the existence of a pathway for synergia-like voiding in the spinal cord.

Although we agree with Rudy's findings, we disagree with the conclusions. We believe that Type 1 and Type 3 DESD are distinct patterns whose audiographic findings are unmistakable. In Type 1 DESD the sphincter relaxation which occurs at the peak of the detrusor contraction is manifest as a sudden and complete silence, whereas in Type 3 there is simply a diminution of the EMG activity at the peak of the detrusor contraction. Moreover, there is often a prodromal increase in EMG activity which precedes the rise in detrusor

FIG. 2.   Type 1 detrusor–external sphincter dyssynergia. There is an increase in EMG activity coincident with the onset of the involuntary detrusor contraction (*upper*). At the peak of the contraction there is sudden and complete electrical silence as voiding occurs (*lower*). B, intravesical pressure; R, abdominal pressure. Each large division on the vertical scale represents 15 cmH$_2$O. (Reproduced with permission from Blaivas et al 1981b.)

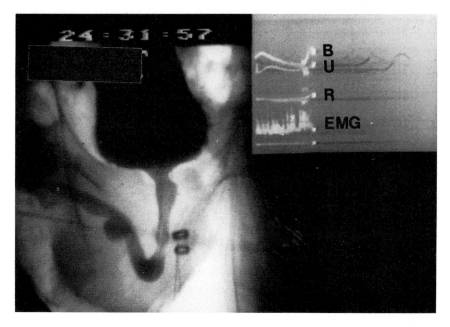

FIG. 3.   Type 2 detrusor–external sphincter dyssynergia. During the involuntary detrusor contraction there are sporadic contractions of the external urethral sphincter. Note the rise in detrusor pressure which occurs each time the external sphincter contracts and the fall in pressure as it relaxes. B, intravesical pressure; U, urethral pressure; R, abdominal pressure. Each large division on the vertical scale represents 15 cmH₂O. (Reproduced with permission from Blaivas et al 1981b.)

pressure, which is also unmistakable to the experienced electromyographer. This distinction is often not apparent on a strip-chart recording of EMG activity and might account for the differences between our data and those of Rudy.

Teleologically, it would appear that patients with Type 3 dyssynergia are at the greatest risk of developing urological complications because they are obstructed throughout the entire course of the detrusor contraction. However, to our knowledge, this hypothesis has not yet been tested in a clinical setting.

Treatment

In patients with sufficient manual dexterity we believe that the most reasonable treatment option for DESD is to abolish the involuntary detrusor contractions (to ensure continence) and then to institute intermittent self-catheterization (in order to empty the bladder) (Diokno 1988). Involuntary detrusor contractions can be abolished pharmacologically with anticholinergic agents such as

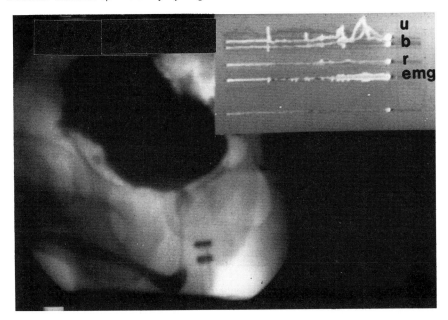

FIG. 4.   Type 3 detrusor–external sphincter dyssynergia. There is a marked increase in EMG activity which persists throughout the detrusor contraction which parallels the rise and fall in detrusor pressure. u, urethral pressure; b, intravesical pressure; r, abdominal pressure. Each large division on the vertical scale represents 15 cmH$_2$O. (Reproduced with permission from Blaivas et al 1981b.)

oxybutinin or by tricyclic antidepressants such as imipramine (Wein 1988). In our experience these medications are effective in about 50% of patients. If they prove ineffective, or the patient is unable to tolerate the side-effects, augmentation enterocystoplasty may be considered. The aim of this procedure is to create a large capacity, low pressure reservoir which can be emptied by intermittent catheterization. A segment of intestine is isolated on its mesentery and incised along its entire antimesenteric border. The detubularized segment is then refashioned into the shape of one half of a sphere. The bladder is also incised in such a way that it is formed into the other half of the sphere and the two structures are sewn together, to form a large spherical augmented bladder.

A number of techniques have been advocated for increasing intravesical pressure to achieve bladder emptying, such as suprapubic percussion, the Credé manoeuvre, and the use of bethanechol chloride, but it has been clearly demonstrated that, at least from a physiological standpoint, these manoeuvres are not merely ineffective, but potentially harmful (Barbalias et al 1983, Yalla et al 1976).

Therapeutic destruction of the external urethral sphincter (external sphincterotomy) is intended to relieve the obstruction caused by the contracting sphincter (Madersbacher & Scott 1975, Whitmore et al 1978, Yalla et al 1977). However, we believe that it should be reserved for quadriplegic patients who have no prospect of recovering function and who are unable to perform intermittent catheterization. It is important to recognize and treat concomitant prostatic or vesical neck obstruction. If prostatic or vesical neck surgery is necessary it can be accomplished at the same time as the sphincterotomy. An external condom catheter is generally necessary after an external sphincterotomy, but total dribbling incontinence is unusual unless the bladder neck and prostatic urethra have also been removed. Failure of sphincterotomy is often due to impaired detrusor contractility, but may also be caused by inadequate incision or unsuspected obstruction at the bladder neck.

Functional electrical stimulation is an exciting new modality in urology for the treatment of neurogenic bladder dysfunction. Simultaneous activation of the external urethral sphincter with the detrusor has been the major difficulty in obtaining synchronized voiding. However, when neural stimulation is combined with peripheral selective neurotomy or neural blockade, satisfactory coordinated voiding can be achieved (Brindley et al 1986, Tanagho et al 1989).

Recently, several avenues of promising research in the treatment of detrusor-sphincter dyssynergia have opened up. Shah et al (1989) have obtained encouraging preliminary results using permanent urethral stents made of metal mesh to keep the membranous urethra open in patients with detrusor–sphincter dyssynergia. This is essentially a non-destructive substitution for external sphincterotomy. Sugaya et al (1988) reported improvement of detrusor–sphincter dyssynergia after transplanting the adrenal medulla to the sacral spinal cord in spinally transected cats.

When all else fails, in-dwelling urethral catheters may be used for short-term bladder management without serious drawback, and occasionally an in-dwelling catheter is the last resort for long-term bladder drainage.

Complications

Without proper treatment, over 50% of men with DESD develop serious urological complications within about five years. The complications include vesico-ureteral reflux, uretero-vesical obstruction, urolithiasis and urosepsis (Blaivas 1982). The primary risk factor is high intravesical pressure (McGuire et al 1981). It is essential to know what the bladder pressures are during filling and during leakage. To avoid damage to the upper urinary tract, the pressure at which bladder emptying occurs should be kept to less than $30\,\text{cmH}_2\text{O}$. Urological complications other than urinary tract infections are less common in women because of lower outlet resistance.

References

Allen TA 1977 The non-neurogenic neurogenic bladder. J Urol 117:232

Barbalias GA, Klauber GT, Blaivas JG 1983 Critical evaluation of the crede maneuver: urodynamic study of 207 patients. J Urol 130:720

Barrington FJF 1915 The nervous control of micturition. Q J Exp Physiol 8:33

Barrington FJF 1921 Relation of hind brain to micturition. Brain 44:23

Barrington FJF 1925 The effect of lesions of the hind- and midbrain on micturition in the cat. J Exp Physiol 15:181

Barrington FJF 1928 The central nervous control of micturition. Brain 51:209

Barrington FJF 1931 The component reflexes of micturition in the cat. Parts I & II. Brain 54:239

Barrington FJF 1933 The localisation of the paths subserving micturition in the spinal cord of the cat. Brain 56:126

Barrington FJF 1941 The component reflexes of micturition in the cat. Part III. Brain 64:239–243

Berger Y, De la Rocha RE, Salinas JM, Blaivas JG 1987 Urodynamic findings in Parkinson's disease. J Urol 138:836–838

Blaivas JG 1982 The neurophysiology of micturition: a clinical study of 550 patients. J Urol 127:958–963

Blaivas JG 1983 Sphincter electromyography. Neurourol Urodyn 2:269–288

Blaivas JG 1988 Techniques of evaluation. In: Yalla S et al (eds) Neurourology and urodynamics: principles and practice. Macmillan, New York, p 155–198

Blaivas JG, Labib KB, Bauer SB, Retik AB 1977 A new approach to electromyography of the external urethral sphincter. J Urol 117:773–777

Blaivas JG, Sinha HP, Zayed AAH, Labib KB 1981a Detrusor–external sphincter dyssynergia. J Urol 125:542–544

Blaivas JG, Sinha HP, Zayed AAH, Labib KB 1981b Detrusor external sphincter dyssynergia: a detailed electromyographic study. J Urol 125:545–548

Bradley WE, Teague CT 1968 Spinal organization of micturition reflex afferents. Exp Neurol 22:504–516

Brindley GS, Polkey CE, Rushton DN, Cardozo L 1986 Sacral anterior root stimulators for bladder control in paraplegia: the first 50 cases. J Neurol Neurosurg Psychiatry 49:1104–1114

de Groat WC 1975 Nervous control of the urinary bladder of the cat. Brain Res 87:201

de Groat WC, Ryall RW 1969 Reflexes to the sacral parasympathetic neurones concerned with micturition in the cat. J Physiol (Lond) 200:87–108

Diokno AC 1988 Clean intermittent self-catheterization. In: Yalla S et al (eds) Neurourology and urodynamics: principles and practice. Macmillan, New York, p 410–416

Elbadawi A 1982 Neuromorphologic basis of vesicourethral function. 1. Histochemistry, ultrastructure, and function of intrinsic nerves of the bladder and urethra. Neurourol Urodyn 1:3

Galeano C, Jubelin B, Germain L, Guenette L 1986 Micturitional reflex in chronic spinalized cats: the underactive detrusor and detrusor–sphincter dyssynergia. Neurourol Urodyn 5:45–63

Garry RC, Roberts TDM, Todd JI 1959 Reflexes involving the external urethral sphincter of the cat. J Physiol (Lond) 149:653

Gosling JA, Dixon JS 1987 Structure and innervation in the human. In: Torrens M, Morrison JFB (eds) The physiology of the lower urinary tract. Springer-Verlag, London, p 1–22

Jolesz FA, Xu CT, Ruenzel PW, Henneman E 1982 Flexor reflex control of the external sphincter of the urethra in paraplegia. Science (Wash DC) 216:1243–1245

Kaplan WE, Firlit CF, Schoenberg HW 1980 Female urethral syndrome. External sphincter splasm as etiology. J Urol 124:48

Kuru M 1965 Nervous control of micturition. Physiol Rev 45:425

Madersbacher H, Scott FB 1975 Twelve o'clock sphincterotomy: technique, indications, results. Urol Int 30:75

McGuire EM, Brady S 1979 Detrusor–sphincter dyssnergia. J Urol 121:774

McGuire EJ, Woodside JR, Borden TA et al 1981 The prognostic value of urodynamic testing in myelodysplastic patients. J Urol 126:205–209

Morrison JFB 1987a Reflex control of the lower urinary tract. In: Torrens M, Morrison JFB (eds) The physiology of the lower urinary tract. Springer-Verlag, London, p 193–236

Morrison JFB 1987b Bladder control: role of higher levels of the central nervous system. In: Torrens M, Morrison JFB (eds) The physiology of the lower urinary tract. Springer-Verlag, London, p 237–274

Morita T, Saeki H, Wada I 1981 Pharmacologic study of the external urethral sphincter throughout recordings of the electromyogram. Jap J Urol 72:559

Pavlakis AJ, Siroky MB, Goldstein I, Krane RJ 1983 Neurourologic findings in Parkinson's disease. J Urol 129:80–83

Raz S, Smith RB 1976 External sphincter spasticity syndrome in female patients. J Urol 115:443

Rossier AB, Fam BA, Lee IY et al 1982 Role of striated and smooth muscle components in the urethral pressure profile in traumatic neurogenic bladders: a neuropharmacological and urodynamic study. Preliminary report. J Urol 128:529–535

Rudy DC, Awad SA, Downie JW 1988 External sphincter dyssynergia: an abnormal continence reflex. J Urol 140:105–110

Salinas JM, Berger Y, De la Rocha RE, Blaivas JG 1986 Urological evaluation in the Shy-Drager syndrome. J Urol 135:741–743

Shah PJR, Milroy EJ, Timoney AG, Eldin A 1989 Permanent external striated sphincter stents in spinal injured patients. Neurourol Urodyn 8:311

Siroky MB, Krane RJ 1982 Neurological aspects of detrusor–sphincter dyssynergia, with reference to the guarding reflex. J Urol 127:953–957

Sugaya K, Nishizawa O, Kohama T, Shimoda N, Tsuchida S 1988 The effect of transplantation of adrenal gland to the sacral spinal cord on the bladder and urethral function in the spinal cat. Neurourol Urodyn 7:254

Tanagho EA, Schmidt RA, Orvis BR 1989 Neural stimulation for control of voiding dysfunction: a preliminary report in 22 patients with serious neuropathic voiding disorders. J Urol 142:340

Torrens MJ 1978 Urethral sphincteric responses to stimulation of the sacral nerves in the human female. Urol Int 33:22–26

Yalla SV, Rossier AB, Fam B 1976 Dyssynergic vesicourethral responses during bladder rehabilitation in spinal cord injury patients: effects of suprapubic percussion, Crede method and bethanechol chloride. J Urol 115:575

Yalla SV, Blunt KJ, Fam BA, Constantinople NL, Gittes RF 1977 Detrusor–urethral sphincter dyssynergia. J Urol 118:1026

Wein AJ 1988 Clinical neuropharmacology of the lower urinary tract. In: Yalla S et al (eds) Neurourology and urodynamics: principles and practice. Macmillan, New York, p 155–198

Whitmore WF, Yalla WV, Fam BA, Gittes RF 1978 Experience with anteromedian (12 o'clock) external sphincterotomy in 100 male subjects with neuropathic bladder. Br J Urol 50:49

Woodburn RT 1968 Anatomy of the bladder and bladder outlet. J Urol 100:474

DISCUSSION

Fowler: Are patients with multiple sclerosis less likely to develop urological complications than patients with spinal cord trauma? I ask this because your work has generated concern as to the precautions we should be taking to look at the upper urinary tract in multiple sclerosis patients. Professor Ian Macdonald, who has seen at least 200 patients a year with multiple sclerosis each year over the course of 15 years, could not recall a patient with multiple sclerosis who had advanced renal failure. It is possible that when such patients become severely ill they go to hospitals for the incurable, and so would not have been seen by him, but it does suggest that severe dyssynergia and spasticity in multiple sclerosis are not always associated with the renal complications that spinal trauma patients have.

Blaivas: The urological complications mainly occur in men, because women wet themselves before the pressure gets too high in the bladder. It is clear that the high pressure generated by the bladder causes the problem, and women become incontinent before that happens. In our studies, approximately 50% of men with multiple sclerosis and persistent bladder symptoms have DESD. But in a population of 200 patients a year, the chances are that 150 or more are women. Of the 50 men, at least half do not have persistent bladder problems; of the remaining 25, half again are likely to have dyssynergia. So out of 200 MS patients that you are looking at, perhaps 12 are really at risk of developing serious bladder or kidney problems. And, of course, renal failure usually develops over many years, rather than suddenly. You may not pick it up until a urinary tract infection or stone develops. So I am not surprised that it is not clinically evident.

Also, I think that a certain amount of the problem is iatrogenic. If a person has detrusor–sphincter dyssynergia but doesn't report it, so no one ever puts in a catheter to make a diagnosis, the chances of developing an infection, or complications, are much less. Once they get into the medical arena of diagnosis, their risk goes up!

Kirby: Coming back to the point about the difference between the neurological reflexes in coughing, as opposed to those involved in the Valsalva manoeuvre, it was our impression from needle electromyography that there might be a difference in the sphincter in the type of muscle activity seen on the EMG during tonic closure of the sphincter compared with that seen when the patient is asked to cough or strain. We thought that this might reflect the type of muscle fibre rather than the neural input, or maybe both. Perhaps the small striated muscle fibres maintaining tonic contraction of the urethra, which increased during bladder filling, were dedicated to maintaining consistent tone over the whole period of the day, while the bigger fast-twitch muscle fibres might be coming in only when the patient coughed. Could the same be true of the anal sphincter?

Blaivas: I think it's entirely likely, and should be easily studied by electromyography. What is really needed, to sort these things out, is for an experienced neurologist, electromyographer, or neurophysiologist to work with a urologist who is interested in the same kind of problem. Then you could do good studies. Meetings like this one are so important because we can exchange new ideas and also generate ideas that can be tested on the same kinds of patients in our different laboratories.

Bartolo: It was fascinating to see your traces in the bladder, because we see a similar phenomenon in the anorectum, which Michael Swash has termed 'anismus'. When we ask patients to defaecate, instead of relaxing their external anal sphincters they contract them. It has been suggested that we are seeing a postural reflex. In your dyssynergic patients, could the effects be related in any way to lack of bladder awareness? We have studied a group of patients with constipation who also have anismus. We try to get them to defaecate, using proctography with simultaneous EMG and manometry. We find a rise in rectal pressure, but instead of relaxing they contract their external anal sphincters. They also have a much higher volume of first rectal sensation than do normal subjects, and a higher threshold of anal sensation. So perhaps they are not relaxing because they lack rectal awareness, so that instead of relaxing they are carrying out a Valsalva manoeuvre.

Blaivas: I would say that rather than a lack of awareness it may be a lack of knowing how to defaecate or urinate properly, and not knowing how to relax, and those things to a large extent can be taught. For example, the vaginal cones mentioned by Dr Swash really do what they are supposed to do; they teach a woman how to contract her vaginal muscles. It would seem to me that you could do the same with your patients, namely to put a cone-like object in the rectum and say to the patient that this is what it is like to contract the anal sphincter muscles; when you let it go and allow it to fall out, that's how you relax the muscle. These things can be taught.

Bartolo: We find with our constipated patients that if we put a different solution into the rectum, for example a very dilute solution of bile acids, rather than saline or barium sulphate, they can relax. And if we do a colectomy on these patients but do nothing to their pelvic floor musculature, they can relax and evacuate stools. So something changes, and we are not retraining them, although Dr Kuijpers can teach them without surgery.

Blaivas: There is no way of knowing which came first. My bias has always been that some of these voiding dysfunctions are learned behaviours and that because of some unpleasant event in the past, patients have lost the ability to relax. I think of the urethral sphincter, and the anal sphincter, as being like a flexor muscle, and when it's trying to avoid pain, it flexes, or contracts. For example, in a urinary tract infection, the subject starts to urinate and as soon as the urine starts to come out it burns, and they stop urinating. That pattern of stopping and starting is exactly what we see in the so-called 'non-neurogenic

neurogenic' bladder, and is probably a subconscious learned behaviour which one hopes can be unlearned. But maybe it is different for the bowel, and not learned there; I don't know.

Swash: I am intrigued by the neurophysiology that must underlie the paradoxical contraction of the external anal sphincter muscle, as if this somatic efferent innervated striated muscle is co-contracting with the visceral efferent innervated smooth detrusor muscle. Is there some failure of inhibition of the switch that Dr de Groat was discussing?

Blaivas: In patients with suprasacral spinal lesions the answer is clearly yes. But I don't know the details of micturition in the reflex described in kittens and in spinally transected adult cats. Do you know, Dr de Groat, if that is a synergistic or dyssynergic kind of micturition?

de Groat: Our view (see Fig. 3 on p 32) is that there is a basic reflex from bladder afferents to the sphincter motor neurons which is excitatory. That reflex is involved in the storage of urine and is called the guarding reflex. This reflex pathway is turned off by the brain during micturition. When the brain has been removed from the circuitry, as in the spinal cord-injured patient, that basic guarding reflex continues to function, even though there is an attempt at a micturition response. So the bladder reflex pathways recover in the spinal animal and trigger a bladder contraction, but the excitatory pathway from the bladder to the sphincter maintains a sphincter contraction, so that urine doesn't flow properly. Therefore lack of inhibition contributes to bladder–sphincter dyssynergia.

The same happens, at least in cats, to the sympathetic pathway; during bladder filling, afferents in the bladder turn on the sympathetic pathway in the hypogastric nerve, and that pathway is active until micturition starts, and is then also normally turned off by the brain. When the spinal cord is cut the brain no longer can turn off the sympathetic pathway, so it remains active during attempts at micturition.

Marsden: Looking at this from the viewpoint of the pontine micturition centre, what instruction does this centre send, in a voluntary micturition?

de Groat: The pontine centre turns off two spinal 'storage' reflexes, namely a bladder-to-sphincter excitatory pathway and a bladder-to-sympathetic inhibitory pathway. The sympathetic reflex causes the urethra and bladder neck to contract; the other reflex causes the external urethral sphincter to contract. Those two pathways are inhibited by the brain during micturition.

Marsden: Is it the same pathway from the brain to both spinal reflexes?

de Groat: We don't know that.

Marsden: You must have separate pathways, surely, to get bladder–sphincter dyssynergia.

Staskin: We find that paraplegic subjects with lesions below the sympathetic outflow do not demonstrate bladder neck dyskinesia, only if the sympathetic outflow is connected to the lower cord; so we do not see this sympathetic problem unless the lesion is above the sympathetic outflow.

de Groat: That is not in disagreement with what I am saying. The sacral afferents from the bladder which excite sphincter motor neurons also project in the cord to the lumbar sympathetic outflow. Bladder distension activates the sympathetic pathways which then initiate contractions of the bladder neck and the proximal urethra, and also inhibition in parasympathetic ganglia.

When this sacral afferent activity increases as the bladder fills further, this information is carried up the cord to the brain. Descending pathways from the brain excite the parasympathetic pathway to the detrusor, causing it to contract, and inhibit the sympathetic and sphincter pathways. What Jerry Blaivas has described in humans is consistent with what we see in the cat. When the brain is disconnected from the spinal cord, he finds that the basic detrusor–sphincter excitatory pathway cannot be inhibited.

Swash: He also finds failure of the detrusor system in some patients, particularly in Parkinson's disease, but also, occasionally, as an isolated problem in patients presenting with retention of urine and inability to micturate. What makes the detrusor system continue to contract, to sustain micturition, in normal individuals?

de Groat: According to our concept there is continued firing of the excitatory pathway from the detrusor to the spinal cord, up to the brain, and back to the detrusor. This is like a switch, and once turned on it stays turned on for a number of seconds.

Blaivas: I am not sure about that. What is incredible is that without any change in sphincter activity you can see fluctuations in detrusor pressure, yet the only way detrusor pressure can change is if the urethra becomes narrower or wider, or for the bladder to contract less or more forcefully. We have documented many patients where detrusor pressure waxes and wanes without any apparent change in urethral resistance. This means that in an abnormal state, there are things that make the same bladders contract better or worse. We don't know what they are, but they clearly exist.

The problem may be myogenic; we don't know that it is neurogenic. But in both neurologically normal and abnormal people we see fluctuations in detrusor pressure that we can only attribute to changes in the contractile force of the bladder, and not to the urethra.

Staskin: We do not see bladder neck closure dyskinesia unless the lesion is above the thoracic outflow. With a C7 lesion, the bladder neck contracts, whereas with a T10 lesion the bladder neck will open.

de Groat: This could be explained by the lesion at T10 interfering with the sympathetic reflex pathway. If the sympathetic pathway is damaged, then it can't close the bladder neck. This is therefore consistent with what we see in the cat.

Staskin: We have actually put catheters into patients and let them void with varying urethral resistance. We have done this in patients with spinal cord injury and in normal subjects. Voiding depends on two different things—facilitation, from a higher centre, most likely, and also some sensory input that tells you, in some way that might become fatigued, whether your bladder is truly empty. In other words, if you void half way and stop, you have a sensation that it is not empty, even after the bladder contraction has finished, whereas if the bladder is being filled to the same volume, you don't feel that urgent sensation. If we put in a catheter and watch a quadriplegic patient void, so that, regardless of what happens to the external sphincter, we are controlling the outlet resistance, the bladder doesn't empty. In normal subjects, with a catheter inserted, we filled them to 300 ml; at the beginning of a bladder contraction we opened the catheter and allowed them to void through a controlled resistance, so that the sphincter muscle would not interrupt flow and only the detrusor muscle determined emptying. At low resistances they could void until emptying, but at higher resistances they thought the bladder was empty although 150–200 ml remained. It might have been sensory fatigue, but there is probably facilitation, and some sensory feedback.

Blaivas: During voiding, I imagine you continue to record afferent discharges from the bladder in the cat, Dr de Groat? So the implication would be that that afferent information is in some way telling the bladder to continue to contract.

de Groat: The afferents from the bladder respond to distension, or to contraction, so they continue to fire during micturition.

Kirby: We all know that to stop voiding midway is a painful experience. During urodynamic studies of patients we ask them to do this. They close the sphincter very tightly, the bladder neck opens up, and the intravesical pressure rises quite steeply and then falls, so presumably the detrusor is being switched off. I have often wondered what is switching the detrusor off in mid-void. The detrusor is programmed to void to completion, to empty the bladder, but obviously it doesn't if you ask people to stop. Is a pontine mechanism turning off the micturition reflex, or is it the fact that the subject is closing the sphincter and this is causing a local inhibition of the detrusor?

de Groat: Ed McGuire and others have shown that afferents from the sphincter muscle, in the pudendal nerve, can inhibit the micturition reflex. So a voluntary contraction of the sphincter muscle will lead to a central inhibition of the reflex pathway to the bladder.

Blaivas: That is the principle underlying electrical stimulation of pudendal afferents to treat detrusor instability.

de Groat: That's right. If you voluntarily contract the sphincter, after a few seconds that leads to an inhibition of the parasympathetic outflow to the bladder. We have done studies (unpublished) similar to those of McGuire, in which we electrically stimulated the nerves to the sphincter muscle to produce a contraction. This inhibited bladder activity. We then administered a neuromuscular blocking agent to the cat. This blocked the contraction of the striated sphincter muscle and eliminated the inhibition of bladder activity.

So these systems are talking to one another: the bladder afferents talk to sphincter motor neurons; sphincter afferents talk to bladder preganglionic neurons. The sphincter-to-bladder pathway is organized in the spinal cord. It's evidently an inhibition of the preganglionic cells.

Blaivas: It is important to emphasize that this reflex does not operate in 50% of the patients that we have studied, and even more of Dr Nordling's. In more than half of our patients, when they have contracted the sphincter and interrupted the stream, it still did not cause the detrusor contractions to abate.

de Groat: Are they normal patients?

Blaivas: Some are neurologically normal; some are not.

Swash: There's a further point about Parkinson's disease. The condition called 'anismus', with so-called paradoxical contraction of the external anal sphincter muscle, occurs in Parkinson's disease and in patients with an idiopathic disorder of defaecation. In some of these patients the abnormality can be switched off by appropriate treatment with L-dopa. When the drug is not given, then they cannot defaecate. Have you any evidence in your studies that the disturbed micturition pattern that you have seen in Parkinsonian patients can be alleviated by dopaminergic medication?

Blaivas: The evidence comes from the Middlesex Hospital near here, in fact! Timothy Christmas used apomorphine to treat the abnormal skeletal muscle activity (Christmas et al 1988). When the patients were on the drug, they voided with much less urethral resistance. Our own data do not really support that, but this was a very nice consistent study. In our study the increased EMG activity seen during voiding did not seem to cause urethral obstruction (Berger et al 1987).

Swash: It is important because it may tell us about the synaptology of the central pathway, presumably at brainstem level.

Marsden: There are two candidates for this effect of dopamine or apomorphine in Parkinson's disease, switching off anismus and also detrusor–sphincter dyssynergia. One is an input onto the pontine micturition centre from the basal ganglia, and the other is the spinal descending dopaminergic pathway. Have you any idea, Dr de Groat, which of those two might be involved?

de Groat: It is paradoxical that dopamine, applied in the pontine micturition centre, facilitates micturition and enhances the reflex pathways to the bladder. One would expect, from the bladder hyperreflexia seen in Parkinson's disease, that dopamine would have the opposite effect. Do Tony Yaksh and Paul Tiseo have data on the effects of dopamine in the spinally transected rat, or effects on the spinal cord in the intact rat?

Tiseo: The only finding, so far as apomorphine is concerned, is that in an intact rat with a morphine blockade of the micturition reflex, when we inject apomorphine both intraperitoneally and intrathecally, the sphincter opens and micturition occurs.

Brindley: As these were intact animals, could an intrathecally administered drug have got up to the pontine micturition centre?

Tiseo: The time course of the effect was against that, because micturition occurs immediately, so I would conclude that the apomorphine did not migrate.

Kirby: Lewin & Porter (1965), in the cat, stimulated the basal ganglia and inhibited the micturition reflex. Conversely, on destruction of the globus pallidum of the basal ganglia they found that the micturition reflex was facilitated (smaller bladder capacities before micturition occurred). That is the opposite of what would be expected from the effect of dopamine on the pontine centre. How do you explain that?

de Groat: We cannot explain it. Their data are consistent with the clinical observation that in Parkinson's disease there is hyperactivity of the bladder. The major question is whether the effect of exogenous dopamine mimics anything that happens under physiological conditions. We have administered haloperidol, a dopamine antagonist, and have not seen any change in the micturition reflex pathway, which implies that under the conditions of our animal model (the decerebrate cat), the dopamine system is not tonically controlling the micturition reflex. So all we have is pharmacological evidence for dopamine receptors in the pontine micturition centre; haloperidol can block the receptors; and activation of those receptors leads to facilitation of the micturition reflex. We do not know whether these observations are physiologically relevant.

Marsden: What is the level of decerebration?

de Groat: At supracollicular level.

Marsden: So it has knocked out your primary basal ganglia system.

de Groat: Exactly. It may require an intact animal to demonstrate these dopaminergic controls.

Marsden: There are no dopaminergic outputs from the basal ganglia, but there are other dopaminergic circuits in the brainstem. The major output of the basal ganglia is GABAergic.

de Groat: Yes. The dopamine neurons within the brainstem project to areas of the mesencephalon, and some of those areas then project back into the pontine micturition centre, and that may be disrupted by decerebration.

References

Berger Y, De la Rocha RE, Salinas JM, Blaivas JG 1987 Urodynamic findings in Parkinson's disease. J Urol 138:836–838

Christmas TJ, Chapple CR, Kempster PA et al 1988 Subcutaneous apomorphine, a potential treatment for voiding dysfunction in Parkinson's disease. Neurourol Urodyn 7:194

Lewin RJ, Porter RW 1965 Inhibition of spontaneous bladder activity by stimulation of the globus pallidus. Neurology 15:1049–1052

General discussion III

Stress urinary incontinence: mechanisms and problems

Burnstock: On an earlier point, I know that clinicians are often imaginative in their use of language, but the 'non-neurogenic neurogenic bladder' was mentioned. What is that?

Blaivas: It is a syndrome described by Terry Allen and Frank Hinman (see Allen 1977). The term describes children whose bladders looked as if they were neurogenic. The syndrome was characterized by infrequent voiding, urinary incontinence, urinary tract infections, and hydronephrosis—all the conditions you see in the neurogenic bladder—yet no neurological lesion is ever detected. These patients were mostly children and were treated successfully with behavioural techniques and hypnosis. I think it is like the patient who starts to urinate, then stops and starts, many times in a single voiding event; some of them present with urinary retention. I think it's a learned behaviour.

Kuijpers: Does incontinence occur spontaneously in animals?

Blaivas: Urinary incontinence occurs in dogs.

Christensen: How can you know that the dog *wants* to resist urination?

Blaivas: Some dogs, trained to be continent until they go outside the house, become incontinent when they get older.

Brading: Our mini-pigs, when they want to urinate, do various behavioural things; they stand up and stretch their back legs. Some of our pigs with unstable bladders occasionally leak urine during unstable contractions without these behavioural changes. We can't say they are incontinent, because we can't ask them, but we assume that this is equivalent to human incontinence.

Blaivas: I see two different points of view about the aetiology of stress incontinence. There is the concept of the paravaginal defect, which is simply a tearing away of the musculo-fascial layers; and the concept of weakness, stretching and denervation of the pelvic floor. Pathophysiologically, they are almost mutually exclusive theories. You would expect that if the nerve became damaged, it would weaken the muscle, and the pelvic floor would sag in the middle—the cystourethrocele. This would be different from when the the fascia becomes detached on the side walls of the pelvis and simply falls because it is no longer held up. How can we investigate this further to see which of the two conditions exist, or whether there are combinations?

Stanton: I suspect there is a combination. I can't visualize the bladder neck slipping at one point. My general feeling is that the whole bladder neck falls down.

Blaivas: There is a difference between falling down because the lateral attachments are detached, as the paravaginal defect hypothesis suggests, and falling because the pelvic floor is weakened and gets stretched. In the former instance, the endopelvic fascia is still strong, but no longer attached.

Swash: One question that should be asked is why stress incontinence sometimes occurs during pregnancy, before delivery. What is the mechanism there? This must be germane to this argument.

Blaivas: Many women have a degree of stress incontinence anyway, that is only apparent during testing or when their bladders are very full. People tend to associate a symptom with some event, and if a person has slight urinary incontinence all the time and they begin to notice it more in the third trimester of pregnancy, it is not necessarily cause and effect. We talked earlier about the possibility of looking at the tension–length relationship of the endopelvic fascia. Has anyone actually done that?

DeLancey: Not that I know, although the techniques for measurement are available. One would like to ask the woman to strain with a certain force and see how much descent occurs for that amount of straining. You wouldn't be able to tell whether the subject was contracting the levator muscles or not, but at least you would have an idea of how much mobility you were getting for the strain.

There are profound changes in the pelvic connective tissue at the end of pregnancy. You can feel with your finger the pubic symphysis move on itself because of a softening of the symphysial ligaments, and that may be one part of the connective tissue change in pregnancy. Also, around the 36th or 37th week, the fetal head descends into the pelvis, which moves the bladder up and makes it an abdominal organ. This dramatically changes the spatial relationships at the end of pregnancy and may be one reason for the incontinence, irrespective of the delivery. So it is difficult to say that even though delivery hasn't occurred, the incontinence is not related to the process of pregnancy. This is hard to sort out because so many changes are going on.

On the question of whether the muscle or the nerve is damaged at birth, there are indirect observations, in that we know that without altering the nerve supply to the urethra we can make women continent after urethral suspension simply by changing the fascial arrangements, so there is a way at least to make a compensatory abnormality, dealing only with fascial tissues. There is also the possibility that I alluded to, that damage to the pelvic floor musculature occurs at the time of birth, and the ligamentous damage then develops over the years afterwards, because it no longer has the assistantce of the muscles in supporting the viscera. An analogy would be that in an individual who has had poliomyelitis and has lost the major muscles in the legs and depends upon locking the knee to maintain joint stability, the ligaments in the knee elongate, over years of taking that daily force. We may be seeing here that the muscular damage at the time of birth leaves the ligaments unsupported, and the ligamentous damage occurs over many years afterwards. When we see these women in their forties, they have the original neuromuscular damage and also the resulting fibrous tissue damage because of lack of the normal resiliency of the pelvic floor.

Blaivas: Then there wouldn't be the paravaginal problem, because instead of pulling away from the side walls of the pelvis, the endopelvic fascia would simply stretch. If it pulls away, the implication is that that tissue is strong enough that when you exert traction on it, for example with a paravaginal repair, the bladder and vesical neck will be pulled back up to their normal position.

Stanton: How do you know that the endopelvic fascia is pulled away? You are making a very black-and-white statement!

DeLancey: There is indirect evidence, in that if you suture the place where the paravaginal tissue has pulled away, the patient's anatomy becomes normal again, with the paravaginal repair, which is done through the space of Retzius, where the edge of the pubocervical fascia is reattached to the arcus tendineus. Mechanical engineers and people who work with composites know that the place where things break is where fibres change direction. For example, you may not be able to break a piece of fishing line by simply pulling it, because it's too strong, but if you put a knot in the middle and change the direction of the flow of force, it will break at the knot. So a weak point will be in an area of stress concentration. The area where the pubocervical fascia comes in to the arcus tendineus or to the pelvic side wall is where there is a change in the direction of the lines of force, and that would be why it would fail at that point rather than in the middle, where the pubocervical fascia is an uninterrupted sheet, where stresses could disperse themselves over a wide area. Whether that happens at the time of childbirth or later on is not known. I like the idea of looking for ways to start measuring some of these things.

Blaivas: I think we have a perfectly plausible explanation for each of these conditions, but we don't know whether one or both are responsible for the descent. Once we understand whether or not there is descent, there is still the clinical problem that people can show equal amounts of descent but not necessarily be incontinent, so there must be a further difference in the urethra. As I said earlier, we really need to key into the pathophysiology in trying to understand which of these factors, or other factors, is important.

DeLancey: It may be that in people with equal amounts of an anatomical descent of the vesical neck, one person has a normally innervated sphincteric mechanism and one an abnormally innervated one. In urinary incontinence, David Warrell's group sorted out patients with genital prolapse, with and without stress incontinence. Those with stress incontinence had nerve conduction deficits, whether or not there was prolapse.

Blaivas: That still does not mean that nerve conduction abnormalities are the cause; it could just as well be the effect! Certainly after pelvic surgery one can always find electromyographic evidence of denervation, whether or not the patient is incontinent. Similarly, the traction and avulsion of a cystocele may stretch the nerves and cause neuropathological changes which are not themselves the cause of the incontinence.

Swash: It's very difficult from clinical observations to prove the hypothesis, as distinct from simply verifying it. When we looked at women who had just had a baby, in a prospective study (Snooks et al 1984), the EMG evidence of reinnervation, implying previous denervation, and the change in terminal motor latency, were most marked in multipara, or after a forceps delivery whether in primipara or multipara, and the pelvic floor was entirely normal afer a Caesarean section. Those women with the most prominent physiological change, particularly an increase in fibre density (chronic partial denervation), were most likely to have a degree of incontinence *post partum*; two had rectal incontinence after the delivery of the first child, both with very marked changes in fibre density and pudendal nerve terminal motor latency.

Blaivas: It would be interesting to see whether we think that ultimately the nerve damage allows the descent of the bladder base, or does that nerve damage some-how destroy the intrinsic property of the urethra to stay closed? All of these things seem to be possible to investigate. The concept of elastance may be a very good way of looking at the natural tendency of the urethra to stay coapted.

Brading: In both systems, if you have abnormalities in the sphincters and nerve damage, how often do you get a functional outflow obstruction, and is there the possibility of secondary changes in the smooth muscle, of either rectum or bladder, as a consequence of that obstruction, which may lead to things like urge incontinence? I am thinking of detrusor–sphincter dyssynergia, which would provide a functional obstruction, so that you might be getting abnormal changes in pressure in the bladder.

Blaivas: The bladders of patients, and animals, that are obstructed are very different from normal, whether the obstruction is mechanical (mainly a prostatic obstruction or a stricture) or dyssynergic. What is clear is that the damage seems to be caused by excessive pressure on the bladder. David Staskin has done nice studies to pull all that together. The higher the pressure and the longer the period for which that bladder sees high pressures, the greater the likelihood of urological complications. The changes haven't been well documented in the human, but in rabbits there are overt changes in the bladder after obstruction—decreased contractility and increased collagen content. In humans you see an excess of collagen, an increase in the spaces between muscle cells, and a decreased number of muscle cells with their replacement by collagen. There are weaker, more poorly sustained detrusor contractions.

Stanton: There's also a sex variation, in that the female bladder does far worse than the male after obstruction. The female bladder tends to fail and be unable to contend with the obstruction far earlier than the male.

Marsden: What about secondary changes to the rectum with anismus?

Bartolo: In faecal incontinence we hardly ever see anismus, but 80% of people with prolapse complain of difficulty during defaecation and 50% of people with so-called idiopathic or neurogenic faecal incontinence complain of incomplete emptying and difficulty, and consequently they strain excessively. We assume that this makes their pudendal neuropathy worse. But what effect it has, in answer to your question, Dr Brading, I cannot say.

Christensen: In people with faecal impactions, incontinence of liquid stool is routine. So true chronic obstruction can lead to faecal incontinence as well.

Swash: The internal anal sphincter is dilated in those patients.

Bartolo: Young patients with idiopathic megarectum, with a solid faecal bolus in the rectum, are usually incontinent; but if you replace that diseased rectum by healthy proximal colon, they generally become continent.

Christensen: Similarly, if you remove a big faecal impaction, frequently the patient returns to normal.

We have been using qualifying adjectives for incontinence—urinary stress incontinence, for instance. This has started me thinking about rectal incontinence. I see two groups of incontinent people, those who pass stool without being aware of it and those who are aware that they need to pass stool but can't prevent its passage. Are those two separate groups, and are we confusing ourselves by studying them as though they were a single group?

Blaivas: I would say that they are two different groups.

Swash: The first group has a sensory disturbance, which is perhaps not found in the second group, which would separate them in functional terms. They don't all have urge incontinence in the way that a urologist would define it, because they have similar electrophysiological features.

Bartolo: That crystallizes it clearly. One group only know they have leaked because of the smell; they can't feel it. Those patients are the worst to deal with. They have bad sensory and motor denervation. Then you see women, classically after obstetric injury, with disruption or partial disruption of the external anal sphincter. They have intense urgency and cannot defer defaecation.

Christensen: Do you agree that there are these two groups?

Bartolo: Absolutely, but there is overlap between the two; that's the problem. I don't know how much overlap there is.

DeLancey: There is also overlap between *urinary* stress and urge incontinence. It's an empirical observation that there are people with both types, whose urge incontinence goes away after operation.

Brading: This might be the result of an outflow obstruction causing the changes that would lead to the urge incontinence?

DeLancey: It actually may be the opposite, in that these patients have a poorly functioning sphincteric mechanism, which gives them their urgency. They can tell that their margin for staying dry is relatively narrow. It is speculated that there is a reflex by which, when urine gets into the proximal urethra, the detrusor is suddenly more active.

Blaivas: That was one of Barrington's reflexes (1931). But there aren't enough people in whom this happens to discover its relevance. It does not occur often enough in the normal stress incontinence patient, at least not in our video studies.

To answer Dr Brading's question on obstruction more specifically, I do not think that obstruction causes *stress* incontinence, but I agree that it clearly produces *urge* incontinence. We see urge incontinence in men with prostatic obstruction and detrusor instability, and in women after urethropexy operations which obstruct them.

Incidentally, and thinking back to Dr Nordling's paper, we have been using the term 'detrusor instability' to imply that this is only a cystometric diagnosis. It is clear to many of us that detrusor instability is also a symptom; people complain of a sudden urge to urinate and they wet before reaching the bathroom. I tend to think that people with that symptom probably have detrusor instability, whether or not it was demonstrated by a cystometrogram. Dr Nordling brought up ambulatory cystometry, implying that because it was a different filling rate, that was the reason for seeing more instability. I would say it is because of measuring over a longer period of time.

Brading: Whatever the reason, the results from ambulatory monitoring are likely to be more meaningful!

Stanton: We demonstrated that with urethral electro-conductance; it was shown by David Holmes that if you measure conductance with the device at the bladder neck over a period of time you will see urine entering the proximal urethra simultaneously with the desire to urinate. That is clear evidence that the bladder neck is opening. Whether the detrusor is contracting is hard to tell, because you may get contractions that are not recordable on your cystometric apparatus. So clearly that is a mechanism for producing urgency.

But it is very difficult to define your patient with stress incontinence and with urge incontinence. A study from Liverpool showed that the number of women complaining of pure stress incontinence with no other symptoms is very low. You have to assign your patients a score as to the relevant weighting of their symptoms. Most women who come with prolapse or with urinary symptoms, if you question them in depth will admit to stress incontinence, urge incontinence, and frequency. You then have to go back to your second line of questioning to define the order of importance.

Blaivas: We did that prospectively in 199 patients with urinary (stress) incontinence (Blaivas & Olsson 1988). We use a voiding diary very similar to Dr Nordling's; we also ask them to write down the time when they get their urge to void, and then they grade the intensity of the urge from one to 10. Then the patients write down the time they actually urinate. Those three parameters tell us how much of the problem is urgency, how much is urge incontinence, and how much is stress incontinence. Many women complain of frequency and urgency, and when they keep the diary, the frequency and the urgency have nothing to do with the sensation. These are social things: 'I am going out, so I must urinate beforehand', and so on.

Stanton: Yes; when such patients come for consultation, they report urgency and frequency, yet they can sit for three hours to avoid missing their consultation, with no suggestion that they have these symptoms.

Kuijpers: Women with an obstetric sphincter rupture do that too; first they have their bowel movements, and then they go to town for shopping; so, in a way, they can handle it socially.

Marsden: Making allowances for that social error, are you all saying that the symptoms of stress incontinence, a feeling of urgency, urge incontinence and frequency occur more or less altogether, in varied proportions?

Stanton: I think they do. Most women in their forties who have had one or two children will have some of these symptoms. It depends on how much you pursue your questioning; you have to be very specific about this, to get the true picture.

Blaivas: We find that half of our 199 stress incontinence patients have a constellation of symptoms; they all had stress incontinence and half also complained of frequency, urgency and/or urge incontinence. The other half voided every three or four hours and denied frequency, urgency or urge incontinence.

Stanton: This is in contradiction to the Liverpool study, which found that very few (2%) people have just stress incontinence.

Blaivas: I know; but in our data, 50% have nothing but stress incontinence.

Brading: Did you do urodynamics on them? What percentage had unstable contractions?

Blaivas: We found that 22% of the patients who did not complain of urge incontinence had detrusor instability. Looking at it the other way, in only 50% of the patients who complained of frequency, urgency, or urge incontinence did we demonstrate instability.

Staskin: I feel partially responsible for this discussion, because I asked earlier whether the gastroenterologists had a classification system for faecal incontinence. It turns out that as soon as you develop one, you will spend most of your time arguing whether it is accurate or not! I think that in a very common condition, namely that you cough and laugh and sneeze, and produce an uninhibited bladder contraction and then leak, which I hesitate to call stress-induced bladder instability, it's common for someone who has uninhibited bladder contractions to perform a stress manoeuvre which provokes a contraction, which is shown during cystometry. I think, though, that everyone would agree that the symptoms are generally mixed, and this is why the urodynamics are useful, to confirm your clinical impression, especially before a surgical procedure. As things become more sophisticated, when we use the term 'stress incontinence' we like to think of under-active sphincter function, if we are making a functional diagnosis, and urge incontinence, which we would like to think means uninhibited bladder contractions.

Blaivas: Are you saying that most people who complain of stress incontinence also have frequency, urgency and urge incontinence?

Staskin: It would not be unusual, depending on the population you look at. The younger the patients, it is more likely that if they cough and laugh and lose a small amount of urine, they have stress incontinence. If they also have frequency and some urgency, it may or may not be related to their desire to empty their bladder. As the population gets older, our conclusion was that if you bring the patients into hospital, no matter how much you question them, the more unreliable their symptoms become in determining what is wrong, because the incidence of bladder instability increases greatly in the elderly population. In fact you are usually right if you make a diagnosis of bladder instability. The diagnosis therefore very much depends on what the population is. A symptomatic classification proves very accurate, but it starts you on subdividing that classification into a functional scheme; so it helps you to understand symptoms but does not help to make a diagnosis.

Bourcier: As a matter of fact, as I become older I find I am taking care of younger women! I am very lucky to deal with such young, nulliparous women and I agree with David Staskin that when they are young, they have just stress incontinence, but less urge incontinence. Later, after childbirth, they have both stress and urge incontinence.

Secondly, when we ask gynaecologists to examine the pelvic floor of very young nulliparous women who wish to use the contraceptive pill, we ask the patient to cough, and we are very surprised by the number of cases of vaginal wall prolapse. I want to ask Stuart Stanton which, among all the risk factors for delivery, is the major factor for becoming incontinent?

Stanton: I don't think that we yet have enough information to be able to make that choice. There is a spectrum of factors which are involved. We need to know much more about the profile of the patient. Nobody has said whether we are talking of black or white patients; there is an enormous difference in the pelvic floor tissues, in terms of the amount of collagen scar tissue formed in a black patient after childbirth. Nobody mentioned the predilection of some patients to collagen defects types I and II, in terms of the ability to support the bladder neck. There is said to be a link between hyperextensibility of the fingers, formation of striae gravidarum, and a deficiency in collagen tissue, and a relationship to urinary incontinence (Al Rawi & Al Rawi 1982). There are so many other factors that come in that we would be naive to select any one factor, just as we are naive if we say there is one operation which will cure incontinence, without taking account of the fact that it's a multifactorial problem.

DeLancey: Another factor is the level of physical activity. Some of our young nursing students realized that they all did the same thing when they went out to run; they ran for five minutes, came back to empty their bladders, and then went out to continue running. We asked a group of 326 patients presenting for gynaecological examinations to fill out a questionnaire about exercise and incontinence (Nygaard et al 1990). It was found that 55% of the women who exercised wore a pad during exercise because of urine leakage. We were amazed that so large a proportion of people who exercise need to wear protection. One therefore wonders whether the sedentary elderly individual may *not* have stress incontinence because she never really gets into an activity that provokes stress incontinence.

Marsden: Perhaps older people don't laugh as much as do young girls who, according to my daughters, commonly experience giggling incontinence!

Stanton: That is a different problem from sphincteric incontinence; it is either detrusor instability, or else the giggling releases your sphincteric control. Perhaps some people grow out of this, but I think this is semi-physiological. We haven't talked either about the concept of coital incontinence, which is either mechanical, or coital incontinence at the time of orgasm.

The other point to make about the elderly is that, sadly, they have been brought up by us as doctors and by our nursing colleagues to think that once you are over 60 or 65, incontinence is something you live with, you don't talk about it, and nothing can be done for it. Therefore many older people won't complain about it unless you question them. The younger generation, because they are into jogging and because we now discuss incontinence, will admit at the age of 18, which they wouldn't do before, that they suffer from it. This trend will continue, and even though our obstetrical performance is improving, with less use of forceps, and fewer babies being born, and so parity is dropping and there is less prolapse, I suspect that the level of incontinence will continue to rise, because people are standing up and saying that it happens and they don't accept this. The other fascinating point, clinically well known, is that no man would suffer the indignity of incontinence for more than 24 hours, whereas women carry on for months and years putting up with it. This is a case for re-education.

Bourcier: We have improved our methods of prevention, so we are seeing fewer patients with incontinence after childbirth. On the other hand, we are now seeing increasing numbers of cases because young women are exercising and jogging and taking up sports. In the future we have to watch more television if we want to improve pelvic floor muscle tone. In countries with 21 TV channels, like Belgium, they are less incontinent!

References

Allen TA 1977 The non-neurogenic neurogenic bladder. J Urol 117:232

Al Rawi ZS, Al Rawi ZT 1982 Joint hypermobility in women with congenital prolapse. Lancet:1439–1441

Barrington FJF 1931 The component reflexes of micturition in the cat, parts I & II. Brain 64:239

Blaivas JG, Olsson CA 1988 Stress incontinence—classification and surgical approach. J Urol 139:727–731

Nygaard I, DeLancey JOL, Arnsdorf L, Murphy E 1990 Exercise and incontinence. Obstet Gynecol, in press

Snooks SJ, Swash M, Setchell M, Henry MM 1984 Injury to innervation of pelvic sphincter musculature in childbirth. Lancet 2:546–550

The physiological evaluation of operative repair for incontinence and prolapse

D. C. C. Bartolo and G. S. Duthie

University Department of Surgery, Bristol Royal Infirmary, Bristol, BS2 8HW, UK

Abstract. Women with incontinence were divided into 30 with anorectal incontinence and 63 with complete rectal prolapse. The former group comprised 14 with a sphincter disruption and the remainder with intact sphincters. After anterior sphincter repair 70% were restored to acceptable continence. Success was associated with a rise in resting and voluntary contraction pressures and improved anal sensation. Patients with prolapse underwent either anterior and posterior rectopexy, or resection rectopexy. Continence was improved in both groups. Postoperatively, 90% following resection rectopexy and 80% following anterior and posterior rectopexy were restored to acceptable continence. Postoperative defaecatory straining and incomplete evacuation were reduced, with no significant differences between the two procedures. Restoration of continence was not associated with any change in sphincter pressures. However, rectal sensory threshold and anal sensation were both improved.

1990 Neurobiology of Incontinence. Wiley, Chichester (Ciba Foundation Symposium 151) p 223–245

Faecal incontinence is a distressing symptom seen commonly in specialized anorectal surgical practice. The majority of cases are due to either sphincter trauma, predominantly obstetric, or rectal prolapse.

There is considerable evidence from histochemical studies (Parks et al 1977), electromyography (Neill et al 1981, Parks 1975, Bartolo et al 1983a,b,c,d, Read et al 1984) and nerve conduction (Kiff et al 1984) studies that most patients with so-called idiopathic faecal incontinence in fact have changes affecting the anal sphincter that are compatible with chronic partial denervation. The most likely causes are obstetric trauma and chronic straining at stool. Studies before and after childbirth have shown that forceps and breech delivery lead to an increase in the external anal sphincter fibre density and pudendal nerve terminal motor latency (Snooks et al 1984). We have recently shown that the sensory threshold in the anal sphincter is increased after vaginal delivery (Cornes & Bartolo 1990). We believe this is the result of damage to the pudendal innervation during parturition. Abnormal defaecatory straining has also been shown to produce changes consistent with chronic partial denervation (Bartolo et al 1983c,d, 1985, 1986a), but there is no conclusive evidence that such patterns of defaecation result in complete rectal prolapse, attractive as such a hypothesis may seem.

The operative approach to severely troubled patients has been to perform a post-anal repair for idiopathic incontinence, a direct repair following surgical or obstetric division, and some form of rectopexy for rectal prolapse. The operation of post-anal repair was developed by the late Sir Alan Parks and based on his concept that continence was predominantly maintained by a flap valve at the anorectal junction (Parks 1975). We questioned the rationale for this operation for the following reasons. Firstly, in videodynamic studies, continence during Valsalva manoeuvres in patients with their rectums filled with liquid was sphincteric with no evidence for a flap valve. Moreover, the anterior rectal wall was always well separated from the top of the anal canal (Bartolo et al 1986b). Secondly, successful post-anal repair does not depend on making the anorectal angle more acute (Bartolo et al 1986b, Miller et al 1988a, Womack et al 1988). On this basis we now use an anterior approach on all patients, which will be discussed in the light of the results.

In patients undergoing successful rectopexy for incontinence related to prolapse the reason for the restoration of continence is unclear. Improved anorectal function, either motor, sensory or both, may contribute. In this paper we present a critical analysis of the outcome after rectopexy for prolapse. We also present an analysis of anterior sphincter repair for idiopathic incontinence using an identical approach to that used for traumatic sphincter injuries.

Methods

Patients

Thirty incontinent female patients with idiopathic or traumatic incontinence were operated on at Bristol Royal Infirmary and all have completed pre- and postoperative assessment. Fourteen had an anterior sphincter defect at surgery; 16 had an intact sphincter. Continence was defined as the ability to contain solid and liquid stool without leakage. We analysed the data from 63 patients with complete rectal prolapse of whom 21 were continent and 42 incontinent. The findings were compared to a control group of 30 patients. Patients with prolapse underwent either anterior and posterior Marlex rectopexy (MR) or resection and rectopexy (RR). We carried out pre- and postoperative studies on 15 incontinent patients in each group.

All patients had our routine detailed history taken, using a standard questionnaire. In addition, each has had intensive physiological and radiological assessment, including manometry, electrosensitivity and proctography.

Manometry

Sphincter length, maximum resting pressure (MRP), and maximum voluntary contraction (MVC) were measured by a closed water-filled manometry system and a station pullthrough technique after precalibration of the recorder for pressures of 0–200 cmH$_2$O (Miller et al 1989a). The patient was examined in the left lateral position and the probe was withdrawn and pressures were recorded at 1 cm intervals. Sphincter length was defined as the detected high pressure zone and the pressure measured at each station. The process was repeated with the patient contracting the sphincter to determine MVC. The recto-anal inhibitory reflex was elicited in all patients. Rectal sensation and pressures were measured using a balloon containing a manometric transducer. The balloon was filled at 150 ml/minute H$_2$O at 37 °C. The volume and pressures at first rectal sensation and maximum tolerable volume were recorded and rectal compliance was measured from the slope of the infusion curve dV/dP.

Anal canal electrosensitivity

The method of Roe et al (1986) was used. After the anal canal length had been defined by manometry, a graduated catheter with two platinum electrodes placed 1 cm apart was introduced into the anal canal and the threshold of anal sensation to minute electrical stimuli was measured in the lower, middle and upper anal canal. These stimuli were delivered from a constant current generator whose output varied between 0 and 25 mA. Three recordings were taken at each site and were averaged to give the electrosensitivity threshold. To permit statistical analysis, those in whom the threshold was not reached, because of lack of sensation, were recorded as having sensitivities of 26 mA.

Proctography

The anorectal angle and perineal descent were measured radiographically during static proctography with the patient in the left lateral position. Measurements were taken with the subject at rest during maximal contraction of the pelvic floor, and while straining as in defaecation. A barium sulphate and starch solution was introduced into the unprepared rectum and the anal canal was delineated by a radio-opaque ball and chain inserted after the barium paste. The anorectal angle was defined as the angle between a line drawn along the chain in the anal canal, and a line bisecting the rectum. Perineal descent was determined from a line drawn from the most distal part of the coccyx to the most anterior part of the pubic symphysis. A perpendicular line was dropped from this to the anorectal angle. An angle lying below the line was recorded as a negative value of perineal descent; measurements above the line were positive. Rectal prolapse patients had the prolapse confirmed by evacuation proctography and clinical observation (Bartolo et al 1988).

Statistics

All values were recorded as medians with ranges in parenthesis. The significance of unpaired data was assessed by the Mann-Whitney U test, and that of paired pre- and postoperative data by the Wilcoxon paired signed rank test. Improvement in symptoms was assessed by χ-squared analysis. For all tests in this study, values of P less than 0.05 were considered significant.

Surgery

All operative procedures were undertaken by one surgeon (D.C.C.B). The technique of sphincter repair for traumatic injury is described elsewhere (Parks & McPartlin 1980), but an additional levatorplasty or posterior colporrhaphy was performed. The space between the rectum and vagina is developed until the space above the levatores is entered. The two limbs of the puborectalis and pubococcygeus are then plicated using two superficial and two deep 2/0 Prolene sutures, in an attempt to augment the length of the anal canal. Through our anterior approach any divided ends of sphincter are identified, isolated, and thereafter plicated with 2/0 Prolene. Those patients without sphincter divisions at operation had the external sphincter divided anteriorly and plicated in exactly the same manner as in the group with disrupted sphincters. Skin closure under tension was avoided and any defect was allowed to heal by secondary intention (usually in under six weeks). No colostomies were fashioned at any operative procedure.

Two different techniques of rectopexy were used in the patients with rectal prolapse. Anterior and posterior Marlex rectopexy (MR), as described by Nicholls & Simson (1986), with full mobilization of the rectum including division of both lateral ligaments, was used in the first group. The resection and rectopexy (RR) procedure was modified from that of Frykman & Goldberg (1969). Mobilization was similar to that for MR but extended to include the descending colon, splenic flexure and left half of the transverse colon. The redundant sigmoid, proximal rectum and distal descending colon were resected to allow an anastomosis without tension between the upper descending colon and rectum at approximately 12 cm from the anal verge. Additionally, four low posterior Prolene sutures were inserted between the rectum and the pelvic fascia at the level of the lateral ligaments to fix the rectum and prevent postoperative prolapse.

Results

The ages of the patients and the duration of follow-up (Table 1) were similar in all groups except for those with traumatic incontinence, who were predominantly younger women with sphincter injuries secondary to obstetric trauma. Those with prolapse and concurrent incontinence tended to be older but this group did not reach statistical significance.

TABLE 1   Clinical details of patients

	Traumatic incontinence	Idiopathic incontinence	Marlex rectopexy	Resection rectopexy
Age (years)	32 (23–49)	66 (36–80)	62 (45–78)	63.5 (23–83)
Postoperative follow-up (years)	5 (1–18)	4 (2–12)	6 (5–15)	5 (3–12)

Idiopathic and traumatic incontinence

Sphincter pressures.   In those with idiopathic incontinence, 69% were improved after repair; success being defined as restoration of continence to solid and liquid stool, and 72% of those with traumatic incontinence were rendered continent (Table 2). Despite the repair, sphincter length (Table 3) was not significantly improved, nor was maximum resting pressure (MRP). Maximum voluntary contraction (MVC) was improved in the trauma group, but not in the idiopathic group overall. However, when those with a successful outcome were considered in this group, MVC was improved (preoperative, 105 (45–190) vs postoperative, 120 (45–233); $P < 0.05$), but this improvement was not seen in MRP. Considering the incontinent group as one, those rendered continent postoperatively did have significantly improved MRP: 60 (10–105), compared with the failures: 40 (10–74), $P < 0.05$ (Mann-Whitney U test).

Mucosal electrosensitivity.   Electrosensitivity thresholds were not significantly altered in the lower or middle anal canal by surgery, but in the upper anal canal there was a marked improvement in both the traumatic and idiopathic groups.

Proctography.   After surgery for a traumatic sphincter injury, the anorectal angle became more acute. Conversely in those without a sphincter disruption the angle actually became *more* obtuse postoperatively.

TABLE 2   Continence: pre- and postoperative sphincter repair and prolapse repair

	Continent preoperative (%)	Continent postoperative (%)
Traumatic incontinent	7	72
Idiopathic incontinent	0	69
Marlex rectopexy	27	80
Resection rectopexy	27	90

TABLE 3 Incontinent patients: pre- and postoperative physiological and radiological data

	Traumatic incontinence		Idiopathic incontinence	
	Preoperative	Postoperative	Preoperative	Postoperative
Sphincter length (cm)	3 (2–4)	3 (1–3.5)	3 (0–4)	3 (0–4)
MRP (cmH$_2$O)	55.4 (28–105)	62 (33–80)	55.5 (0–100)	56 (30–137)
MVC (cmH$_2$O)	80 (50–115)	115 (75–290)**	107 (5–200)	117 (45–230)
Mucosal electrosensitivity (mA)				
Lower anal canal	6.3 (4.3–17.6)	8 (4–11)	7 (4–16.6)	8 (4–25)
Mid anal canal	6.8 (4–20)	6.3 (3–19)	9 (3–25)	8 (3–25)
Upper anal canal	17 (4–25)	10.7 (1.6–25)*	24 (3.3–25)	9 (6–25)*
Anorectal angle				
Rest	107 (83–134)	98 (83–117)	105 (86–152)	118 (95–180)*
Squeeze	100 (84–134)	91 (60–112)*	97 (71–153)	113 (85–165)
Strain	119 (108–135)	110 (90–136)*	123 (89–152)	125 (101–180)
Perineal descent (cm)				
Rest	−0.7 (−2.6 to 0.2)	−1.0 (−2.7 to 0.9)	−2.1 (−3.2 to 0)	−2.4 (3.4 to 0)
Squeeze	−0.3 (−2.2 to 0.8)	−0.4 (−2.1 to 0.9)	−1.6 (−3.2 to 0.6)	−1.7 (−2.7 to 0)
Strain	−2.2 (−5.7 to −0.1)	−3 (−6.3 to 0)	−3.5 (−8.2 to 1.2)	−4.2 (−7 to 0)

*$P < 0.05$
**$P < 0.005$ } Wilcoxon paired signed rank test.

Prolapse patients: continent and incontinent

Sphincter pressures (Table 4).   Incontinent patients with rectal prolapse had significantly shorter sphincters than the remaining patients. A significant reduction was also seen in MRP and MVC compared with the controls for both groups, which were significantly lower in the incontinent group than in the continent patients with prolapse.

Mucosal electrosensitivity.   There were significantly higher thresholds for anal canal electrosensitivity at all levels in the anal canal in both patient groups, but notably in the upper anal canal sensation was poorer in those with incontinence and prolapse.

Rectal sensation.   Appreciation of rectal filling was better in incontinent patients, who had a lower volume of first rectal sensation.

Proctography.   Radiological studies showed that the anorectal angle was significantly more obtuse at rest, on contraction and on straining in all patients with prolapse. Similarly, perineal descent was greater in both patient groups than in controls.

Prolapse repair: comparison of Marlex and resection rectopexy

The prolapse was corrected in all patients postoperatively. Both operative procedures were associated with significant improvement in continence (Table 2). Despite this, neither operation improved sphincter length, or resting or voluntary contraction pressures (Table 5).

Radiological data showed no consistent changes that were associated with improved continence, in relation to either the anorectal angle or perineal descent.

Function

With regard to symptoms of postoperative constipation, the incidence of excessive straining at stool (MR, preoperative 66.5% vs 33.5% postoperative: RR, 89% vs 11%), a feeling of incomplete emptying (MR, 66.5% vs 33.5%: RR, 66.5% vs 33.5%) and call to stool (MR, 88% vs 72%: RR, 80% vs 72%) were not significantly altered, despite a trend towards improvement in bowel habit overall. Bowel frequency was similarly not significantly altered.

Electrosensitivity thresholds in the anal canal were significantly improved by resection rectopexy but not by Marlex rectopexy, although the group considered as a whole was improved ($P < 0.01$). Rectal sensitivity was significantly improved in both groups. There were no anastomotic leaks in patients undergoing a colorectal anastomosis.

TABLE 4 Prolapse: physiology of continent patients, incontinent patients and controls

	Control (n = 30)	Prolapse continent (n = 21)	Prolapse incontinent (n = 42)
Age (years)	55.5 (38–83)	66 (32–85)	73 (23–90)
Sphincter length (cm)	3.5 (2–4)	3.0 (2–4)	2.5 (1–4)‡
MRP (cmH$_2$O)	85 (60–115)	45 (5–160)†	25 (0–90)†‡
MVC (cmH$_2$O)	200 (110–290)	120 (15–675)†	85 (5–350)†‡
Mucosal electrosensitivity (mA)			
Lower anal canal	4.85 (3–7)	8.5 (3–26)†	8.25 (3–26)
Mid anal canal	4.3 (2–6)	8.6 (2–26)†	11.65 (4.3–26)†
Upper anal canal	5.65 (3.3–7.4)	20 (3–26)†	26 (8–26)†‡
Rectal sensation			
Volume to first rectal sensation (ml)	67.5 (35–145)	77.5 (40–250)*	47.5 (20–165)†
Anorectal angle			
Rest	92.5 (78–102)	101 (77–154)†	111 (73–140)†
Squeeze	86 (70–130)	94 (71–140)†	96 (76–143)†
Strain	111 (80–130)	125 (97–189)†	125.5 (89–154)†
Perineal descent			
Rest	0 (−1.1 to 1.0)	−0.8 (−3.2 to 1.5)†	−1.6 (−6.4 to 1.0)†
Squeeze	1 (−1.1 to 2.2)	−0.3 (−3.2 to 2.5)†*	−1.2 (−7.4 to 3.0)†
Strain	−1.7 (−4.3 to 0.9)	−4.6 (−8.4 to −1.1)†	−4.6 (−9.1 to 0.4)†

*P<0.05 cf. incontinent prolapse.
†P<0.05 cf. continent prolapse.
‡P<0.05 cf. controls.

TABLE 5 Prolapse: pre- and postoperative physiological and radiological data

	Marlex rectopexy		Resection rectopexy	
	Preoperative	Postoperative	Preoperative	Postoperative
Sphincter length (cm)	3 (2–4)	3 (2–4)	3 (2–4)	3 (2–4)
MRP (cmH$_2$O)	65 (20–160)	50 (20–125)	45 (12–145)	60 (25–185)
MVC (cmH$_2$O)	170 (45–265)	190 (30–225)	125 (30–215)	112.5 (50–230)
Mucosal electrosensitivity (mA)				
Lower anal canal	6.5 (3–20)	8 (1–14)	10 (6–26)	6.5 (4–12)
Mid anal canal	8 (3–26)	9 (3–17)	11 (6–18)	7 (3–15)
Upper anal canal	18 (3–26)	13 (3–26)	15 (10–26)	13 (1–19)†
Rectal sensation				
Volume to first rectal sensation (ml)	77.5 (30–415)	50 (25–301)*	55 (20–250)	32.5 (20–70)*
Anorectal angle				
Rest	101 (81–123)	125 (98–138)	106 (95–146)	118 (110–135)
Squeeze	91 (72–116)	105 (95–138)	105 (83–137)	119 (95–130)
Strain	121 (76–140)	137 (74–160)‡	114 (104–148)	140 (121–144)
Perineal descent (cm)				
Rest	−1.1 (−2.2 to 0)	0 (−2.7 to 0.7)*	−0.9 (−2.6 to 1.8)	−1.5 (−4.5 to 0)
Squeeze	−1.2 (−3 to 0.2)	−0.2 (−3.7 to 1.2)	−1.2 (−2 to 0)	−1.5 (−3.1 to −1)
Strain	−4.5 (−6.6 to −1.5)	−2.7 (−6.8 to −0.1)	−3.6 (−9.7 to 2.1)	−4 (−6.3 to −2.2)

*P<0.02
†P<0.05 ⎫ Wilcoxon paired signed rank test.
‡P<0.01 ⎭

Discussion

When faced with a new female patient with faecal incontinence we obtain a detailed obstetric history to ascertain whether there has been a sphincter tear during parturition. During physical examination we look carefully for rectal prolapse, complete or incomplete. This may entail digital examination with the patients straining to defaecate, watching them empty their rectums, or using proctography to define an internal or external prolapse. If rectal prolapse is confirmed we offer an abdominal rectopexy, since this operation in our hands yields the best improvement in continence. In the absence of a sphincter division many Units in the UK would proceed to post-anal repair. Indeed, normal continence was restored to 59% of patients treated in our Unit using this approach (Miller et al 1988a).

Since success did not depend on improving the anorectal angle we wondered whether using an anterior approach, together with plication of the levators in front of the rectum, would achieve similar restoration of continence. Anatomically this approach is attractive, because the anal sphincter, while well supported posteriorly by the puborectalis and levators, is in women a fairly slender structure, anteriorly made up only of the external and internal sphincters. Plicating the levators in front of the rectum may work by elongating the functional anal canal, but in this study we could not show that the resting anal canal length was significantly altered by the operation. This is hardly surprising, since we should have addressed sphincter function under stress or during a maximal voluntary contraction. Under these conditions we may have demonstrated a change postoperatively. Despite this, continence was restored to 69% postoperatively in those without a sphincter tear. In these patients, resting anal pressures did not change significantly after surgery. On the other hand, maximum voluntary contraction pressures rose significantly in those with a successful outcome. As in our previous studies (Miller et al 1988a), continence was restored without improvement in the anorectal angle. Indeed it actually became more obtuse, which adds further evidence to refute a flap-valve theory of continence based on an acute anorectal angle. The extent of perineal descent was likewise not significantly altered by the procedure.

It was notable that anal mucosal sensitivities were significantly reduced in the upper anal canal after operation. We suggest this is due to lifting the sensitive richly innervated transitional zone back up into its normal place in the anal canal. This would allow improved conscious awareness of rectal contents during anorectal sampling (Miller et al 1988b,c) thereby allowing the women either to take appropriate action and defaecate, or to make more effective and co-ordinated use of their defective, neuropathic anal sphincter musculature.

Our results of repair of traumatic sphincter divisions are comparable to those reported by others (Laurberg et al 1988). There was a non-significant trend towards improved resting pressures. Voluntary contraction pressures, on the other hand, improved to a very significant degree. The anorectal angle did not change significantly but the squeeze angle became more acute. Since this is a function of voluntary sphincter activity, this change is compatible with the improvement in voluntary contraction pressures. Anal sensation was improved in the proximal anal canal, reflecting restoration of normal anal anatomy (Miller et al 1989b).

The surgical management of patients with complete rectal prolapse involves correcting the actual prolapse, restoring continence and resolving the underlying defaecatory disorder. The physiological assessment of the group of prolapse patients as a whole indicates that the distinction between the continent and incontinent patients is that the latter have shorter sphincters and significantly lower resting and voluntary contraction pressures. Both groups have excessive perineal descent at rest on straining. They also have similarly impaired anal sensation, although the upper rectum is significantly less sensitive in the incontinent patients.

The role of rectal sensation is more difficult to evaluate. Clearly, if one can appreciate small volumes, appropriate measures can be taken to avoid accidental incontinence. There are a small group of incontinent patients who soil because they lack rectal awareness. The significance of a lower volume of first rectal sensation in the incontinent group is not obvious.

The outcome after rectopexy is reasonably satisfactory, in that we came close to achieving our objectives delineated above. All patients have had their prolapse corrected. Whereas 27% of patients were continent before surgery, this figure rose to 80% and 90% respectively in the two treatment groups. Finally, there has been a trend towards improvement in the underlying defaecatory disorder.

The mechanism by which continence is restored to normal is uncertain. Obviously, it is likely to be multifactorial and our relatively unphysiological assessment may be too crude to detect the subtle changes which tip the balance in favour of continence. We could find no evidence that resting or voluntary contraction pressures altered significantly. Nor were there any significant changes in anorectal angulation, which if anything became more obtuse.

There was a significant reduction in the volume of first rectal sensation, which may mean that the subject's rectal awareness has been improved, allowing the continence mechanism to be more efficient.

We were concerned that Marlex rectopexy would lead to an increase in postoperative constipation, as reported by others (Watts et al 1985). Stool frequency was not altered, while the incidence of straining at stool, together with the sensation of inadequate emptying, was decreased following surgery. We were left with 34% in whom these symptoms persisted, and we questioned whether a resection rectopexy would have been a better option. One mechanism by which rectopexy may work is by inducing postoperative constipation, although in our hands this did not appear to be the case. If, however, this mechanism were important, as suggested by others, we might expect a resection to lead to diarrhoea and thus be less effective in restoring normal continence. On the other hand, by avoiding artificial implants we would reduce the reaction to them by the rectum, which may be advantageous. Continence rates were slightly better, at 90% after resection rectopexy. Moreover the trend was towards even better resolution of the underlying defaecatory disorder, with 89% straining at stool preoperatively and only 11% following surgery. Thus the trends, albeit non-significant, have favoured resection rectopexy as practised by Watts et al (1985) from the Minnesota group. Furthermore, this procedure does not involve insertion of foreign material with its attendant risks of infection. The disadvantage is the potential for anastomotic leakage. This has not been a problem in this series.

There are many options when the surgery of rectal prolapse is being considered. In planning the optimum procedure the surgeon should tailor the operation to the individual patient's needs. Since we do not know precisely how rectopexy restores continence there is clearly a need for further work to try to determine the mechanisms. We are currently measuring anal and rectal pressures, combined with sphincter electromyography, in ambulatory patients. Thus, the patients are away from the artificial laboratory environment and recordings should be more physiological. Moreover, we will be able to analyse the response to spontaneous rises in rectal pressure, passing flatus and defaecation. We believe that improvements in outcome will come from careful evaluation of patients' objective physiological variables, before and after surgery.

References

Bartolo DCC, Jarratt JA, Read NW 1983a The use of conventional electromyography to assess external anal sphincter neuropathy in man. J Neurol Neurosurg Psychiatry 46:1115–1118

Bartolo DCC, Jarratt JA, Read NW 1983b The cutaneo-anal reflex: a useful index of neuropathy? Br J Surg 70:660–633

Bartolo DCC, Read NW, Jarratt JA, Read MG, Donnelly TC, Johnson AG 1983c Differences in anal sphincter function and clinical presentation in patients with pelvic floor descent. Gastroenterology 85:68–75

Bartolo DCC, Jarratt JA, Read MG, Donnelly TC, Read NW 1983d The role of partial denervation of the puborectalis in idiopathic faecal incontinence. Br J Surg 70:664–667

Bartolo DCC, Roe AM, Virjee J, Mortensen NJMcC 1985 Evacuation proctography in obstructed defaecation and rectal intussusception. Br J Surg 72(Suppl):S111–116

Bartolo DCC, Roe AM, Mortensen NJMcC 1986a The relationship between perineal descent and denervation of the puborectalis in continent patients. Int J Colorectal Dis 1:91–95

Bartolo DCC, Roe AM, Locke-Edmunds JC, Virjee J, Mortensen NJMcC 1986b Flap valve theory of anorectal continence. Br J Surg 73:1012–1014

Bartolo DCC, Roe AM, Virjee J, Mortensen NJMcC, Locke-Edmunds JC 1988 An analysis of rectal morphology in obstructed defaecation. Int J Colorect Dis 3:17–22

Cornes H, Bartolo DCC 1990 The effect of vaginal delivery on anal canal sensation. Br J Surg 77:in press

Frykman HM, Goldberg SM 1969 The surgical treatment of rectal procidentia. Surg Gynecol Obstet 129:1225–1230

Kiff ES, Barnes PRH, Swash M 1984 Evidence of pudendal neuropathy in patients with perineal descent and chronic straining at stool. Gut 25:1279–1282

Laurberg S, Swash M, Henry MM 1988 Delayed external sphincter repair for obstetric tear. Br J Surg 75:786–788

Miller R, Bartolo DCC, Locke-Edmunds JC, Mortensen NJMcC 1988a A prospective study of conservative and operative treatment for faecal incontinence. Br J Surg 75:101–105

Miller R, Lewis G, Bartolo DCC, Cervero F, Mortensen NJMcC 1988b Sensory discrimination and dynamic activity in the anorectum: evidence using a new ambulatory technique. Br J Surg 75:1003–1007

Miller R, Bartolo DCC, Cervero F, Mortensen NJMcC 1988c Anorectal sampling: a comparison of normal and incontinent patients. Br J Surg 75:44–46

Miller R, Bartolo DCC, James D, Mortensen NJMcC 1989a Air-filled microballoon manometry for use in anorectal physiology. Br J Surg 76:72–75

Miller R, Orrom W, Cornes H, Duthie GS, Bartolo DCC 1989b Anterior sphincter plication and levatorplasty in the treatment of faecal incontinence. Br J Surg 76:1058–1060

Neill ME, Parks AG, Swash M 1981 Physiological studies of the anal sphincter musculature in faecal incontinence and rectal prolapse. Br J Surg 68:531–536

Nicholls RJ, Simson JNL 1986 Anteroposterior rectopexy in the treatment of solitary rectal ulcer syndrome without overt rectal prolapse. Br J Surg 73:222–224

Parks AG 1975 Anorectal incontinence. Proc R Soc Med 68:681–690

Parks AG, McPartlin JF 1980 Surgical repair of the anal sphincters following injury. In: Rolo C, Smith R (eds) Operative surgery. Butterworth Scientific, Sevenoaks, p 245–248

Parks AG, Swash M, Urich H 1977 Sphincter denervation in anorectal incontinence and rectal prolapse. Gut 18:656–665

Read NW, Bartolo DCC, Read MG 1984 Differences in anal function in patients with incontinence to solids and in patients with incontinence to liquids. Br J Surg 71:39–42

Roe AM, Bartolo DCC, Mortensen NJMcC 1986 New method for assessment of anal sensation in various anorectal disorders. Br J Surg 73:310–321

Snooks SJ, Setchell M, Swash M, Henry MM 1984 Injury to the innervation of the pelvic floor musculature in childbirth. Lancet 2:546–550

Watts JD, Rothenberger DA, Buls JG, Goldberg SM, Nivatvongs S 1985 The management of procidentia. Dis Colon Rectum 28:96–102

Womack NR, Morrison JFB, Williams NS 1988 Prospective study of the effects of post anal repair in neurogenic faecal incontinence. Br J Surg 75:48–52

DISCUSSION

Kuijpers: We recently finished a study on faecal incontinence. We studied 212 patients with disorders of continence: 156 were incontinent with no control for solid stools; 31 had insufficient function, meaning no control for liquid stools and/or gas; and 25 had soiling, which means the loss of small amounts of mucus.

Anal resting and squeeze pressures varied widely in the different groups. There was a huge overlap. Mean resting and squeeze pressures were 9.5 kPa and 9.4 kPa respectively in normals. In the soiling group, mean resting pressure was decreased by 50% (4.8 kPa), while external sphincter function was normal (10.3 kPa). In the insufficient group, internal sphincter function was decreased to 7.1 kPa and external sphincter function to 6.1 kPa. Sphincter functions were even lower in the incontinent group (5.1 and 2.7 kPa respectively). Most differences in sphincter functions were statistically significant. We concluded that the external sphincter determines the degree of continence, whereas the function of the internal sphincter is to retain small amounts of mucus.

Can we use manometry in a clinical setting? Manometry is a suitable procedure for determining anal sphincter function. But there is a wide variation, both in normals and in patients; resting pressures vary from 4.1 to 18.0 kPa in normals and squeeze pressures from 0.0 to 21.1 kPa in incontinent patients. So manometry is not of great help in determining the exact degree of continence.

The causes of faecal incontinence were neurogenic in 109 patients, obstetric trauma in 33 and iatrogenic in 59. We compared the complaints of the three groups and noticed that soiling mainly occurred in the iatrogenic group, which suggested that anorectal surgery can impair internal sphincter function.

Comparing the incontinent patients in the neurogenic and obstetric groups, we found that, of course, all patients in the obstetric group were females, and that 93% in the neurogenic group were females. So neurogenic incontinence is a typical female disease. About 25% of these women were virgins, had no constipation, and did not strain, so it really is 'idiopathic neurogenic'.

We looked at the incidence of prolapse, either present at the time of investigation or previously treated. A low incidence was found in the obstetric group (3%), but a 64% incidence in the neurogenic group, suggesting a relation between prolapse and pelvic floor denervation. The iatrogenic group had an incidence of 20%. We therefore believe that prolapse is caused by pelvic floor denervation; impaired pelvic floor function diminishes the supportive function with prolapse as a result.

DeLancey: Were these cases of rectal prolapse, or genital prolapse?

Kuijpers: These were urological, gynaecological and colorectal prolapses. In doing anorectal surgery, internal sphincter function can be impaired in some patients, while in others pelvic floor denervation can occur.

We also looked at the occurrence of the feeling of urge—the call to stool. It was absent in 70% of females with neurogenic incontinence, compared to 3% in the obstetric group.

Neurogenic faecal incontinence can be treated by post-anal repair. During this procedure the puborectalis and the external sphincter are plicated behind the anorectum. We looked at the results in 39 patients after three months; 15% had complete restoration of continence, 28% had good results, with an accident only once a week or less, 26% had no ability to retain faeces, but the feeling of urge had been restored, and 31% did not improve. So about 50% of the patients were able to retain faeces and in nearly 70% the feeling of urge had been restored. We did manometry in these patients and found no change between preoperative and postoperative results, neither for resting pressures nor for squeeze pressures, and neither for the total group nor for the different subgroups. So resting and squeeze pressures are not useful markers for predicting surgical outcome. Thus restoration of neurogenic faecal incontinence is not caused by the restoration of sphincter function. It is more likely that it is caused by restoration of the local anatomy.

Swash: I completely agree with what you say. We have studied a group of patients with idiopathic anorectal incontinence some years after post-anal repair. The longer such patients are followed, the less good are the results and the more disappointing the procedure appears to be. The striking point in our study (Laurberg et al 1990) was that the indices of denervation, namely changes in EMG and the anal sphincter squeeze pressures, were far worse postoperatively, some months or years later, than they had been preoperatively, but these observations did not correlate with the functional benefit. Some patients were still continent, but they had far worse denervation than in the studies made preoperatively some years before. We concluded that either the operation makes the denervation worse, presumably by causing fibrosis and interfering with local anatomy, or the progressive neurogenic change underlying sphincter denervation had continued. There was no very strict correlation of these results with the functional result, so whatever the surgeon is doing, he is restoring some anatomical–pressure relationship that is not dependent upon the underlying role of an innervated pelvic floor musculature in achieving a satisfactory clinical result.

Dr Kuijpers, I assume that the 25% of patients in whom there was no identified local cause probably had a cauda equina or lower pelvic cause for their denervation?

Kuijpers: Maybe; we didn't check that.

Marsden: So what is this anatomy that surgeons are restoring?

Bartolo: We don't know!

Swash: One explanation is that the anal canal has been lengthened.

Bartolo: The problem there is that we have always done the wrong test. We measure resting anal canal length, whereas we should be measuring voluntary contraction sphincter length. Norman Williams' group in a very small series produced an elongation of anal canal length but didn't change any of the other variables, and his results are slightly at variance with mine and with Hans Kuijpers' results, and with others. But until we start to change the methods of testing, we won't be able to see whether a levatorplasty helps.

Swash: The only thing that is clear is that the mechanism of continence in these patients is different from the mechanism in normal subjects.

Kuijpers: David Bartolo's procedures may affect rectal capacity, rectal compliance and rectal sensitivity. This may influence the increase in continence seen after the posterior rectopexy procedure.

Bartolo: In the prolapse repairs we reduced the volume at first sensation, and that may be the effect; but I wondered if we were doing something to the autonomic nerves, because clearly we cause a lot of disruption; we are, I think, dividing the sacral parasympathetic nerves, which come in with the lateral ligaments, and in all of those patients I have gone right down to the anus and completely divided those ligaments. A surgeon at St Marks, James Thompson, does not divide the lateral ligaments when he does rectopexy, and I know from anecdotal data from David Lubowski that his constipation rate after rectopexy is the lowest in the hospital.

Burnstock: Something that is now emerging is that when you cut or damage nerves, those that remain undergo compensatory changes in expression of transmitters. The time course of change in your patients would be interesting to know, because these trophic changes in expression take time. Have you any information on the time course of these events?

Bartolo: The measurements were done approximately 3–6 months after surgery. The improvement is seen much earlier. A few people take 2–3 weeks to get better, but most patients leave hospital after about 10 days and are continent from then on.

Burnstock: Six to eight days is the minimum time for trophic changes in a number of models that we have examined, which is compatible with your 10 days.

Wong: I agree with Mr Bartolo's statement. Our patients, by the time they are ready for discharge after 7–10 days, have already noticed a significant difference in control. With respect to rectal prolapse repairs, we looked at our last 23 patients with abdominal proctopexy and sigmoid resection. Our findings were similar, with the only exception being that we have found a significant improvement in squeeze pressure postoperatively. But the pressure measurements preoperatively may have been lower in our group of patients than yours were, Mr Bartolo, because our pressures tend to be lower in that group.

Christensen: The patients you treat really have two problems: incontinence and rectal prolapse. Which comes first? Are they incontinent for months or years before the prolapse occurs, or do these things seem to happen simultaneously?

Bartolo: It's often difficult to know. We see some young people, often male patients, with complete rectal prolapse, who have had prolapse for many years and have been completely continent for most of that time. They come for treatment only when they become incontinent. These patients presumably have an anatomical disorder; they have rather lax supporting tissues surrounding the rectum. Most of the prolapse patients whom we see are incontinent and it is difficult to analyse which came first. Many are nulliparous women, so obstetric factors are not as relevant as in what I call anorectal or idiopathic neurogenic incontinence.

Christensen: One can visualize that the sphincter simply gets loose and lets the rectum fall out, so that the incontinence would progress and lead to the prolapse. Conversely, perhaps when the prolapse has occurred, the sphincter cannot work effectively because there is a big plug of tissue in there. If so, then everybody with a prolapse should be incontinent, but it sounds as if that's not true. Can you explain?

Bartolo: There are alterations in manometric measurements in the prolapse patients; if we compare continent patients with rectal prolapse to incontinent ones, the continent patients have lower pressures than normal controls, but much higher pressures than the incontinent patients. But I am confused by the incontinent patients with incomplete rectal prolapse, who have near-normal pressures that are higher than those of the continent patients with complete prolapse. So clearly it is not just a barrier effect; there is something about the sheer presence of the prolapse, or the intussusception, that is affecting the sphincter mechanism.

Christensen: Dr Swash said something a few minutes ago that started me thinking. He said that what is wrong might be that the anal canal has become too long. Perhaps rectal prolapse and sphincter function have little to do with each other; maybe the *rectum* itself has become too long and so it's loose in the available space and some of it gets caught in the sphincter, and so prolapse occurs. If that's the case, the fundamental problem might lie with the longitudinal muscle layer of the rectum, which is surely what keeps the rectum within a reasonable range of length. That raises the question of what is the function of that longitudinal muscle layer in the rectum, and the answer is that no one knows. Nevertheless, I suspect that in the rectum, where the longitudinal layer is uniformly distributed around the circumference, this probably has a good deal to do with regulating the length of that segment and perhaps that's where the disease begins, in the function of that muscle layer.

Swash: That is what Sir Arbuthnot Lane thought in 1900, when he was perfecting colectomy. He thought that the colon was redundant and could therefore be removed. It became a socially acceptable operation, and he was lampooned, in George Bernard Shaw's *The Doctor's Dilemma*!

Burnstock: Isn't the longitudinal muscle coat in the human rectum thicker, relative to the circular coat, than in any other region of the gut? If this were so in humans, as it certainly is in many other mammals, you would expect it to have an important role.

Christensen: Yes. This coat is relatively very much thicker in the rectum than elsewhere in the gut. It is about equal in thickness to the circular layer in the rectum, whereas in the small intestine it is only about one-fifth the thickness of the circular muscle layer.

Wong: We don't see a longer rectum in patients with rectal prolapse, but we do see a lot of laxity of the lateral ligaments and a long rectal mesentery. There is redundancy higher up, certainly in the sigmoid and proximal colon, in many prolapse patients. This may tie in with the work John DeLancey described with respect to smooth muscle and collagen abnormalities in the more anterior structures in female patients with weak pelvic floors. These abnormalities may also be occurring in rectal prolapse patients with loss of smooth muscle or collagen. We see very flimsy lateral ligaments in these patients.

Christensen: What we call lateral ligaments are really small bundles of smooth muscle, aren't they?

Wong: They are condensations of endopelvic fascia, which do contain smooth muscle.

Marsden: Michael Swash said earlier that if you ask them, many of the people with apparently isolated rectal incontinence prove to have urinary symptoms as well. This provokes the question of what happens to urinary incontinence after surgery for rectal incontinence.

Bartolo: Some get better and some get worse! Many improve. We have tried to do urodynamics on patients and it has been somewhat difficult, so I haven't got the data.

Marsden: Those who get better do so despite, presumably, no improvement in the denervation of their urethral sphincters, or even perhaps a worsening?

Swash: Yes, but that recovery might be a mechanical effect of the surgery; a number of the gynaecological procedures used for treating urinary incontinence have a stabilizing effect on the pelvic floor.

Marsden: Do I take it that the operation that David Bartolo does for rectal incontinence is called something different, but really is the same operation as Mr Stanton does?

Stanton: I wouldn't do a post-anal repair; it's far too specialized! I operate on posterior wall prolapse of rectum into vagina, without incontinence or mucosal or rectal prolapse. The only similarity comes in the last part that David Bartolo described, when we pull together the levator ani muscle, which is after you have done your main surgery.

Kirby: The lateral ligaments are where the pelvic nerves to the bladder sweep round the side of the rectum to go in underneath the trigone, so you would expect there to be a parasympathetic decentralization from a neuronopraxis, either from the traction on these or from an actual division of the nerves. Do the patients not get bladder dysfunction? After gynaecological operations of that type, urinary retention is common.

Bartolo: It depends how the operation is done. Some surgeons simply put their hand behind the rectum and pull very hard; they inevitably divide all the autonomic nerves. But you can do a careful anatomical dissection, preserving all the nerves, and finally divide the lateral ligament close to the rectum; so we hope we do not damage the autonomic nerves to the bladder, or make the patients impotent, or divide the nervi erigentes. These can occasionally be seen running lateral to the lateral ligaments. I assume we are dividing the parasympathetic output to the rectum.

Kuijpers: You don't see constipation after a low anterior resection, which is strange. You mobilize the rectum, and yet do not see any constipation.

Bartolo: Many surgeons do observe very severe constipation after rectopexy.

Kuijpers: I know; we have a 50% incidence.

Swash: Is that associated physiologically with slow transit through the lower part of the gut?

Kuijpers: Yes, colonic slow transit.

Wong: Many prolapse patients have pre-existing constipation, to the point that one of my colleagues states that if you don't improve the constipation, in your treatment of these patients, then you don't help the patient. He (Dr Stanley M. Goldberg) will do a subtotal colectomy in addition to rectopexy in patients with combined slow colonic transit and rectal prolapse.

Christensen: It's worth pointing out that the vagal innervation of the colon extends in some mammals well beyond the caecum, so when you resect distal to the mid-colon, you are resecting the part that you have denervated.

Bartolo: But what is the effect of doing that? You would expect that if you left the left colon in, all your patients would be constipated, if you have divided the parasympathetic nerves.

Christensen: It would depend on whether you divided them all.

Bartolo: I don't know where they are, unfortunately.

Christensen: The question is whether all the parasympathetic innervation of the left colon comes in at the level of the rectum and then ascends in the shunt fascicles or ascending colonic nerves, or whether there is a component from the pudendal nerves or other pathways.

Bartolo: But where do they come in?

Christensen: I don't know where parasympathetic nerves come in, in man! In cats they enter the colon at the top of the rectum, at the level of the recto-sigmoid junction, fairly high up (Christensen et al 1984, Christensen & Rick 1987).

Bartolo: So they come in with the sympathetic nerves?

Christensen: I don't know, because I haven't looked at the sympathetic nerve pathways.

Brindley: Could you not tell whether you have denervated the rectum by the results of rectal manometry? Do the rectums that you fear you have denervated respond by contraction when you fill them?

Bartolo: All I can say is that the volume of first sensation, recorded by infusion manometry, falls after Ivalon retropexy. One could argue that this is a reaction to the foreign material placed around the rectum (Ivalon is a potent inflammatory agent). But in patients in whom we haven't put in an implant (suture retropexy) we still see a reduction in this volume at first sensation. I am therefore keen to do ambulatory studies, because in a physiological setting, or the closest we can get to it, we may see changes in rectal motor activity. So far, we have been unable to look at proper rectal evoked contractions.

Brindley: In this investigation, you fill the rectum with liquid and ask the patients whether they feel it. You also record pressure, so were there pressure responses before and after the operation?

Bartolo: We are not looking at rectal contractility; we just look at the crude pressure generated by infusing liquid into the rectum.

Brindley: But if you fill the normal rectum quickly, it gives contraction waves. Does it do so in these patients?

Bartolo: It depends how you do it. If you put 50 ml into the rectum you see a rectal contraction which then relaxes. But we have given a constant infusion, so all we see is a straight line.

de Groat: The follow-up of the improvement of sensation is important to evaluate. It would be nice to know whether sensations in the rectum, in the anal canal and in the various other structures that are left untouched do change in a parallel way, after surgery.

Does the denervation after some of the surgical procedures involve the pudendal innervation of the pelvic floor? If you damaged that innervation, you would also interfere with anal canal sensation, which is probably mediated through the pudendal nerve. Do anal canal sensation and rectal sensation change? Do you think that because of the rectal prolapse, there may be damage to those nerves, and that by suspending the intestine you allow some of those nerves to grow back into that region, or extend to that region, and that this contributes to improvement in sensation? Or is there expansion of the pudendal afferent system from the anal canal along into the rectum which has been denervated by your surgical procedure?

Perhaps, as Michael Swash has suggested, the sensation is not occurring from mucosal afferents, or even afferents in the wall of the rectum, but from afferents in the striated muscle or the pelvic floor muscles which surround the rectum. Do you have any feelings about whether the sensation is intramucosal, within the wall, or extra-rectal? And have you looked at the various sensations in the different parts of the bowel that remain?

Bartolo: All we have done is looked at rectal sensation in the way I described and at anal canal sensation. There is evidence to suggest that a lot of rectal sensation is in the pelvic floor musculature, but there is no doubt that when the rectum is removed and replaced by ileum, patients still have an awareness of rectal filling, but it isn't the same as that induced by the normal rectum. So there must be an element of sensation induced from the rectum itself; but I can't say more than that.

de Groat: If you remove the rectum and put ileum in its place, I presume that the rectal-to-internal anal canal reflex will be eliminated. I believe the myenteric plexus is like the brain, in that reinnervation is limited. Does the loss of reflex connections from the bowel into the internal anal region have any role in the reduction of symptoms that you see in these patients?

Bartolo: This was one of the most disappointing things about these studies. I had wondered if we would alter the threshold of recto-anal inhibition, because we did the tests on all patients. They all had a recto-anal inhibitory reflex, but the volume producing complete inhibition didn't change after surgery. I had hoped that we were perhaps removing a bolus from the rectum, a prolapse, and so the internal sphincter was recovering and was no longer relaxing, as it was preoperatively. But we have no evidence for that.

Maggi: I wonder whether the nerve lesions that you may produce during surgical intervention may lead to the formation of neuromas. It is known that if you cut a somatic nerve you can induce them. The properties of the neuroma are very different from those of a normal sensory nerve terminal, with differences in the electrical properties and possibly the expression of new receptors which are not normally present on nerve terminals and give abnormal excitation. Could this occur in a visceral nerve? If so, perhaps an abnormal afferent input generated at the level of the neuroma could be the cause of the functional disturbances.

Marsden: Does one get neuromas with autonomic nerves?

Burnstock: Sympathetic hyperinnervation occurs at severed nerve stumps. ATP receptors are present on sensory neurons (Krishtal et al 1983) and sympathetic nerves release ATP in addition to noradrenaline (see Burnstock 1988). Guanethidine, which prevents the release of ATP as well as noradrenaline, is particularly effective in preventing long-term pain or causalgia, whereas the adrenoreceptor antagonists are less effective.

I am concerned by the way people talk of a 'denervated' rectum. The rectum is loaded with nerves, including large numbers of intrinsic neurons; so there is no way of denervating it, either chemically or surgically. You can sympathetically denervate the rectum, or denervate it of parasympathetic preganglionic fibres, but you are only removing a small proportion of the total innervation in this way.

Stanton: Would 'decentralized' be a better term?

Burnstock: Yes, although this is not always easy to achieve surgically, because of the number of small as well as large nerve bundles that enter the organ.

Brindley: The word has always been used by physiologists to mean cutting the external nerve connections, rather than any internal nervous structures.

Burnstock: People who transplant hearts often neglect to take into account the fact that the heart contains many intrinsic neurons that may proliferate and replace extrinsically denervated target sites. Many people sometimes fail to recognize that there are intrinsic neurons in the airways and in the bladder too.

de Groat: We tend to think of the pudendal nerve as a somatic nerve and the pelvic nerve as a parasympathetic nerve, and we talk in humans about the presacral nerves being sympathetic. It is probably not true that these nerves are so homogeneous. The pelvic nerve of many mammals contains thousands of sympathetic postganglionic fibres that come from the sympathetic chain ganglia, so it's a mixed nerve, both sympathetic and parasympathetic. In addition, in the pudendal nerve there are many sympathetic postganglionic axons that come from the sympathetic chain. Geoff Burnstock mentioned sympathectomy; it is important to realize, however, that following transection of sympathetic nerves, if the pudendal and pelvic nerves are intact, sympathetic axons from these nerves could grow back into the organs and reinnervate them. Thus it might be very difficult in this region of the viscera to produce a sympathectomy surgically, because of all the nerves carrying sympathetic fibres.

Swash: When the gut has been transected at gut resection, do the Auerbach and Meissner plexuses re-grow, re-form their connections and function as normal? Does the recto-anal reflex occur again, and does peristalsis occur normally?

Burnstock: I am not aware of many modern studies of this kind. Judging by the reinnervation of aganglionic colonic segments in Hirschsprung's disease, sympathetic fibres appear to grow readily into the aganglionic areas, but the intrinsic neurons seem reluctant to send collateral sprouts into these sites. This may be because appropriate nerve growth factors for peptidergic nerves are not produced.

Brading: Perhaps there is some link through the smooth muscle cells. Movement could trigger sensory nerves, so that you get reflex activity propagated past a block.

If I had to undergo an operation such as David Bartolo was discussing, I would be very careful for months afterwards with my diet, and my bowel habits. In other words, how much of the improvement that you see is purely the result of psychologically induced changes in behaviour?

Bartolo: This is a very good point. All our data are generated by either a physiology technician or a research fellow; it is very important that the surgeon doesn't ask the patient the question about improvement, because all our patients want to please us, and it is important that someone totally objective and independent asks the questions. We had a control group receiving biofeedback in our previous study of post-anal repair, and we had very poor results from biofeedback therapy for incontinence, so purely psychological effects seem unlikely.

Christensen: One particular mammal, I believe the Brazilian opossum, recently introduced into the USA as an experimental animal, regularly develops fatal rectal prolapse unless given a particular diet. Do any other species develop rectal prolapse on abnormal diets?

Bartolo: Many horses develop it. I don't think they need treatment. It's very common.

Kuijpers: Prolapse is normal during defaecation in horses.

Christensen: But that is not a permanent prolapse, whereas it is in the Brazilian opossum, in which it becomes infected and causes death.

Bartolo: The same would happen in humans: most people push their prolapse back, or it returns spontaneously. If you don't, it becomes gangrenous.

References

Burnstock G 1988 Sympathetic purinergic transmission in small blood vessels. Trends Pharmacol Sci 9:116–117

Christensen J, Rick GA 1987 The distribution of myelinated nerves in the ascending nerves and myenteric plexus of the cat colon. Am J Anat 178:250–258

Christensen J, Stiles MJ, Rick GA, Sutherland J 1984 Comparative anatomy of the myenteric plexus of the distal colon in eight mammals. Gastroenterology 86:706–713

Krishtal OA, Marchenko SM, Pidoplichko VI 1983 Receptor for ATP in the membrane of mammalian sensory neurones. Neurosci Lett 35:41–45

Laurberg S, Swash M, Henry MM 1990 Does postanal repair accelerate neurogenic damage to the pelvic floor? Br J Surg, in press

Surgical approaches to anal incontinence

W. Douglas Wong and David A. Rothenberger

Division of Colon and Rectal Surgery, University of Minnesota Medical School, Box 450, Mayo Building, 420 Delaware Street SE, Minneapolis, MN 55455, USA

Abstract. Primary repair of acute anal sphincter injuries by direct apposition of the severed external sphincter without tension is advisable whenever feasible. However, the majority of patients who are candidates for surgical treatment of anal incontinence will undergo a secondary repair, the type of which will depend on the underlying aetiology and the surgeon's preference and experience. The most successful of these procedures is sphincter reconstruction with or without levatoroplasty for a disrupted anal sphincter (due to surgical, obstetrical or other trauma) in the absence of underlying neurological damage. Success rates are reported at 80–90%. Post-anal repair is advocated for patients with a poorly functioning sphincter with an obtuse anorectal angle, most of whom have a neurogenic basis for their incontinence. Success rates vary from 60 to 75% of cases but long-term results have been less satisfactory. Rectal procidentia is associated with faecal incontinence in 65–75% of cases. Abdominal repair (we favour suture rectopexy with sigmoid resection) restores continence in 50–80% of such patients. Patients with persisting incontinence are candidates for post-anal repair. Anal encirclement with an elastic, Dacron®-impregnated Silastic® sleeve has a limited role in selected patients. For more severe incontinence, muscle transfers (gracilis, gluteus maximus, etc.) can achieve some success but continence is less than perfect. We are currently assessing the use of an artificial anal sphincter (a modification of the AMS 800™ urinary sphincter). For patients who fail all therapeutic options, a stoma will provide a better lifestyle than coping with the consequences of faecal incontinence.

1990 Neurobiology of Incontinence. Wiley, Chichester (Ciba Foundation Symposium 151) p 246–266

Anal incontinence can be a severely incapacitating, albeit benign, disorder, which can devastate the lives of afflicted individuals. While properly directed medical therapy improves a considerable number of patients, there remain a subgroup who do not respond well enough to carry on a normal lifestyle. Many of these will be candidates for one of a variety of surgical approaches, depending on the assessment of the patient's general condition and the underlying aetiology of the incontinence. Those who are significantly incontinent of normal formed stool are most likely to benefit from surgery (Henry 1987). A thorough working knowledge of anorectal and pelvic floor anatomy and physiology is essential for any surgeon undertaking a surgical repair for anal incontinence. A classification of surgical procedures is tabulated in Table 1.

I. Primary repair

An acute, traumatic sphincter injury should be repaired primarily whenever possible by direct suture apposition with 2-O polyglycolic acid horizontal mattress sutures. Those patients with extensive local trauma and significant tissue loss, and those with concomitant life-threatening injuries, are best treated with debridement, colostomy and delayed sphincter repair.

TABLE 1 Surgical therapy for anal incontinence

I. Primary repair
   Apposition versus overlap ± temporary colostomy

II. Secondary repair
   Imbrication sphincteroplasty
      Overlapping repair
      Levatoroplasty with overlapping repair
      Plication repair
   Post-anal repair

III. Correction of underlying disease or condition
   Rectal procidentia
      Rectopexy with sigmoid resection ± levatoroplasty
      Perineal rectosigmoidectomy ± levatoroplasty
      Delorme procedure ± levatoroplasty
   Carcinoma—restorative resection
   Infection—drainage/antibiotics
   Radiation—restorative resection
   Inflammatory bowel disease—restorative resection

IV. Encirclement procedures
   Foreign material
      Thiersch procedure
      Dacron®-impregnated Silastic®
      Artificial bowel sphincter
   Muscle transfer
      Gracilis and other skeletal muscles
      Free muscle transplants

V. Stoma procedure (colostomy)

Adapted from Rothenberger 1989.

II. Secondary repair

A. *Imbrication sphincteroplasty*

This is the procedure of choice for the secondary repair of disrupted anal sphincter injuries. After a complete whole-gut lavage with polyethylene glycol solution and administration of prophylactic antibiotics, the severed ends of the external sphincter are mobilized from the scar and surrounding tissues (Fig. 1). At this point a decision is made as to the best method of reconstructing the sphincter mechanism.

1. Overlapping repair (Fig. 1).   This procedure is chosen if the sphincter injury was distal and the ends of the muscle are completely divided. Fang et al (1984) have emphasized the importance of retaining the scar on the two ends of the severed muscle. After these two scarred ends have been mobilized, the muscles

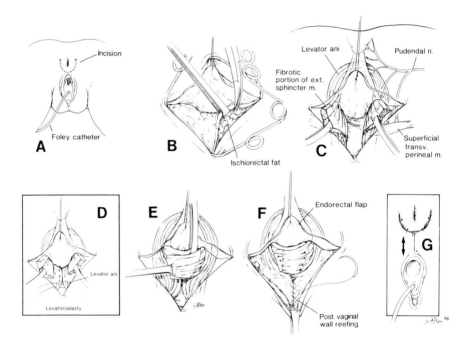

FIG. 1.   Imbrication sphincteroplasty. (A) The patient is in the prone jack-knife position. A curvilinear incision is made over the sphincter defect which is usually anterior. (B) A flap of anoderm, mucosa, and submucosa is raised and the external sphincter dissected. (C) The external sphincter ends with adjacent scar tissue are completely mobilized. (D) For severe injuries, an anterior levatoroplasty is performed. (E and F) An overlapping sphincteroplasty is performed using horizontal mattress sutures. (G) The flap of anoderm and mucosa is loosely tacked over the reconstructed muscle, and perineal body skin coverage is achieved vertically.

are overlapped and sutured with two rows of 2-O polyglycolic acid horizontal mattress sutures which are placed in the preserved scar tissue, which holds the sutures more securely than the soft muscle. The sutures are then tied to achieve a snug repair which should feel tight to the fifth digit.

2. Levatoroplasty with overlapping repair (Fig. 1D).   For more severe injuries in which the entire sphincter mechanism has been disrupted, a plication of the anterior levator muscles is performed before the overlapping sphincteroplasty. The purpose of adding this levatoroplasty in such injuries is to both strengthen and lengthen the anal canal, which we believe improves continence.

3. Plication repair.   In less severe injuries, after mobilization of the sphincter it may be evident that the muscle is not completely divided but rather attenuated anteriorly. In this instance, rather than dividing the splayed out, but intact muscle, a plication of the intact muscle and scar is achieved using horizontal mattress sutures rather than the conventional overlapping repair.

After any three of these modifications of imbrication sphincteroplasty the wound can be left open and packed lightly with Nu gauze® or, in selected cases, closed primarily. We do not feel that it is necessary to perform a stoma procedure when undertaking such repairs. Motson (1985) made a survey of various authors performing sphincter repair and noted that surgeons in North America rarely use a colostomy, while those in Australia and the United Kingdom use it more frequently. He noted, however, that there were significant differences in the patient populations, with the majority being obstetrical injuries in North America and operative injuries in the United Kingdom.

Results of imbrication sphincteroplasty

Fang et al (1984) had previously reported the results at the University of Minnesota with an overall 90% success rate with imbrication sphincteroplasty. Other centres have reported similarly satisfactory results with sphincter repair (Browning & Motson 1983, Corman 1985). It should be noted that a concomitant rectovaginal fistula, which accompanies such injuries in a significant number of female patients, can be directly repaired using this imbrication sphincteroplasty.

The causes of failure of this sphincteroplasty procedure consist largely of early postoperative sepsis, fistula formation, and pelvic floor neuropathy (Browning & Motson 1983, Yoshioka & Keighley 1989). Laurberg et al (1988) have emphasized the importance of ruling out a neurological deficit in those patients sustaining a birth injury. They reported that 47% of 19 patients with obstetrical injury had an associated neurological deficit, as determined by EMG assessment. Of nine patients with an associated neurological deficit, only one achieved an excellent or good result with sphincteroplasty. On the other hand, of 10 patients with no identifiable neurological deficit, eight achieved excellent or good postoperative results. This emphasizes the need for preoperative physiological assessment in patients with such injuries.

Yoshioka & Keighley (1989) were unable to demonstrate any significant change in the maximum anal resting pressure or maximum squeeze pressures when assessed both preoperatively and postoperatively in patients undergoing a sphincter repair. They did note, however, that those patients with higher pre-operative squeeze pressures generally achieved better continence postoperatively.

We have compared the preoperative and postoperative manometric assessment of anal sphincter function in 12 women sustaining birth-related injuries. After sphincteroplasty all 12 patients described some improvement of their continence, when a subjective assessment was compared pre- and postoperatively. Nine of the 12 patients were totally continent or only very rarely incontinent to flatus after surgery (Group 1). Three patients, however, remained partially incontinent (Group 2). When the preoperative and postoperative manometric assessments on these two groups were compared, the nine patients in Group 1 who had achieved total continence all had at least a 1.5-fold increase in their maximum voluntary contractions at two consecutive 1 cm intervals within the anal canal. Eight of the nine patients had a similar 1.5-fold increase in their resting pressures postoperatively. Of the three patients classified as a poor result (Group 2), two had improvement in maximum voluntary contractions greater than or equal to 1.5 times the preoperative manometric pressures. However, it may be of some importance that none of the patients in this group of three had any significant improvement in their greatest resting pressure. This would suggest that in order for a satisfactory postoperative result to be achieved, improvement in both maximum voluntary contraction and resting pressure is needed. It was also demonstrated that a lengthening of the effective high pressure zone by the repair appeared to correlate with better postoperative function (M. Lawrence et al 1989, unpublished work).

B. Post-anal repair

The post-anal repair was originally proposed by Parks (1975) for patients with anal incontinence who have an intact but poorly functioning sphincter and a wide anorectal angle. The intention as first proposed was to restore the anorectal angle and lengthen the anal canal by performing a posterior levatoroplasty through an intersphincteric approach. Candidates for this procedure are those with neurogenic incontinence; patients with obstetrical injuries in which there has not been disruption of the sphincter ring, but rather prolonged labour and a secondary pelvic floor neuropathy with subsequent incontinence; patients who fail an imbrication sphincteroplasty; and patients who failed to have their continence restored after repair of a rectal prolapse. The technique is outlined in Fig. 2.

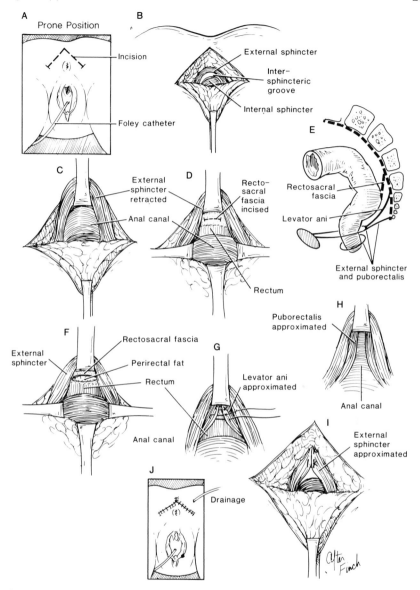

FIG. 2. Parks' post-anal repair. (A) The patient is in the prone jack-knife position. An incision is made as shown. (B) The intersphincteric plane is dissected. (C) The external sphincter is retracted. (D and E) The rectosacral fascia is incised. (F) Perirectal fat is swept off laterally to expose the levator ani muscles. (G and H) The levators are approximated with horizontal mattress sutures. (I) Plicating sutures are placed in the external sphincter muscle. (J) The incision is closed over a closed suction drain. (Reproduced with permission of B. C. Decker Inc. from Rothenberger DA Anal Incontinence. In: Cameron JL (ed) Current surgical therapy, 3rd edn. Toronto: B. C. Decker, 1989.)

Initial restoration of faecal continence has been reported at about 80% after post-anal repair (Parks 1975, Womack et al 1988). At the University of Minnesota we have not been able to duplicate these results. Our results are similar to those reported by Miller et al (1988), with 59% achieving a successful repair. A long-term follow-up of patients undergoing a post-anal repair by Yoshioka et al (1988) has indicated that only about 34% of patients become completely continent.

Most patients with anal incontinence will have diminished anal canal pressures, diminished anal sphincter length, and an obtuse anorectal angle. The post-anal repair was predicated upon the belief that the flap-valve theory played a significant role in continence. The operation was therefore designed to restore the anorectal angle and increase sphincter length by plication of the posterior pelvic floor muscles. Physiological studies after post-anal repair have been somewhat contradictory. Browning et al (1984) have reported an increase in anal canal length and resting and squeeze pressures after post-anal repair. Preston et al (1984) have reported that the anorectal angle is accentuated in patients undergoing a successful post-anal repair. On the other hand, Miller et al (1988) documented no change in the anorectal angle, although resting and squeeze pressures improved. Other studies have failed to demonstrate any alteration either in the anorectal angle or in resting or squeeze pressures (Yoshioka et al 1988, Womack et al 1988). These findings therefore cast doubt on the validity of the flap-valve theory and the role, if any, of the anorectal angle in maintaining continence. Womack et al (1988) have concluded, on the basis of their results, that post-anal repair should not be restricted to patients with widening of the anorectal angle, because the beneficial effects of the surgery do not appear to be related to any reduction in this parameter. Several authors have documented a consistent increase in anal canal length in those patients achieving a satisfactory result after post-anal repair (Browning & Parks 1983, Womack et al 1988, Yoshioka et al 1988).

It is unclear why some patients benefit from post-anal repair and others do not. It would seem evident that the beneficial effect is not due to any reduction of the anorectal angle and that a wide anorectal angle is not necessarily a prerequisite for this procedure. Parks' proposal that the beneficial effect was due to increased efficiency of function of the voluntary anal sphincter muscles would not seem to be substantiated by the failure of two major studies to show any improvement in either basal or maximum voluntary contraction. The increase in the anal canal length appears to be the one factor that is consistently improved and that may correlate with a successful outcome.

III. Surgical procedures directed at an underlying condition

Patients with rectal procidentia have an associated anal incontinence rate of about 65–75% (Broden et al 1988, Yoshioka et al 1989). Surgery for their incontinence is best directed at the underlying prolapse in the first instance.

For good-risk patients we prefer an abdominal rectopexy and sigmoid resection. In our hands this procedure restores continence in over 50% of patients (Watts et al 1985). For poor-risk patients we prefer a perineal rectosigmoidectomy or alternatively a Delorme procedure. However, restoration of continence is less likely after a perineal procedure than after an abdominal procedure. If preoperative anorectal physiological assessment has revealed a short anal canal with low pressures, consideration may be given to concomitant levatoroplasty when either the perineal rectosigmoidectomy or Delorme procedure is performed.

Broden et al (1988) reported on 15 patients with rectal prolapse repaired by a Ripstein technique. Sixty-seven per cent of the patients (10/15) were incontinent preoperatively, while postoperatively continence was restored in the majority with only 20% (3/15) remaining incontinent. Broden et al (1988) noted an improvement in resting pressures when postoperative pressures were assessed and compared to preoperative pressures. Those patients in whom continence was not restored continued to have very low resting pressures.

Yoshioka et al (1989) reported on 12 patients with overt rectal prolapse, nine of whom were incontinent. Six of these were subsequently rendered continent by abdominal rectopexy. The authors noted preoperative diminished resting pressures and maximum squeeze pressures and an obtuse anorectal angle in these patients, by comparison with normal controls, and were unable to demonstrate any change in these parameters after rectopexy.

At the University of Minnesota we have studied 23 patients with rectal prolapse, before and after surgical repair. Fourteen of the 23 patients were incontinent preoperatively, whereas only five remained so after repair. In the whole group there was a significant increase postoperatively in both resting anal pressure and maximum voluntary contraction pressure (J. G. Williams et al 1989, unpublished work).

If significant incontinence persists for six months or so after procidentia repair, a post-anal repair is advocated, with the expectation that up to 50% of these patients will have continence restored.

IV. Encirclement procedures

Some patients with anal incontinence have insufficient functional muscle mass to allow a secondary repair. Other patients have such severe neurogenic incontinence despite an intact sphincter muscle that total incontinence is present. In such instances, alternative procedures making use of an encirclement procedure with either skeletal muscle transfer or synthetic material may be considered.

A. Muscle transfers

When a direct repair is impossible, or for those patients in whom multiple attempts at repair have failed and who refuse a colostomy, a muscle transfer may be considered as a last resort. The two muscles commonly used for this are the gracilis muscle or alternatively the gluteus maximus muscle. Although our experience is limited, we prefer the gracilis muscle at the University of Minnesota. The technique is outlined in Fig. 3. Pickrell et al (1952) proposed the transplantation of a gracilis muscle with its retained vascular and nervous supply to surround the anal canal. The results of this operation, however, have been variable. Leguit et al (1985) reported on 10 patients with a six-month to 17-year follow-up. Ninety per cent of patients were continent to formed faeces, whereas one patient was worsened after the procedure. Yoshioka & Keighley (1988) reported six cases treated with a gracilis muscle transplant with poor functional results in all patients, all of whom were ultimately treated with colostomy. They found no objective improvement in resting or voluntary pressure postoperatively in their patients.

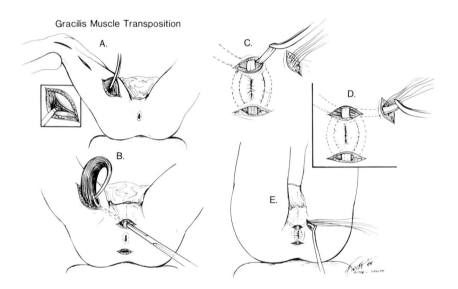

FIG. 3.   Gracilis muscle transposition. (A) The patient is in a modified lithotomy position. Three incisions are used to mobilize the gracilis muscle. (B) Two incisions are made posterior and anterior to the anus to expose the midline raphe. A tunnel is developed between the anterior perianal incision and the proximal thigh incision. The gracilis muscle is brought through the tunnel. (C) The gracilis muscle is passed under the anterior raphe around and under the posterior raphe and around to the anterior incision behind the muscle belly. (D) The fascia overlying the contralateral ischial tuberosity is exposed. Sutures are placed in this fascia, and the tendinous portion of the gracilis muscle is pulled through a tunnel to this site. (E) The leg is adducted, the tendon is pulled taut, and sutures are used to secure the gracilis tendon to the ischial tuberosity. (Reproduced with permission of B. C. Decker Inc. from Rothenberger DA Anal incontinence. In Cameron JL (ed) Current surgical therapy, 3rd edn. Toronto: B. C. Decker, 1989.)

Implantation of a neuromuscular stimulator has been reported to increase the function of a gracilis muscle transposition (Baeten et al 1988).

The use of muscle transfers to restore continence has a limited role in the surgical approach to incontinence. In properly selected, motivated patients, who are particularly anxious to avoid a colostomy, this operation may achieve a successful result, although continence is generally less than perfect.

B. Synthetic encirclement procedure

1. Dacron®-impregnated Silastic®. The use of a Dacron®-impregnated Silastic® sheet as a modified Thiersch procedure for the correction of rectal prolapse and anal incontinence was first reported by Labow et al in 1980. The Silastic sheet is cut into a 2 cm strip. A tunnel is developed through two lateral incisions over the ischiorectal fossae and the Silastic material is placed so as to encircle the anal canal. The Lahey clinic have reported their experience in 11 patients undergoing this procedure, six of whom obtained improved faecal continence. They reported a 25% extrusion and infection rate (Horn et al 1985). Despite the elasticity of this material, the anal canal does not gain any dynamic function after implantation and there is a significant incidence of infection and extrusion. We currently do not use the Silastic sling for anal incontinence.

2. Artificial anal sphincter. In order to provide an alternative for patients who either fail traditional surgical repair or are not candidates for procedures to restore their continence, the concept of a totally implantable artificial bowel sphincter has been tried in animals and humans since the advent of medical-grade silicone. We are currently taking part in a three-centre clinical trial to test an artificial sphincter device designed to provide continence to faeces and to allow defaecation at will. This American Medical System's bowel sphincter will be similar to the AMS Sphincter 800™, an artificial urinary sphincter prosthesis which is currently in commercial distribution. Modifications to the device have been made to allow for its use in the anal region.

The success of the artificial urinary sphincter, which was first implanted in 1972, has stimulated much interest in its use to control faecal incontinence. The artificial urinary sphincter has been implanted in over 4000 children and adults and experience has shown that it is safe, well tolerated, and very effective.

The AMS Sphincter 800™ was designed for use in both adults and children and consists of three main parts: (A) a pressure-regulating balloon; (B) a control pump; and (C) an occlusive cuff (sphincter) (Fig. 4). When implanted this prosthesis simulates normal sphincter function by opening and closing at the control of the patient. When the patient wishes to evacuate, he/she simply squeezes the control pump, which has been implanted in the scrotum or labium, several times. This causes fluid to move from the pressurized cuff into the pressure-regulating balloon and thus deflates the cuff to allow evacuation to

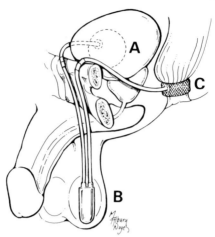

FIG. 4.   Artificial anal sphincter in a male patient. (A) Pressure-regulating balloon.
(B) Control pump. (C) Occlusive cuff. Repeated squeezing of the control pump (B) causes
fluid to move from the pressurized cuff (C) into the pressure-regulating balloon (A),
thereby deflating the cuff to allow defaecation. The fluid then slowly returns to the cuff
from the balloon over the ensuing 7–10 minutes.

occur. Over the next several minutes the balloon then automatically repressurizes
the cuff and continence is again restored. The control pump is designed to allow
the implanted device to be deactivated for extended lengths of time without
additional surgery.

Patients undergo a complete bowel washout with Colyte®, and antibiotic
prophylaxis is instituted. Two lateral circumferential incisions approximately
3 cm long are made over the ischiorectal region bilaterally. These are deepened
into the ischiorectal fossae on either side and a tunnel is created around the
anal canal outside the external sphincter. Pulleys are established, utilizing the
raphe of the transverse perinei muscle anteriorly and the anococcygeal raphe
posteriorly. This allows the cuff to be placed in the correct position around
the anal canal and will maintain it in position cephalad enough to prevent erosion
distally. The connecting tubing from the cuff is tunnelled subcutaneously into
the suprapubic region and the pump is tunnelled subcutaneously into one side
of the scrotum or labium majora. The pressure-regulating balloon is placed into
the space of Retzius through a small Pfannenstiel incision. The two connections
between the pressure-regulating balloon and the pump and the cuff and the pump
are made subcutaneously in the suprapubic region. All wounds are meticulously
closed. The system is left deactivated postoperatively, with the first activation
of the device planned for about six weeks postoperatively.

Christiansen & Lorentzen (1989) have recently reported on their initial
experience with five patients with neurogenic incontinence treated with the

TABLE 2 Results of installation of an artificial anal sphincter in two female patients

Age (years)	Pre-existing stoma	Aetiology	Continence			Complications	Follow-up (months)
			Solid	Liquid	Gas		
32	Yes	Obstetric injury (multiple failed repairs)	Yes	Yes	Yes	None	5
42	No	Obstetric injury (multiple failed repairs)	No	No	No	Seroma Dehiscence Secondary infection Removal of device	2

artificial 800 urinary sphincter placed around the anus. These five patients ranged in age from 25 to 67. The device was activated early in the postoperative period, generally between 10 and 14 days. The authors noted that the system worked with solid or semi-solid stool but less satisfactorily when diarrhoea was present. One of their five patients was a failure because of infection, which necessitated removal of the system. Of the remaining patients, three have achieved good results, with one fair result.

In Minnesota we have performed this procedure on two patients so far, both female. One patient has been extremely successful; however, the other developed a seroma early in the postoperative period which drained spontaneously and subsequently became infected, requiring total removal of the device. The successful patient had an existing stoma at the time her device was implanted. After activation of the device and colostomy closure she has been totally continent of stool and gas. The follow-up to date in this patient is relatively short, only five months. The results of our two patients are shown in Table 2.

The artificial urinary sphincter has been very successful for urinary incontinence, with a very low mechanical failure rate and infection rate. From this experience it is reasonable to believe that the risk of mechanical failure and infection should be acceptable when the device is used in the anal region for anal incontinence. The preliminary results with implantation of an artificial bowel sphincter for anal incontinence are encouraging. Several modifications to the device are currently being made which are expected to better adapt this device for our purposes. Long-term follow-up with respect to function and complications will be critical to the ultimate success of this procedure. It is far too early in our experience to make any judgements. It is hoped that the three-centre trial in which we are now participating will establish this as a viable option for patients who have no other alternative but a stoma procedure for the devastating consequences of anal incontinence.

V. Stoma procedure

When the surgical repairs discussed in this chapter either have failed or have no reasonable chance of succeeding, it should be remembered that a stoma will provide the patient afflicted with anal incontinence with a much better quality of life and a more satisfactory lifestyle than suffering the daily ravages of faecal incontinence. An end-sigmoid colostomy is the preferred stoma whenever feasible.

References

Baeten C, Spaans F, Fluks A 1988 An implanted neuromuscular stimulator for fecal continence following previously implanted gracilis muscle—a report of a case. Dis Colon Rectum 31:134–137

Broden G, Dolk A, Holmstrom B 1988 Recovery of the internal anal sphincter following rectopexy: a possible explanation for continence improvement. Int J Colorectal Dis 3:23–28

Browning GGP, Motson RW 1983 Results of Parks' operation for faecal incontinence after anal sphincter injury. Br Med J 286:1873–1875

Browning GGP, Parks AG 1983 Postanal repair for neuropathic faecal incontinence: correlation of clinical result and anal canal pressures. Br J Surg 70:101–104

Browning GGP, Rutter KRP, Motson RW, Neill ME 1984 Postanal repair for idiopathic faecal incontinence. Ann R Coll Surg Engl (Suppl):30–33

Christiansen J, Lorentzen M 1989 Implantation of artificial sphincter for anal incontinence. Dis Colon Rectum 32:432–436

Corman ML 1985 Anal incontinence following obstetrical injury. Dis Colon Rectum 28:86–89

Fang DT, Nivatvongs S, Vermeulen FD, Herman FN, Goldberg SM, Rothenberger DA 1984 Overlapping sphincteroplasty for acquired anal incontinence. Dis Colon Rectum 27:720–722

Henry MM 1987 Pathogenesis and management of fecal incontinence in the adult. Gastroenterol Clin North Am 16:35–45

Horn HR, Schoetz DJ, Coller JA, Veidenheimer MC 1985 Sphincter repair with a Silastic® sling for anal incontinence and rectal procidentia. Dis Colon Rectum 28:868–872

Labow S, Rubin RJ, Hoexter B, Salvati EP 1980 Perineal repair of rectal procidentia with an elastic fabric sling. Dis Colon Rectum 23:467–469

Laurberg S, Swash M, Henry MM 1988 Delayed external sphincter repair for obstetric tear. Br J Surg 75:786–788

Leguit P Jr, van Baal JG, Brummelkamp WH 1985 Gracilis muscle transposition in the treatment of fecal incontinence; long-term follow-up and evaluation of anal pressure recordings. Dis Colon Rectum 28:1–4

Miller R, Bartolo DCC, Locke-Edmunds JC, Mortensen NJMcC 1988 Prospective study of conservative and operative treatment for faecal incontinence. Br J Surg 75:101–105

Motson RW 1985 Sphincter injuries: indications for, and results of sphincter repair. Br J Surg 72(Suppl):S19–S21

Parks AG 1975 Anorectal incontinence. Proc R Soc Med 68:681–691

Pickrell KL, Broadbent TR, Masters FW, Metzger JT 1952 Construction of a rectal sphincter and restoration of anal continence by transplanting the gracilis muscle. Ann Surg 135:853–862

Preston DM, Lennard-Jones ME, Thomas BM 1984 The balloon proctogram. Br J Surg 71:29–32

Rothenberger DA 1989 Anal incontinence. In: Cameron JL (ed) Curent surgical therapy, 3rd edn. B. C. Decker, Philadelphia, p 185–194

Watts JD, Rothenberger DA, Buls JG, Goldberg SM, Nivatvongs S 1985 The management of procidentia—30 years' experience. Dis Colon Rectum 28:96–102

Womack NR, Morrison JFB, Williams NS 1988 Prospective study of the effects of postanal repair in neurogenic faecal incontinence. Br J Surg 75:48–52

Yoshioka K, Keighley MRB 1988 Clinical and manometric assessment of gracilis muscle transplant for fecal incontinence. Dis Colon Rectum 31:767–769

Yoshioka K, Keighley MRB 1989 Sphincter repair for fecal incontinence. Dis Colon Rectum 32:39–42

Yoshioka K, Hyland G, Keighley MRB 1988 Physiological changes after postanal repair and parameters predicting outcome. Br J Surg 75:1220–1224

Yoshioka K, Hyland G, Keighley MRB 1989 Anorectal function after abdominal rectopexy: parameters of predictive value in identifying return of continence. Br J Surg 76:64–68

DISCUSSION

Bartolo: One view is that a maintained anal sphincter pressure of about 70 mmHg should render that sphincter mucosa ischaemic, yet we see people with anal fissures with much higher pressures than that. With the artificial sphincter, is there any danger of ischaemic necrosis? Presumably we normally relax our sphincters spontaneously to allow adequate perfusion of the anus. What sort of problem is likely to arise?

Wong: This is certainly something that we have considered when setting up the protocol for the artificial sphincter. I think that the anal area itself is accustomed to a fairly high pressure, say 40–80 mmHg, but you are right that we tend to relax the sphincter intermittently. In animal studies, a pressure of up to 70 mmHg around bowel alone has been tolerated. The urologists have used the device around the bowel in patients with a neosigmoid bladder, and they developed some atrophy in the bowel itself with pressures up to 70 mmHg. Several of their patients had to be be revised because of atrophy due presumably to ischaemia. Subsequently they had no further problems with atrophy. We haven't seen that yet in our one patient with the artificial sphincter (or in Dr Christiansen's five patients), but if we exceed a pressure of 70 mmHg, that may be a problem.

Staskin: Dr Wong, how long do you wait after implantation of the sphincter before activating the compression around the bowel segment?

Wong: In our one patient we left it for four weeks before we activated this device.

Staskin: We wait at least six weeks after implantation before we activate the cuff. As a result of this delay, a scar has formed around the Silastic cuff.

I should add that the high cost of these devices (the urinary one costs two to three thousand dollars just for the device) makes this option prohibitive, particularly for national health services.

Kirby: I am surprised, Dr Wong, that if you are using a urethral artificial sphincter you have a long-enough cuff to get sufficient dilatation of the anus for voiding. I would have expected this to give a severe risk of obstruction. In the urethra, even when the cuff is fully relaxed, there is still some constriction, but enough fluid gets through and the sphincter works reasonably effectively.

Wong: Two of Dr Christensen's patients did have obstructive problems. He used the urinary cuff; we have used a modification of that. We worked with the company before starting the clinical trials and modified the cuff with them, in terms of both length and width and adding some reinforcing material to strengthen it.

Nordling: Presumably you have to move much larger volumes of fluid from the cuff with the bowel sphincter?

Wong: Yes.

Kirby: Generally the feeling is that bowel is much less tolerant of constant pressure being put on it than is the urethra.

Wong: That is certainly true of bowel above the anal sphincter level. We believe that the anus is different, because it is accustomed to a high pressure. At night, the patients with the artificial sphincter do very well, if we leave the cuff deflated. Intermittent deflation may be one answer to the problems of possible ischaemia and atrophy. Certainly initially we didn't activate the device continuously, even during the daytime hours.

Burnstock: May I suggest here that whenever you get human material, besides sending it to the pathologists for analysis, you send it also to pharmacologists and to neuroscientists who can study receptor localization by autoradiography, and also use immunofluorescence to study transmitter localization. Such tools are now available and much could be learned about the plasticity of autonomic nerves and changes in expression of transmitters and receptors.

Marsden: What are the indications for the use of the device that you discussed, Dr Wong?

Wong: At present we are using it only as an alternative to colostomy; but, as I said, we have not been happy with the results of post-anal repair, and in the future, if our clinical success rate with the sphincter device proves to be good, patients whom we now consider suitable for post-anal repair for neurogenic incontinence could receive this device.

Kuijpers: Our results of post-anal repair after three years are down to 50%, but this is still quite good. Could you implant the device even after post-anal repair?

Wong: Yes. I don't think that a post-anal repair will interfere with implantation in any adverse way. I have a patient who has had two gracilis muscle transpositions. Technically it may be difficult to insert a device in such a patient, but post-anal repair should not present a problem for subsequent artificial sphincter implantation.

Kuijpers: There is another new development in which a gracilis muscle is encircled around the anal canal and is then stimulated continuously with a pacemaker.

Wong: Yes. We may hear about this in Dr Brindley's paper.

Marsden: For urinary purposes, how long have these devices been implanted for?

Staskin: Some patients have had them for at least ten years. There is probably a mechanical failure rate of about 10% per year. For example, the cuff experiences shear forces at its corners, when it is inflated and deflated, which can cause leakage. The reservoir usually maintains its pressure, but this does decrease as the reservoir expands a little. For one reason or another there is an approximately 10% revision rate per year.

Kirby: Artificial urinary sphincters have been implanted since 1972, and some have been unmodified since then. There have, however, been modifications since those early days, and the latest figures suggest that they are now 80–90% effective and that their functional half-life is about ten years. They work especially well in men with incontinence after prostatectomy. But in my experience they work less well in women with unsuccessful surgery for stress incontinence, usually because these patients have had so many previous operations. The female urethra, perhaps like the bowel, seems less tolerant than the male urethra of a constant pressure being placed on it. However, in some patients you have no other option, apart from a urinary diversion or a long-term catheter.

Staskin: I don't put artificial sphincters into women at all, but that is because I believe 'sling' surgery to be the better operation. If you enter the vagina or urethra, when you place the cuff around the urethra there will be erosion into the vagina or through the urethra. With the sling operation, even if a woman has a non-contractile bladder and will need to use intermittent catheterization, I would prefer that to putting in an artificial device, because of the problem of erosion; whereas in men it works very well for urinary incontinence. In children, the device is put around the bladder neck, not around the perineal urethra, because of the small urethral size, so it becomes an intra-abdominal procedure.

Brindley: In adults, do you sometimes use the bladder neck rather than urethra? Theoretically you might expect that above the urethra the cuff is not subject to abdominal pressure, and we know that in the AMS device the transfer of abdominal pressure within the device is slow, so there should still be stress incontinence when they cough, with the cuff around the bulbar urethra. Some patients with cauda equina lesions have cuffs around the urethra and it is not safe to inflate them strongly enough to avoid stress incontinence completely. If they could be put around the bladder neck, in theory they would be all right.

Nordling: Your theory is quite right. If you put the cuff around the bulbar urethra, patients remain only mildly incontinent. If you put it round the bladder neck, they will be completely continent.

Brindley: You do it around the bladder neck, then?

Nordling: We do both, depending on the aetiology of incontinence and on the patient's condition.

Kirby: That's my experience also. It is better to put the cuff around the bladder neck, because you have more tissue for the cuff to rest around, and there is less tendency for it to erode. The operation is more difficult, but I think that's the optimum site. In men it doesn't interfere with ejaculation either, in that site, so it doesn't lead to sexual dysfunction. However, the main indication in men is for incontinence after prostatectomy, when the bladder neck cannot be used because it has already been scarred and destroyed by the prostatectomy, so you have to put the cuff round the bulbar urethra. The trouble there is that you can feel the device when you sit on it, and can also sometimes deflate the cuff inadvertently and become 'incontinent'.

Bartolo: Dr Staskin mentioned the high cost of the device, but this is open to debate. If the artificial sphincter costs 2000–3000 dollars, we are treating young women with obstetric injury who have had failed surgery, and the only other option is a colostomy. If you consider the expense of one or two colostomy plugs per day, if you use irrigation, or bags for a period of 40 years on National Health Service prescription, that will cost more than this device. So although there is a short-term expenditure, there is also a long-term gain.

Staskin: You are speaking to the converted; I agree entirely. Unfortunately, not everyone who listens to that argument is as reasonable as I am!

Christensen: Your device has a half-life of only about ten years, though. You might need two devices or more over a 40-year lifespan.

Brading: But with more devices, the cost should come down?

Kuijpers: Another alternative to colostomy is daily colonic irrigation. I am using this in a number of patients; they do it themselves, and it works quite well. It takes only about 45 minutes each morning.

Bartolo: I have not been very successful with this. Either the patients won't do it, because of the inconvenience, or they fail to retain the balloon.

Wong: The possibility of a combined urinary and faecal continence device has been raised, with one pressure-regulating balloon and one control pump, but two cuffs, for patients with double incontinence. Has anyone had experience of patients with both types of incontinence, where this might be applicable?

Kirby: I have never heard of anybody having both devices, but there is no reason why you shouldn't. It certainly is not uncommon to have urinary and faecal incontinence.

Staskin: There are people with urinary sphincters and artificial penile prostheses, but fortunately they have two different pumps!

Wong: We have a patient waiting for an artificial urinary sphincter who also needs an artificial bowel sphincter. The question is whether to put two different units in at once; this raised the question of designing the dual anal device.

Staskin: When you say you grade faecal incontinence, is this done by what would seem to be a reasonably objective method? We constantly argue about what 'improved', 'very improved' and so on mean. How do you follow up these patients?

Wong: We use a scoring system that was proposed by David Bartolo, based on the frequency of the incontinence, and the type of leakage (gas, liquid or solid). The scoring system runs up to 18 and gives us an objective means of scoring incontinence.

Staskin: We do an objective pad test; the patient puts on a pad and goes through various manoeuvres in a one-hour or three-hour test. The pad is weighed. I am not sure whether this test is applicable to faecal incontinence.

On another point, the ureterosigmoidostomy is a form of urinary diversion where the ureters are implanted into the sigmoid colon. When this procedure is done in patients with bladder cancer, a problem arises with continence of very liquid stool when urine and faeces are mixed together. Perhaps the more objective tests used by colorectal specialists can be applied to urology patients to determine whether they would have a problem with the more liquid stool. A common practice in urology is to give an enema of 500 ml of oatmeal and ask the patient to walk around for an hour; if patients can hold this, they usually do well after this procedure.

Bartolo: Nick Read's saline continence test is probably as objective a test as any. When I worked in his laboratory we found that some patients said they were faecally incontinent but didn't leak in this test. We tried to make it more 'physiological' by infusing a dilute solution of bile acid, which seemed to correlate better with faecal incontinence. You have to consider the properties of the liquid that you are putting into the rectum; I don't know how urine reacts with rectal mucosa, but it won't necessarily be the same as saline. That's as near as we can get.

Kirby: This question of the rectum being used as a reservoir for a mixture of urine and faeces is interesting, because most patients in whom this procedure is done must walk around with a rectum full of fluid, yet the majority are continent. This comes back to the question of the internal anal sphincter, which is designed to open when the rectum is full, as it is in these patients. One wonders whether their internal anal sphincters are constantly open. They certainly get nocturnal leakage of urine during sleep; that may be because the external striated sphincter intermittently relaxes in sleep. Has anyone looked to see whether the internal anal sphincter is closed when the rectum is full of fluid?

Bartolo: In ambulatory studies with long-term monitoring there are periods of relaxation of the external anal sphincter. The Mayo group showed that during REM sleep the external sphincter relaxes quite profoundly, so perhaps during these periods your patients are leaking at night. We know that the external sphincter is tonically active, during both day and night, but clearly there are periods, apparently during REM sleep, when it relaxes.

Swash: The point being raised is that the recto-anal reflex is inhibited in these patients, by some mechanism.

Bartolo: I can't comment on that. Nick Read said that if the rectum is slowly inflated with liquid, the internal sphincter remain closed; urinary flow rates are very slow, so perhaps they can cope with a small trickle.

Swash: What happens to the compliance of the rectum when it is being studied in this way?

Kirby: The patients don't obviously develop great rectal distension. The thick smooth muscle coat, discussed earlier, probably prevents it. Other segments of bowel used as urinary reservoirs do undergo some degree of distension.

Marsden: Do the striated external urethral sphincter and anal sphincter behave like the rest of the striated muscle during REM sleep, namely become silent?

Swash: Except in studies by Floyd & Walls (1953), where there was no indication of external anal sphincter relaxation at any stage of sleep.

Marsden: This is not what the Mayo findings suggest, according to David Bartolo.

Kuijpers: Didn't Sir Alan Parks demonstrate that the external anal sphincter works even during sleep, continuously?

Swash: Yes. That goes back to work by Gowers in the last century.

Fowler: The urethral sphincter is certainly active under light anaesthesia. Surely the abductors of the vocal cords remain active during sleep?

Marsden: One would hope so! I would be fascinated to know, from studies in which sleep stages are monitored, what happens to the external urethral and anal sphincters.

Fowler: This has probably been looked at, for the explanation of nocturnal enuresis. This doesn't particularly occur during REM sleep (see Inoue et al 1987).

Marsden: If the received wisdom is that the external sphincter does go to sleep on occasions, if not completely, during REM sleep, like the rest of the skeletal muscle, one must depend entirely on the internal anal and urinary sphincters for continence during those periods.

Kirby: There is an interesting parallel there; when we remove the bladder and prostate and use a bowel substitute for their replacement, the patient is now dependent on the external striated muscle sphincter for urinary continence. Most patients are continent by day but by night they nearly all leak. We see this as being due to loss of the internal smooth muscle sphincter and bladder neck sphincter and reliance on the external striated sphincter to give urinary continence by day, but not by night.

Nordling: That's not completely right. There is probably some relaxation of the sphincter. We have tried to make measurements of urethral pressure in these patients at night, and it doesn't drop very much during sleep, so there must be some active sphincter muscle at that time. Incontinence is normally due to bowel contractions during the night, which overcome the resistance in the urethra.

Kirby: Why should that occur only at night?

Nordling: Because when you are awake you can contract your striated sphincter against this. With low pressure reservoirs incontinence is not seen before the volume of the bladder is 500 ml, so in these patients incontinence is first seen as overflow incontinence.

Burnstock: We have not yet discussed sensory impulses originating from the mucosal lining of the colon, yet there are many nerves in the submucosal area and at the bases of the mucosal epithelium. I suspect that the internal anal sphincter would be very much affected by sensory-initiated reflexes within the gut. If urine is introduced into the rectum, as in this particular procedure of implanting ureters into the sigmoid colon, I would be surprised if reflexes were not initiated which would influence the internal anal sphincter.

References

Floyd WF, Walls EW 1953 Electromyograph of the sphincter ani externus in man. J Physiol (Lond) 122:599–609

Inoue M, Shimojima H, Chiba H, Tsukahara N, Tajika Y, Taka K 1987 Rhythmic slow wave observed on nocturnal sleep encephalogram in children with idiopathic nocturnal enuresis. Sleep 10:570–579

Treatment of urinary and faecal incontinence by surgically implanted devices

G. S. Brindley

MRC Neurological Prostheses Unit, Institute of Psychiatry, De Crespigny Park, London SE5 8AF, UK

Abstract. Three kinds of implant to treat incontinence are considered. The sacral anterior root stimulator (with sacral posterior rhizotomy) is already effective in urinary incontinence due to spinal cord injury, and will have wider application. The conditional pudendal nerve stimulator and the conditional gracilis nerve stimulator are, respectively, almost untried and entirely untried devices; but they show promise, and if successful may help very many patients.

1990 Neurobiology of Incontinence. Wiley, Chichester (Ciba Foundation Symposium 151) p 267–282

The surgical implantation of manufactured objects, especially artificial sphincters, is well established in the treatment of urinary incontinence. It has been tried, and some success claimed, in the treatment of faecal incontinence.

The present paper will say nothing about implants that are well established, but will consider just three kinds that are not. The first of them, the sacral anterior root stimulator, has given great benefit to a few hundreds of patients. The second, the conditional pudendal nerve stimulator, has been tried in only three patients. The third, the conditional gracilis nerve stimulator, has not yet been tried at all.

Sacral anterior root stimulator

Papers already published (references given in Brindley 1988) give much information about clinical aspects of this implant, and a conference in Le Mans in November 1989 will assemble much more. I can therefore, after a brief description, concentrate on its scientific basis.

Description

The sacral anterior root stimulator allows independent electrical stimulation of three or four spinal nerve roots or pairs or groups of such roots, the electrical power for stimulating being conveyed across the skin by three or four radio-frequency inductive links. Commonly there are three rather than four such links, and one is allotted to both S2 anterior roots, one to both S3 anterior roots and the third to both S4 (or both S4 and both S5) anterior roots. The anterior roots are usually trapped intrathecally at about the level of the 5th lumbar vertebrae, and the corresponding posterior roots are usually cut at the same time. In a few patients, where the intrathecal approach is clearly contra-indicated, an extradural approach through the sacrum is used. This approach is easier and quicker for mere access to the roots, but much less favourable for accurate and safe posterior rhizotomy.

Application

This is chiefly to patients with spinal injuries who are troubled by urinary incontinence, persisting or recurrent urinary infection associated with high residual urine volume, or low bladder compliance endangering the upper urinary tracts. The benefits, though substantial for men, are even greater for women, because incontinence is more burdensome to them. Most patients treated up to now have complete spinal cord transections, but those with incomplete lesions can also be treated. A few patients with multiple sclerosis are suitable. Though the main purpose of the implant is urinary, there are often collateral benefits for defaecation and penile erection.

Basic anatomy

The S2 to S5 anterior roots carry the whole of the excitatory motor nerve supply to the detrusor muscle of the bladder, the main part (perhaps the whole) of the excitatory motor nerve supply to the rectum, pelvic colon and descending colon, and an important part of the erectile nerve supply to the penis. They also carry the whole of the somatic motor nerve supply to the pelvic floor and extrinsic and intrinsic urethral rhabdosphincters, and some somatic nerve supply to lower limb muscles.

The S2 to S5 posterior roots carry all or nearly all the sensory and reflex-afferent fibres from the bladder and rectum. The distinction between 'all' and 'nearly all' can be an important one, and it is difficult or impossible to make this distinction by ordinary anatomical techniques. A substantial and fast-growing contribution to our knowledge about it comes from observations on patients with sacral anterior stimulators and sacral posterior rhizotomy.

Permanence of bladder areflexia after sacral posterior rhizotomy

Many surgeons have tried to treat reflex urinary incontinence by cutting the bladder nerve supply close to the bladder or within its wall, or by injecting alcohol or other poisons near the trigone or in the sacral foramina or the lower part of the sacral canal. The effect of these procedures have been found, at least in most cases, to last only a few months. The nerve fibres, both motor and sensory, regenerate and resume their function.

Spinal roots within the sub-arachnoid space, both anterior and posterior, regenerate anatomically if cut or injured, as Cajal showed 70 years ago. In implanting sacral anterior root stimulators we fairly often damage one or more anterior roots. These damaged roots look normal at the end of the operation, respond to stimulation for three or four days after the operation, are unresponsive at seven or eight days, respond again after a delay of four to eight months, and thereafter remain responsive. The unresponsiveness at eight days must indicate Wallerian degeneration, and the renewed responsiveness after a few months must indicate that some of the degenerated fibres have regenerated, found their proper destinations, and made effective connection with striated or smooth muscle.

After similar accidental damage to sacral posterior roots, or after intentional posterior rhizotomy, there seems to be no such recovery of function. Posterior rhizotomy of all segments from S2 to S5, or posterior rhizotomy of S3 to S4 with crushing of the unsplit S5 roots, has been done only since 1986; before that year we wrongly supposed that the risks of separating the anterior from the posterior root in S4 and S5 outweighed the benefits. Most of the patients who in the years 1986–1988 have had radical posterior rhizotomy have lost all pelvic floor and bladder reflexes and have not recovered them in up to 32 months, despite well-preserved pelvic floor and bladder function driven through the implant. Thirty-two months is already much longer than peripheral denervations commonly last. We can get still longer follow-ups if we include early patients who appear to have had accidental posterior root damage. Four patients who had sacral anterior root stimulators implanted in 1982–1984 and became continent, having previously had severe reflex incontinence (numbers 12, 38, 43 and 50 of Brindley et al 1986), had cystometry done in 1988 or 1989 primarily in order to check their voiding pressures. All four were found to have areflexic bladders up to 500 or 600 ml filling, and normal compliance.

This empirical evidence does not yet suffice to prove that the effects of sacral posterior root section or damage in suppressing detrusor reflex activity are permanent, but they clearly point in this direction, and further evidence is accumulating year by year.

It is not in the least surprising that the effects of anterior root damage should be temporary and those of posterior root damage permanent. Nerve fibres probably regenerate about equally well in both, but the cells of origin of the anterior root fibres lie in the spinal cord, so that regeneration must be towards the periphery, and the new synapses that must be formed are on muscle cells. In many parts of the body these are known to be formed fairly efficiently. The cells of origin of the posterior root fibres lie in the spinal ganglia, so that regeneration towards the cord is required. The regenerating fibres must continue to grow within the cord and make appropriate new synapses. Most of the many investigations in which such regeneration in the central nervous system has been examined have found that only a small minority of fibres grow, and of these fibres only a few make anatomical synaptic connexion. *Appropriately functioning* synapses may be rarer still.

Urinary uses of the implant

Somatic motor fibres are large myelinated, and preganglionic parasympathetic fibres are small myelinated, with no overlap in their distribution of size. It is therefore possible by weak stimulation to activate all the somatic fibres in a spinal root and none of the parasympathetic fibres. A few patients use such stimulation to activate the urethral rhabdosphincters and pelvic floor, and thus avoid stress incontinence. Most patients become continent without such sphincter activation. Their only urinary use of their implant is for micturition. This is achieved by stimulating the roots (usually all three pairs) with bursts of strong pulses. The bursts last about three seconds and are separated by gaps of about seven seconds. Each pulse typically generates an impulse in every somatic fibre and every parasympathetic fibre of each stimulated root. During a burst, the rhabdosphincters are strongly activated. The bladder reacts much more slowly, and the peak of detrusor pressure caused by each burst comes during the following gap, when the rhabdosphincters, in a favourable case, are fully relaxed.

Pelvic afferent fibres that do not run in sacral posterior roots

Two possible paths for such fibres have to be thought about: lumbar or lower thoracic roots, and sacral anterior roots.

Lumbar or lower thoracic roots.   The T11 to L2 anterior roots certainly carry sympathetic (efferent) fibres to most of the pelvic viscera. It would not be surprising if the posterior roots of the same segments carried some pelvic visceral afferent fibres, though if so they seem to be of small importance compared with the pelvic visceral afferent fibres that enter by sacral posterior roots.

It is stated in anatomical textbooks that no visceral afferent fibres run in the L4 to S1 roots, but the evidence for such statements seems to be weak.

Sacral anterior roots.   Doubts are from time to time expressed (e.g. Coggeshall et al 1975, Floyd et al 1976) about the exact and invariable truth of the

Bell-Magendie law that all anterior root fibres are efferent and all posterior root fibres afferent. Practical implications if the Bell-Magendie law were not true might be (1) the electrical stimulation of sacral anterior roots might be painful, or might trigger autonomic dysreflexia; (2) even the most radical posterior rhizotomy might be insufficient to make the bladder perfectly areflexic.

At present there are no final, complete answers either to the scientific questions about pelvic afferent fibres in non-sacral roots and sacral anterior roots, or to the practical questions about the sensory and reflex effects of anterior root stimulation and posterior rhizotomy. The practical questions are less difficult to answer than the scientific ones, and our knowledge of the answers, though incomplete, is steadily growing.

Of 22 patients with preserved pelvic pain sensitivity who have had sacral anterior root stimulators implanted since 1978, two have always been unable to use their implants because attempts to do so are excessively painful. One other experienced moderate pain when she used the implant, and now no longer uses it because she can empty her bladder by straining and fist pressure. Three experience very mild pain which they find no deterrent to use of the implant. In the remaining 16 patients stimulation of anterior root is entirely painless. The painlessness in 16 patients proves that in them the S2 to S4 anterior roots contain no myelinated pain fibres. It does not prove the absence of unmyelinated pain fibres, because the stimuli needed for micturition may not be strong enough to stimulate unmyelinated fibres. The pain, severe or mild, experienced by six patients does not prove that their anterior roots contain pain fibres, for two reasons: first, the surgeons could accidentally have included some posterior root bundles in what seemed to be anterior roots; and secondly, even if (as is likely) the anterior roots were correctly separated from the posterior, the pain could be due to synchronous activation of recurrent collaterals of numerous motor fibres.

As to pelvic afferents entering the cord by roots above the S2, the patients 12, 38, 43 and 50 of Brindley et al (1986) cited above, and patients 1, 2, 3, 5, 6 and 7 of Madersbacher et al (1988) and patients 1–6, 10 and 12 of Egon et al (1989), illustrate that operative intervention restricted to the S2 and lower roots can convert detrusor hyperreflexia into detrusor areflexia. There are, however, a few patients in whom complete detrusor areflexia is not achieved, despite a posterior rhizotomy that seemed to include S2 and all lower roots bilaterally. Further experience will probably make it clear whether these are patients in whom, despite intra-operative appearances, the posterior rhizotomy was incomplete; or whether some detrusor reflex afferents in some people enter the cord by roots above S2, or by anterior roots. Similar questions about afferent fibres responsible for sensation and for autonomic dysreflexia are likewise not yet fully answered, but are beginning to be answered. I can, for example, say that no patient from the centres well known to me whose sacral posterior rhizotomy seemed to be complete has subsequently had a severe autonomic dysreflexic attack triggered by sacral root stimulation or overfilling of the bladder, and very few have had mild attacks.

The conditional pudendal nerve stimulator

Patients with severe reflex incontinence but normal or nearly normal sensation in the sacral dermatomes will usually not consent to being treated by sacral posterior rhizotomy, with or without implantation of a sacral anterior root stimulator. Anticholinergics usually help such patients, but often fail to achieve complete continence or have side-effects that the patient will not tolerate.

Electrical stimulation through anal or vaginal electrodes and a battery-driven external stimulator has often been tried in such patients, usually with partial success, but often not with enough success to compensate for the discomfort and inconvenience of wearing the device. Such stimulation seems to work chiefly by inhibition of the reflex detrusor contractions, as described by Fall et al (1977). The commercially available anal and vaginal devices stimulate few if any of the motor fibres of the pudendal nerves. They cause brief reflex pelvic floor contractions when first switched on, but little or no sustained increase in pelvic floor activity.

By a specially designed anal plug (Brindley et al 1974) it is possible to achieve electrical stimulation of all alpha motor fibres in both pudendal nerves. Such stimulation is moderately but not severely painful, the pain coming chiefly from stimulation of the skin of the anal canal. The special anal plug is useless for treating incontinence, but can be used to diagnose whether, if a less uncomfortable device were made that would at appropriate times stimulate the pudendal nerves and nothing else, it would be likely to achieve continence. We find in normal volunteers that pudendal nerve stimulation by the special anal plug during micturition stops the flow in less than a second. This is much too fast to be due to inhibition of the detrusor contraction, and evidently depends on rhabdosphincter activation. Whether this activation is of the extrinsic and intrinsic rhabdosphincters or only the extrinsic is unknown.

In patients with severe reflex incontinence from spinal cord injury or multiple sclerosis, similar stimulation of the pudendal nerves inhibits reflex detrusor contractions. The inhibition begins about two seconds after the beginning of the burst of stimulation. Complete detrusor relaxation, if achieved at all, is achieved in about seven seconds. It is not achieved in all trials in all patients, but there are some patients in whom it fails only when the bladder is extremely full. At least in these patients a *conditional pudendal nerve stimulator implant* (Brindley & Donaldson 1986) is a rational remedy for incontinence. This implant stimulates both pudendal nerves at a frequency and strength set by external equipment but at times determined by a sensor of bladder pressure. The aim is that when a reflex detrusor contraction occurs, the stimulator will be switched on, the resulting rhabdosphincter contraction will prevent leakage of urine during the first few seconds, and the inhibition of the detrusor contractions will prevent it thereafter. There are two probable advantages in stimulating the pudendal nerves only during detrusor contractions: first, the stimulation causes mild pain, which is tolerable for a short time but unpleasant if it has to be suffered all day; secondly, we find in tests with the special anal plug that continence can be maintained up to a larger bladder volume by stimulation switched on only when a bladder contraction occurs than by continuous stimulation.

The sensor that controls the conditional pudendal nerve stimulator implant is an applanation tonometer sewn on to the dome of the bladder. Its threshold can be adjusted after implantation by injecting or withdrawing saline into or from a self-sealing capsule. Only four conditional pudendal nerve stimulators have been implanted, three in 1984 and 1985 into women with multiple sclerosis, and one in February 1990 into a woman whose severe reflex incontinence was due to an incomplete lower thoracic spinal cord injury. The recent patient and one of the earlier patients use their implants regularly, and are continent when using them.

The only part of this implant that is novel from an engineering point of view is the sensor of bladder pressure. In one patient this still works well, four years after implantation. It contains no manufactured component that is likely to fail within 20 years. The kinds of failure that we feared were partial detachment from the bladder or walling off from the bladder by an inflexible thick layer of fibrous tissue. By analogy with other kinds of implant in human patients and experimental bladder sensors in animals, these are unlikely to occur late if they have not occurred in the first year. Thus the chief question about the conditional pudendal nerve stimulator is whether there are sufficiently many patients, identifiable in advance, in whom it will give good enough urinary continence to justify a substantial surgical operation.

The conditional gracilis nerve stimulator

Transposition of the gracilis muscle, leaving its upper attachment, nerve supply and main blood supply intact and wrapping its lower end around the anorectal junction, is a fairly old remedy for faecal incontinence, sporadically practised for years but not with enough success to become popular. One way to make it more effective is to use an implanted stimulator to activate the muscle, except during defaecation (Stricker et al 1988, N. Williams & S. Watkins, personal communication). But skeletal muscles exert only small forces when activated constantly for many hours, even if their properties have been altered favourably by previous long-term low frequency stimulation. Better results could probably be obtained by stimulating the nerve to the gracilis muscle at very low frequency for most of the day and night, but at higher frequency when the rectum is full. A sensor of rectal filling could be analogous to the long-term implantable intracranial pressure sensor of Brindley et al (1983), consisting of a radio-frequency-tuned circuit and a piece of ferrite whose distance from the tuned circuit alters its resonant frequency. The virtues of this kind of sensor are simplicity, durability (expected implanted lifetime at least 20 years) and the facility for interrogation either by implanted circuitry, or by an external device. One would expect to use external sensing and an inductively powered stimulator with early implants where the optimum design is not yet achieved, but internal sensing and an implanted power supply in fully developed implants. The tuned circuit of the rectal filling sensor will use a figure-of-eight coil implanted behind the rectum, and a ferrite flux guide implanted in front of the rectum.

Implantation of such sensors into animals has begun in 1989, and it is hoped that the first implantations into patients will follow in 1990.

References

Brindley GS 1988 The actions of parasympathetic and sympathetic nerves in human micturition, erection and seminal emission, and their restoration in paraplegic patients by implanted electrical stimulators. Proc R Soc Lond Biol Sci 235:111–120

Brindley GS, Donaldson PEK 1986 Electrolytic current-control elements for surgically implanted electrical devices. Med & Biol Eng & Comput 24:439–441

Brindley GS, Rushton DN, Craggs MD 1974 The pressure exerted by the external sphincter of the urethra when its motor nerve fibres are stimulated electrically. Br J Urol 46:453–462

Brindley GS, Polkey CE, Cooper JD 1983 Technique for very long-term monitoring of intracranial pressure. Med & Biol Eng & Comput 21:460–464

Brindley GS, Polkey CE, Rushton DN, Cardozo L 1986 Sacral anterior root stimulators for bladder control in paraplegia: the first 50 cases. J Neurol Neurosurg Psychiatry 49:1104–1114

Coggeshall RE, Applebaum ML, Fazen M, Stubbs TB, Sykes MT 1975 Unmyelinated axons in human ventral roots, a possible explanation for the failure of dorsal rhizotomy to relieve pain. Brain 98:157–166

Egon G, Colombel P, Des Roseaux F, Philippi R, Herlant M 1989 Electrostimulation des racines sacrées antérieures chez le paraplégique. A propos de 13 observations. Ann Réadaptation Med Phys 32:47–57

Fall M, Erlandson BE, Sundin T, Waagstein F 1977 Intravaginal electrical stimulation: clinical experiments on bladder inhibition. Scand J Urol Nephrol Suppl 44:41–48

Floyd K, Koley J, Morrison JFB 1976 Afferent discharges in the sacral ventral roots of cat. J Physiol (Lond) 259:37–38P

Madersbacher H, Fischer J, Ebner A 1988 Anterior sacral root stimulator (Brindley): experience especially in women with neurogenic urinary incontinence. Neurourol Urodyn 7:593–601

Stricker JW, Schoetz DJ, Coller JA, Veidenheimer MC 1988 Surgical correction of anal incontinence. Dis Colon Rectum 31:533–540

DISCUSSION

Swash: The notion behind the gracilis nerve stimulator sphincteroplasty was that the muscle should have its normal physiological contraction characteristics altered to a more 'tonic' type, before construction of the sphincter (Hallan et al 1990). This is achieved using continuous low level electrical stimulation, and has to be maintained indefinitely to achieve a satisfactory sphincteric function. A major problem with this muscle transposition procedure is that the muscle is a long way from its neurovascular bundle and undergoes considerable avascular necrosis. So the attempt by Williams and his colleagues (Hallan et al 1990) to make it into a lively sphincter is a new approach. In preliminary experiments, using sartorius in the dog, we found that considerable lengths of the muscle implanted as a sphincter were necrotic, or even replaced by fibrous tissue and regenerating myoblasts; only the proximal part, still in the thigh, retained function. It becomes critically important, therefore, to make sure that enough muscle is alive in the thigh to pull on the rather inelastic fibrous connective sling that is now around the anal canal. There are therefore technical problems at present, which must not be forgotten.

Brindley: Much depends on the continued success of the present stimulated gracilis transpositions and on whether they really work better when the stimulators are on than when they are off. If they do, and they continue to work, then to continue to use the technique and improve on it seems justified.

Bartolo: I did a gracilis transplantation and was impressed that although there is a lovely muscle in the thigh, the bit that was wrapped round the anal sphincter was just tendon, at the time of implantation.

Doug Wong spoke about the use of the AMS sphincter for faecal continence. It worries me that you say you would need to have the gracilis stimulator running at a relatively high frequency all the time. Could you combine this technology with a device like the silicone AMS sphincter so that the stimulator could respond to changes in intra-rectal pressure?

Brindley: There may be a way of doing that, but on the whole it is better to control a mechanical device like the AMS sphincter mechanically, rather than electrically.

Brading: If you use the gracilis muscle to wrap round the anal sphincter, it might be useful to make it more of a 'tonic' muscle *in situ* in the thigh before you dissect it. If you stimulate a 'fast' twitch muscle continuously at the right frequency it gets a much increased vascularization, as well as taking on other properties of the 'slow' twitch muscles. This would take only a week or ten days.

Kuijpers: The problem in neurogenic incontinence is the denervation of the pelvic floor, as we have discussed. Would it be possible to stimulate the floor itself, continuously, by some device, to strengthen the muscle?

Brindley: People have used electrical stimulation of a weak pelvic floor, but the results are rather poor.

Kuijpers: You could mobilize the rectum through a laparotomy and then leave some stimulation device for constant stimulation of the striated muscle?

Brindley: External stimulators do train the pelvic floor muscles, and I don't think you could train them better by an implant; where most of the motor nerve fibres are lost it isn't promising. It has been tried by external stimulation and was not very successful.

Kuijpers: But stimulation for 24 hours a day has not been tried?

Marsden: Direct electrical stimulation to muscle is very painful, however. What about pelvic splanchnic nerve stimulators?

Brindley: They have no advantage over sacral anterior root stimulation.

Marsden: And what about conus medullaris stimulators?

Brindley: This is just a bad way of doing what we do better with sacral anterior root stimulation!

Marsden: Do you dismiss the use of direct electrical bladder stimulation?

Brindley: It is not useless, but it has a very small field of application. If the cauda equina is completely destroyed, most patients have adequate bladder emptying by straining or by expression, but some don't, or it is not a satisfactory management. If they also have no pelvic pain sensation, one could consider a direct bladder stimulator. This is a very small number of patients, however.

de Groat: With electrical stimulation via the anterior root stimulator, are there differences in the threshold for activation of the bladder and bowel? (I am thinking in terms of the intensity of stimulation rather than frequency.)

Brindley: If there are threshold differences they are tiny. We don't need to use different strengths of stimulus for micturition and defaecation. The control box of the sacral anterior root stimulator has provision for the separate adjustment of voltage and pulse duration for different programmes. That facility is used for erection; the erectile nerve fibres are evidently smaller than the bladder fibres and we need stronger stimuli for erection than for micturition. For defaecation we don't, because bowel fibres seem to be of the the same average diameter as bladder fibres.

de Groat: In the cat, the preganglionic fibres to the bladder are myelinated B fibres, whereas the fibres to the bowel area unmyelinated C fibres. The threshold intensities are about five times greater for bladder than bowel.

Brindley: That is clearly not so in man. As you say, the difference between a small myelinated and an unmyelinated fibre in threshold for short pulses is huge; the longer the pulse the less that difference. But we use short pulses. It would be easy to measure strength–duration curves and prove that bowel fibres are myelinated; but merely from the thresholds for our 100 µs pulses there's no doubt that this is so. And even the erectile nerve fibres, though they have higher thresholds, are myelinated fibres, rather than unmyelinated, in man.

de Groat: What are the differences in threshold for anal sphincter activation versus bladder activation, with sacral root stimulation?

Brindley: About a factor of three.

Kirby: I gather it is no longer true that you can only use sacral root stimulators in patients with complete spinal lesions?

Brindley: We have put 33 into patients with incomplete cord lesions, or with multiple sclerosis. Of the 33 patients with incomplete lesions, six with multiple sclerosis and the rest with incomplete cord injuries, into whom sacral anterior root stimulators were implanted, 22 had pelvic pain sensitivity. As I said, two of those 22 are unable to use their implants because attempts to stimulate the anterior roots are very painful. In one of those two, we know that the pain is really due to anterior root stimulation, because the patient had a complete L5–S5 posterior rhizotomy at the conus medullaris. In the other patient it could perhaps be a surgical error, some posterior root strands being accidentally included with the anterior roots.

Of the 22 patients who had preserved pelvic pain sensitivity, 13 use their implants with no pain at all and four use them although each use causes brief mild pain. There are five non-users among the 22—the two just mentioned, and three with reasons for non-use other than pain.

Marsden: Were the 22 patients with incomplete cord lesions all deafferented?

Brindley: Not all. In the first 50 patients with sacral anterior root stimulators we never did a thorough deafferentation; we didn't know we could safely separate the anterior from the posterior root in S4 until 1985, so the early ones were nearly all incompletely deafferented or not deafferented at all. One or two may have been completely deafferented by accidental intraoperative damage to posterior roots. Some of these first 50 patients had incomplete lesions; for example, two of our six multiple sclerosis patients were among the first 50.

Kirby: The possibility suggests itself of implanting stimulators into some of the many patients with acontractile bladders who self-catheterize themselves and yet have no apparent neurological cause for it.

Brindley: You would have to make sure that transrectal stimulation of the pelvic splanchnic nerves makes their bladders contract. If it does, they may be suitable for this procedure, though some may experience pain on stimulation, especially if you don't cut the posterior roots.

Kirby: Some of these patients get so fed up with self-catheterization, because of infections and urethral pain, that they go on to have a urinary diversion and stoma, which is an extreme way of managing the problem. For those patients, sacral anterior root stimulation might be an alternative.

Brindley: Send such a patient to me for trial of transrectal stimulation, to see whether we can produce any bladder pressure; if we can, I could discuss with the patient whether he or she wants this remedy considered.

Fowler: This group of patients have atonic bladders as a result of having impaired relaxation of the sphincter, so presumably they have sustained damage to the innervation of the bladder secondary to that effect, and therefore I would not expect them to respond.

Brindley: I had thought that these patients didn't have sacral root innervation to the bladder, from previous discussions? But we can find this out by transrectal stimulation. If they retain a parasympathetic innervation, they are in principle suitable for a sacral root stimulator.

Kirby: I haven't operated on many of these patients, but when I do, the detrusor muscle looks reasonably normal, macroscopically and microscopically.

Brindley: After a cauda equina lesion, the bladder also looks reasonably normal; it has muscle which is apparently maintained in a healthy state.

Kirby: I expected a reduction in the amount of cholinergic innervation, although there will still be postganglionic nerve present, but these patients with atonic bladders didn't seem to be profoundly denervated or decentralized, so some of them might be suitable for stimulation. It would be of great interest to test their response to transrectal stimulation of the pelvic splanchnic nerve.

Burnstock: We have been implanting electrodes on autonomic fibres, the hypogastric nerve in the guinea pig and the great auricular nerve of rabbits. We compared the effects of high activity for eight days (by chronic stimulation of these nerves), to the effects of low impulse activity by decentralization. Some rather remarkable things happen. We already know that autonomic fibres show much more plasticity than motor fibres. We looked at the guinea pig vas deferens, which is supplied by the hypogastric nerve, and there was nearly a doubling of the number of varicosities per unit length of autonomic fibres after chronic stimulation. Furthermore, the rate of regeneration was increased 10–20-fold by chronic stimulation of the cut fibres.

Brindley: So you stimulated preganglionically and you improve regeneration postganglionically?

Burnstock: Yes.

de Groat: The NIH is now awarding contracts for the development of microstimulation in the spinal cord to do the things you are doing with root stimulation. Do you see any advantages of microstimulation in the spinal cord over root stimulation?

Brindley: Not in the kinds of patients we are now treating. This is a totally new idea to me. Microstimulation in the visual cortex of the brain to enable blind people to see makes a certain amount of sense, but I can't see where spinal microstimulation would be useful in bladder control. But it will be interesting to learn why the NIH is supporting this; there may be some justification.

Stanton: What exactly is microstimulation?

de Groat: This is stimulation using very small metal electrodes so that a limited area of the spinal cord, a nucleus for example, can be stimulated, as opposed to gross stimulation of the entire cord or of multiple tracts. The goal is to attempt to stimulate the autonomic nucleus selectively, rather than to stimulate the sphincter and the autonomic outflow together.

Brindley: One reason for my initial scepticism is that voiding with bursts and gaps works so well. The bladder pressures are not excessively high; the residual volumes are tiny. It works so well that there seems to be no need to improve on it.

de Groat: That is why I asked the question!

Kirby: Suppose one were to put a microstimulator in the brainstem pontine nucleus, one might expect to be able to stimulate the detrusor and inhibit the pudendal innervation simultaneously, from your work?

de Groat: You can in cats and rats.

Kirby: We have been using a magnet to stimulate the motor cortex in certain patients and get the pelvic floor to contract. I don't think we know whether we are getting bladder contractions as well, but there is no sign of incontinence with magnetic stimulation. If we measured the pressure inside the bladder, we might find a pressure rise. Would microstimulation up in the motor cortex have any role, to selectively stimulate perhaps the pelvic floor or even the detrusor?

Brindley: I tend to be sceptical about this.

Marsden: I am even more sceptical, because in all the neurological conditions that one is trying to deal with there is damage to the efferent pathways, whether in the spinal cord itself or in the descending pathways.

Brindley: But there are people with urge incontinence who clearly have no neurological lesions.

Marsden: Except those with frontal lobe damage that leads to loss of control of urinary continence. One might conceive of activating their intact pontine micturition centre; but unfortunately they usually are demented.

Swash: The necessity for deafferentation seems to me to be a problem in the further development of implanted stimulator procedures. How are we to get round this necessity?

Brindley: Capsaicin will perhaps be an answer. One might be able to deafferent the bladder permanently by putting capsaicin into it. If that failed, one could apply capsaicin to the posterior root ganglia and so make the extradural procedure safer, because the extradural approach is surgically simpler, except for the deafferentation.

Swash: Selective peripheral deafferentation would be a nice approach.

Marsden: What are the survival rates of the intradurally applied electrodes versus the extradural electrodes?

Brindley: There is no difference in how long the implants last. At present the mean time to failure is 16.8 years (42 failures in 706 implant-years), but it will go up as the proportion of implants with modifications to improve reliability increases. All but two of the 42 failures were repairable, and the two unrepairable implants have been replaced by new ones.

Marsden: And what is the possibility of mechanical improvements in artificial urethral sphincters?

Brindley: In a man, if you put the cuff round the bulbar urethra, he is likely to have stress incontinence with the standard AMS device because the transfer of abdominal pressure to the cuff is very slow, much too slow to cope with the effect of a cough. In my Unit we have developed artificial sphincters in which transfer is exceedingly rapid. In theory they should be the complete answer to the artificial sphincter where for reasons of previous surgical damage to the bladder neck you must put the cuff on the bulbar urethra. There are other advantages of the new device; you can regulate the pressure non-invasively after it is implanted.

de Groat: This clinical experiment described by Professor Brindley is fascinating. There are many things one could do (given patients willing to go along with the experimentation). One thing, to carry on from Geoff Burnstock's suggestion, is to examine the possibility of long-term modulation of function either through continuous electrical stimulation, or by withholding stimulation. For example, if a patient were stimulated for several months in the way Professor Brindley described, the functions of the synapses in the periphery might be enhanced. If then stimulation were withheld (e.g. in a patient where a stimulator stopped functioning), when stimulation was resumed it is possible that there would be an initial reduction in the effectiveness of the stimulation. Do you have any experience with this type of experiment?

Brindley: This reduction doesn't happen, at least in 2–3 weeks. We know this because implants fail and it is often two or three weeks before we are able to repair them. They then work instantly as well as they did before. But we have one patient who has been self-catheterizing for three years with a failed implant and now wants us to mend the implant. We might find that it makes a difference that his bladder hasn't been used normally for three years. On the other hand, urological experience tends to go against this. When people with anuria who are on dialysis for a long time receive renal transplants, the very day they have the new kidney, the bladder functions perfectly normally although it hasn't been filled for years and probably hasn't contracted, because most bladders if not filled don't contract.

Brading: The smooth muscles contract all the time. It is just that they are not synchronous, so you don't get an increase in internal pressure.

Brindley: In that case it could be that the patients with unused implants are in the same state, and that's why we see no change in performance when they are not used for a time.

Fowler: Do I gather from your work that the status of the S5 root is in doubt?

Brindley: There are some patients in whom we don't see an S5 root, but in others we do. I know of one German patient in whom the S5 root gave over $20\,cmH_2O$ bladder pressure. Whenever we seen an S5 root that gives a pressure of $5\,cmH_2O$ or less, we crush it, because so small a root is very difficult to separate into anterior and posterior. The theory is that after crushing, the anterior root fibres will ultimately regenerate and any innervation of the anal sphincter will return; the posterior root fibres will regenerate, but make no functional connexions when they reach the spinal cord.

de Groat: You mentioned the pudendal nerve stimulator and said that it could inhibit unstable detrusor contractions. In regard to earlier discussion on the peripheral, smooth muscle or central origin of unstable contractions, what does their inhibition tell you about their origin?

Brindley: Impulses are coming out along the sacral anterior roots at the time of the contraction. The active intermediate horn cells are presumably driven by synaptic bombardment, at least in part coming from bladder afferents. I don't think one can say anything more than this.

Brading: Presumably if you can inhibit the unstable contractions by pudendal nerve stimulation, they must be driven through the spinal cord. But the contractions that can't be inhibited by this means may be myogenic. This might be a good way of telling whether the unstable contractions are in the bladder or are genuinely hyperreflexic.

Brindley: I don't recall any patient in whom there was *no* inhibition of detrusor contractions by pudendal stimulation; the question is whether it is complete and reliable, in which case one is justified in putting in a stimulator, or erratic and not quite complete, as it is in about half the patients I have seen.

de Groat: Thus it would be important to know the percentage of the detrusor contractions that are inhibited by the electrical stimulation. To carry that a step further, in terms of using selective microstimulation in the cord, it would be possible in theory to stimulate inhibitory areas of the cord and turn off the unstable contractions which are centrally mediated. Whereas Professor Brindley is attempting to activate pelvic organs using the stimulation, and this works well with electrical stimulation of a peripheral nerve, if there is activity that is unwanted and that is centrally generated, then microstimulation in the spinal cord or brain should be an effective way to turn that activity off. So this would be one justification for developing the microstimulation technique.

Staskin: What about using stimulators for sensory problems—for pain syndromes or bladder syndromes?

Brindley: Posterior column stimulators certainly help some patients with pain, probably including bladder pain.

Marsden: You are developing mechanical implants to allow defaecation by restoration of the anorectal angulation. In the light of discussion at this symposium, is that something you will pursue?

Brindley: This is David Rushton's project in my department. Although I have heard things here that make me a little less enthusiastic about this kind of mechanical implant than I was—I mean suggestions that anorectal angulation is not as important as was formerly supposed—I am not convinced that the puborectalis muscle is unimportant, and I think the project remains a good one. David Rushton's implant is a low-risk one, because it doesn't endanger the blood supply of any organ.

Swash: We have to remember that there are a number of ways in which faecal continence can be achieved, either by inflating some form of cuff around the anal canal at its caudal end, or by contracting the anal sphincter, the puborectalis or the whole pelvic floor. It doesn't really matter how you do it, so long as it works. Another point to remember is that the operations and other forms of treatment all seem to achieve faecal continence by methods other than the normal physiological method—whatever that is!

Marsden: All these surgical approaches have the consequence of inducing fibrosis around the bottom ends of the urinary and faecal outlets.

Wong: If we are operating on a chordoma and we have to remove the sacrum, including S2, in such patients, thereby rendering them faecally incontinent, should we put in the implant at the time of surgery, or later?

Brindley: If sacral segmental nerves have to be destroyed surgically within the sacrum, a stimulator applied to these nerves more peripherally will be ineffective, because all the nerve fibres will degenerate within 10 days, and they are unlikely to regenerate.

Reference

Hallan RI, Williams NS, Hustan MRE et al 1990 Electrically stimulated sartorius neosphincter: canine model of activation and skeletal muscle transformation. Br J Surg 77:208–213

General discussion IV

Effects of denervation: smooth muscle hypertrophy and nerve regeneration

Swash: In some patients with faecal incontinence in whom there is marked denervation of the pelvic floor, the internal anal sphincter is markedly hypertrophied. It is particularly prominent in people with pelvic floor denervation due to myelomeningocele or poliomyelitis, or other long-standing neurogenic problems. What are the factors that lead to smooth muscle hypertrophy?

Burnstock: An increase in pressure, whether in a blood vessel, in the gut or in the bladder, soon leads to hypertrophy of smooth muscle cells. The bladder is very quick to show hypertrophy. Presumably, increased pressure in the rectum leads to hypertrophy of smooth muscle too?

Swash: Only a few patients develop this response to this functional abnormality or load, so it's not a universal finding. I saw it in a patient who had a hypertrophied internal anal sphincter and in whom haemorrhoidectomy had been followed by devastating faecal incontinence because the pelvic floor was weak, and the patient had presumably been relying previously on the internal anal sphincter for continence.

Burnstock: Is there hyperplasia as well as hypertrophy?

Swash: There is hyperplasia as well. There are more fascicles and more muscle fibres, as well as fibre hypertrophy.

Burnstock: There is much current interest in the trophic factors that control smooth muscle proliferation.

Brindley: It is known that obstructed bladders hypertrophy, and so do bladders that are over-active after spinal injuries. The question of under-active bladders also arises. According to David Thomas, who does cystoscopies on patients with complete cauda equina lesions, they sometimes have trabeculated bladders just like those of patients with over-active bladders. Why should this be so?

Staskin: People often claim to find hypertrophy where in fact the spaces between the muscle fibres are increased and therefore it looks as if the muscle fibres are bigger. Patients who are peripherally denervated after an abdominal-perineal resection for rectal carcinoma may go on to develop flaccid, very compliant bladders, or develop a 'Christmas tree' type of neurogenic bladder (named after its appearance on cystography) which is extremely thickened and trabeculated and non-complaint. Some say that bladder thickening is the result of chronic infection and other sequelae of bladder denervation, but that is not the way the patients present clinically. One wonders whether an alternative neural

283

pathway has been activated and doesn't cause a contraction, but does cause smooth muscle activity in an uncoordinated fashion throughout the bladder, which might be responsible for the hypertrophy.

Brindley: I was assured by David Thomas that patients with areflexic bladders of good compliance, with complete cauda equina lesions, looked hypertrophied, at least on cystoscopic appearances, so they may be misleading.

Kirby: That is right. We have looked at patients with cauda equina lesions with pelvic nerve injury and patients with multiple system atrophy (Shy–Drager syndrome). All those patients are decentralized, if not denervated. The bladder looks hypertrophied on cystoscopy, yet it is atonic and areflexic and has loss of compliance on filling. These patients also lose their voluntary bladder contractions. It really begs the question, whether denervation or decentralization causes hypertrophy. Alison Brading found that the opposite is true; didn't you show that hypertrophy causes denervation?

Brading: Only that they can occur together (Speakman et al 1987).

Kirby: Perhaps part of the problem in prostatic bladder outflow obstruction is first denervation, then hypertrophy, rather than the other way around?

Swash: There is hyperplasia as well, in incontinent patients.

Kirby: Yes; in obstructed patients John Gosling has shown hyperplasia as well as hypertrophy in the detrusor muscle (Gilpin et al 1985). The muscle fibres are bigger and become more numerous.

Brading: We have some indications of mini-pig bladders that have nerve damage but are not hypertrophic, so I don't know that denervation and hypertrophy always go together.

Burnstock: What was the evidence that the innervation was reduced in the hypertrophic bladder? For example, assays calculated according to nerve density per unit weight can give a distorted picture if there is hypertrophy of muscle.

Brading: We have a standard procedure using sections taken at intervals through the bladder and stained for acetylcholinesterase. We also use electron microscopy to count nerve profiles. The nerve counts are corrected to allow for hypertrophy (Speakman et al 1987). The actual number of nerves in the total bladder is greatly reduced, by up to 90%.

de Groat: Are we discussing denervated or areflexic bladders? The former are also called autonomous hyperactive bladders. These occur with conus lesions. They are not very compliant and generate relatively high pressures.

Kirby: It's difficult to be certain clinically, because the lesions are usually incomplete, but they are patients who complain of inability to void and are self-catheterizing. It is usually due to a conus or cauda equina lesion, produced by a prolapsed intervertebral disc or a tumour.

de Groat: The patients with autonomous hyperactive bladders are at some risk because they store urine at very high pressures. Patients with myelomeningocele exhibit this type of bladder disorder.

Kirby: Myelomeningocele is more complicated because it is an incomplete denervation. But patients with pure cauda equina lesions generally have raised intravesicular pressures during bladder filling.

de Groat: We have conducted studies in cats to examine the mechanisms involved in the development of the autonomous hyperactive bladder (de Groat & Kawatani 1989). The experimental animals have an intact afferent innervation, but the preganglionic axons are interrupted. Under these conditions we have detected local reflexes where the C fibre afferents make short-loop connections with the ganglion cells. In theory, when the bladder is distended in these lesioned animals, afferent activity could generate a discharge in the postganglionic neurons and feed excitation back to the bladder.

Thus the areflexic bladder is not necessarily inactive; it may be receiving a tonic excitatory input from local circuits in the peripheral nervous system. Under these conditions the bladder doesn't store urine properly and holds urine at a high pressure. These local circuits may be formed by sprouting of afferent axons to reinnervate the denervated postganglionic neurons.

Brading: And the parasympathetic ganglia are very often in the bladder wall, so the input doesn't have far to go.

de Groat: Yes, the neurons could be in the bladder wall. In some species, such as the guinea pig, as Geoff Burnstock has described, these kinds of local connections may be present in normal conditions and accentuated by denervation, to produce a more prominent local reflex pathway. One wonders whether drugs can be developed that interfere with this system at various points, so that the autonomous hyperactive bladder can be treated pharmacologically rather than neurosurgically. In one report, these patients were treated by removal of the sacral dorsal root ganglia. Bladder activity was reduced, implying that in patients the afferent system may be important in triggering this hyperactivity.

Maggi: If your hypothesis is correct, it would be worth trying intravesical capsaicin to block a fraction of sensory nerves and see whether you can reduce the bladder hyperactivity.

de Groat: This would definitely be worth investigating.

Andersson: It has been said that these autonomous waves of contraction in parasympathetically decentralized patients with overflow incontinence are susceptible to α-receptor blockers (Norlén & Sundin 1978). If this is the case, it suggests that the postganglionic neuron is adrenergic.

de Groat: Unfortunately, those studies used phenoxybenzamine as the α-blocking agent, and this drug has an atropine-like action. Our studies in the cat were designed to examine the adrenergic hypothesis. We concluded that the early investigators misinterpreted their data and that they used phenoxybenzamine at such high concentrations that it was blocking the muscarinic receptors in the bladder smooth muscle. We saw very little evidence for α-adrenergic mechanisms in this model.

Maggi: There are short adrenergic neurons in the pelvic ganglia, so I don't think there is necessarily any disagreement here. A neuropeptide released locally in the pelvic ganglia could release noradrenaline from these adrenergic neurons. Both tachykinins and CGRP have been shown to excite elements in sympathetic ganglia (Saria et al 1987, Dun & Mo 1989). Therefore a local reflex mediated by sensory nerves in the bladder might well lead to activation of adrenergic elements in the ganglia.

de Groat: In the cat, VIP is present in 25–30% of the bladder afferents, and is present only in C fibres. When VIP is administered to denervated ganglia it has an excitatory effect. I think Geoff Burnstock also saw a slow depolarization by VIP in intramural ganglia from the guinea pig. Therefore not only substance P but other peptides could be the excitatory transmitters in this system.

Andersson: When we tried prazosin on patients with parasympathetic decentralization and increased outflow resistance, we also noted an effect on the autonomous waves (Andersson et al 1981). This means that it's not completely certain that the effects of phenoxybenzamine were mediated through receptors other than α-adrenoreceptors.

de Groat: One other complication is that these parasympathetic ganglion cells have α_1 excitatory receptors, and their firing is facilitated by α_1-adrenergic mechanisms.

Maggi: Studies in animals have shown that the tachykinins, such as substance P, are very important, but this is not necessarily the case for the human bladder. In other visceral organs, such as ileum or colon, we have evidence that capsaicin releases VIP from human tissue (Maggi et al 1989), so there may be important organ-related and species-related differences in the expression of neuropeptides in sensory nerves.

Kirby: Didn't Sundin also show an overgrowth of sympathetic nerve terminals in denervated cat bladders?

de Groat: Yes. There are various kinds of reinnervation after damage to the parasympathetic nerves. The bladder ganglia in the cat also receive inputs from hypogastric sympathetic nerves, and we confirm the earlier findings of Sundin and coworkers that stimulation of the hypogastric nerve in animals with parasympathetic lesions will lead to a bladder contraction (Sundin & Dahlström 1973, Sundin et al 1977). This seems to be mediated not through an adrenergic activation of smooth muscle, but through cholinergic activation of the ganglion cells. It is blocked by atropine rather than by phenoxybenzamine.

Burnstock: Prostaglandins are very important in the bladder; one only has to mechanically disturb the bladder and prostaglandins are produced which have potent local effects. Furthermore, when the pelvic nerve is stimulated, in some species, 30–60% of the contractile response is blocked by indomethacin, an inhibitor of prostaglandin synthesis. This may be important in surgery and during other manipulations.

Stanton: We have given intravesical prostaglandin, in an attempt to overcome postoperative urinary retention, following the study of Bultitude et al (1976). But one can't conceive of one dose of prostaglandins producing activity in a bladder that has been quiescent for years. We were unable to produce effective bladder contractions. There was a response, but not a sustained contraction. We wondered how much of the prostaglandin was getting back across the epithelium into the bladder muscle.

Maggi: Were those bladders areflexic?

Stanton: They weren't showing any response to bladder filling.

Maggi: In my view, major targets of prostanoids delivered into the bladder are the sensory nerves. There is clear evidence that prostanoids can sensitize or stimulate sensory nerves in the bladder (Maggi et al 1988); they can contract the muscle, but it is a very weak effect and it may also contribute to sensitizing sensory nerves. But if there were no reflex on which to work I don't see how prostaglandins could facilitate anything.

Andersson: Which prostaglandins did you use?

Stanton: We used E2 and also $F_{2\alpha}$. But we haven't used the methyl analogue, which may be more effective.

Andersson: There are differences in the actions of the prostaglandins between bladder and urethra (Andersson et al 1977). Prostaglandin $F_{2\alpha}$ contracts both; prostaglandins E2 and E1 relax the urethra and contract the bladder. We tried to facilitate bladder emptying in women with difficulty in this by applying PGE2 into the urethra (Andersson et al 1978), and it also leaked into the bladder. We recorded a small decrease in intraurethral pressure and an increase in bladder pressure; there were vesical pain sensations, urge, and also dysmenorrhoea-like pains, but there was no effective increase in bladder pressure that would improve emptying.

Staskin: I shall be discussing the use of prostaglandins in my paper (see p 300).

Stanton: We went on to use flurbiprofen in high doses for instability, to the extent that people were getting side-effects. This wasn't effective either. But it may be worth looking at again.

Burnstock: Have you used prostacyclin at all?

Stanton: No.

Burnstock: I should also mention that ATP is a potent initiator of prostaglandin and prostacyclin synthesis!

References

Andersson K-E, Ek A, Persson CGA 1977 Effects of prostaglandins on the isolated human bladder and urethra. Acta Physiol Scand 100:165–171

Andersson K-E, Henriksson L, Ulmstrom U 1978 Effect of prostaglandin E_2 applied locally on intravesical and intraurethral pressures in women. Eur J Urol 4:366–369

Andersson K-E, Ek A, Hedlund H, Mattiasson A 1981 Effects of prazosin on isolated human urethra and in patients with lower motor neuron lesions. Invest Urol 19:39–42

Bultitude MI, Hills NH, Shuttleworth KED 1976 Clinical and experimental studies on the action of prostaglandins and their synthesis inhibitors on detrusor muscle in vitro and in vivo. Br J Urol 48:631–637

de Groat WC, Kawatani M 1989 Reorganization of sympathetic preganglionic connections in bladder ganglia of the cat following parasympathetic denervation. J Physiol (Lond) 409:431–449

Dun NJ, Mo N 1989 CGRP evokes distinct types of excitatory response in guinea-pig coeliac ganglion cells. Brain Res 476:256–264

Gilpin SA, Gosling JA, Bernard RJ 1985 Morphological and morphometric studies of the human obstructed, trabeculated urinary bladder. Br J Urol 57:525–529

Maggi CA, Giuliani S, Coute B et al 1988 Prostanoids modulate reflex micturition by acting through capsaicin-sensitive afferents. Eur J Pharmacol 145:105–112

Maggi CA, Sauticioli P, Del Bianco E et al 1989 Release of VIP- but not CGRP-like immunoreactivity from the human isolated small intestine. Neurosci Lett 98:317–320

Norlén L, Sundin T 1978 Alphaadrenolytic treatment in patients with autonomous bladders. Acta Pharmacol Toxicol 43 (Suppl II):31–34

Saria A, Ma RC, Dun NJ, Theodorsson-Norheim E, Lundberg JM 1987 Neurokinin A in capsaicin-sensitive neurons of the guinea-pig inferior mesenteric ganglia: an additional putative mediator for the non-cholinergic excitatory postsynaptic potential. Neuroscience 21:951– 958

Speakman MJ, Brading AF, Gilpin CJ, Dixon JS, Gilpin SA, Gosling J 1987 Bladder outflow obstruction—a cause of denervation supersensitivity. J Urol 138:1461–1466

Sundin T, Dahlström A 1973 The sympathetic innervation of the urinary bladder and urethra in the normal state and after parasympathetic denervation at the spinal root level. Scand J Urol Nephrol 7:131–149

Sundin T, Dahlström A, Norlén L, Svedmayer N 1977 The sympathetic innervation and adrenoreceptor function of the human lower urinary tract in the normal state and after parasympathetic denervation. Invest Urol 14:322-328

Urinary incontinence: classification and pharmacological therapy

David R. Staskin,* Alan J. Wein† and Karl-Erik Andersson‡

*Division of Urology, Harvard University School of Medicine, Beth Israel Hospital, 330 Brookline Avenue, Boston, MA 02215, USA, †Department of Urology, University of Pennsylvania School of Medicine, Hospital of the University of Pennsylvania, 3400 Spruce Street, Philadelphia, PA 19104, USA and ‡Department of Clinical Pharmacology, University Hospital of Lund, S-221 85 Lund, Sweden

Abstract. Pharmacological therapy has been developed which can have significant impact in the management of many forms of urinary incontinence and voiding dysfunction. In general the clinical laboratory studies which have supported or challenged the efficacy of many of the commonly prescribed drugs for voiding dysfunction are often difficult to interpret and contradictory. The available clinical studies often do not demonstrate a lack of bias. Nor do they include an adequate number of subjects, use appropriate and sensitive methods of evaluation, employ double-blind placebo-controlled design, or appear statistically valid. Although the contribution of laboratory research has been of unquestionable value in the development of our current knowledge of lower urinary tract pharmacology it is difficult to interpret the results of *in vitro* pharmacological studies because of the array of experimental models used and the need to extrapolate to *in vivo* activity. This paper utilizes a functional scheme which classifies agents by their effects on urinary storage and emptying. The purpose of this review is to promote discussion of the application of uropharmacological investigation to the development of newer, more efficacious forms of drug therapy.

1990 Neurobiology of Incontinence. Wiley, Chichester (Ciba Foundation Symposium 151) p 289–317

Pharmacological therapy now exists which can have a significant impact on the management of many forms of urinary incontinence and voiding dysfunction. We shall review general physiological and pharmacological concepts and the indications for specific medications, and will offer practical caveats concerning the use of some of the commonly prescribed agents within a functional classification.

Lower urinary tract function can be divided into two phases—urinary storage and bladder emptying. Lower urinary tract anatomy can be divided into two functional areas—the bladder and the bladder outlet (Wein 1981). Efficient bladder filling and urinary storage require (1) the accommodation of increasing volumes of urine by the bladder smooth musculature and connective tissue at a low intravesical pressure, with the absence of involuntary bladder contractions and with appropriate sensation, and (2) a closed bladder outlet which provides sufficient resistance through smooth and skeletal musculature components to prevent the loss of urine during increases in intra-abdominal pressure. Efficient bladder emptying requires (1) a coordinated contraction of adequate magnitude by the vesical smooth muscle to accomplish complete bladder emptying, (2) concomitant lowering of resistance at the level of the smooth and striated muscle sphincters, and (3) the absence of anatomical obstruction (observed primarily in the male patient with prostatic enlargement).

Although urinary incontinence should seemingly be classified primarily as a disorder of urinary storage, poor bladder emptying may commonly be the underlying cause which precipitates lower urinary tract storage dysfunction. Currently accepted methods of pharmacological manipulation of the urinary tract include drugs which exert their effect on either the over-active (inappropriately elevated pressure during filling) or under-active (inadequate generation of pressure during emptying) bladder, or the over-active (inappropriately elevated resistance during emptying) or under-active (inadequate resistance during storage) bladder outlet.

The clinical and laboratory studies which have supported or challenged the efficacy of many of the drugs commonly used for voiding dysfunction are often difficult to interpret and are often contradictory. Laboratory research has undoubtedly contributed to the development of our knowledge of lower urinary tract pharmacology, but the results of *in vitro* studies may be affected by the difficulty of interpreting data from the array of experimental models and the need to extrapolate to *in vivo* activity. The available clinical studies do not always demonstrate a lack of bias, include an adequate number of subjects, use appropriate and sensitive methods of evaluation and double-blinded placebo-controlled design, or appear statistically valid. Selected clinical studies will be reviewed in order to illustrate some of these pitfalls.

At the outset it should be noted that despite the rational use of pharmacological therapy, although great improvement is often observed, restoration to normal voiding status is seldom achieved. In some instances an alternative means of emptying the bladder such as intermittent self-catheterization must be acceptable, when the goal of therapy is to precipitate a degree of urinary retention in order to attain continence.

In addition, most if not all clinically useful pharmacological agents have some side-effects. In general the simplest and least hazardous form of treatment should be tried first, and interactions with other medications, or specific contraindications to drug therapy because of other medical conditions, must be considered. The relative cost of medications will not be reviewed here but may be a consideration. Many drugs used to treat unrelated conditions may have a detrimental effect on voiding function if their mechanism of action affects bladder or bladder outlet function, the pattern of urinary production (e.g. diuretics), or the physical or behavioural skills necessary to perform toileting functions (e.g. sedatives). An acute change in continence status, especially in the elderly, always requires a thorough review of current prescription and non-prescription medications.

Therapy designed to facilitate urinary storage

Treatment of abnormalities of storage is directed towards inhibiting bladder contractility or decreasing bladder tone during filling, or towards increasing outlet resistance.

The *over-active bladder* (elevated intravesical pressure) during filling may result from identifiable discrete involuntary contractions or low compliance of the bladder wall, alone or in combination. Involuntary bladder contractions are most commonly seen in association with neurological disease or after neurological injury (detrusor hyperreflexia) with inflammatory or irritative processes in the bladder wall, or with bladder outlet obstruction, or may be idiopathic (detrusor instability). Decreased compliance during filling may be secondary to the sequelae of neurological injury or disease, but may also result from any process that destroys the viscoelastic properties of the bladder wall. Sensory urgency (the sensation of the need to void without a true increase in intravesical pressure) may result in inefficient storage manifested by frequent voiding and may occur secondary to inflammatory, infectious, neurological, psychological, or idiopathic causes.

The *under-active bladder outlet* (decreased outlet resistance) may result from a weakening of anatomical support of the bladder neck and proximal urethra, or urethral dysfunction. Urethral dysfunction may follow physical (surgical or mechanical) damage to the bladder neck or urethral mechanisms, or physiological changes (neurological disease, or hormonal or vascular changes associated with ageing) which affect the innervation or structural elements of the sphincteric mechanism. Classical genuine stress incontinence in women results primarily from anatomical support deficiencies which prevent the normal transmission of increases in intra-abdominal pressure to the bladder neck and proximal urethra. Genuine stress incontinence in the male patient is associated primarily with iatrogenic damage to the sphincteric mechanism during prostate surgery and may be exacerbated by underlying distal sphincteric dysfunction.

Drugs which decrease bladder contractility or increase compliance

Anticholinergic (antimuscarinic) agents. A major portion of the neurohumoral stimulus for physiological bladder contraction is acetylcholine-induced stimulation of postganglionic parasympathetic cholinergic receptor sites on bladder smooth muscle. There are reasons to believe that muscarinic receptors mediate not only normal bladder contractions but also the main part of contractions in hyperactive bladders. Atropine and atropine-like agents are known to produce almost complete paralysis of the normal bladder when injected intravenously. However, despite the ability of the antimuscarinic agents to produce significant clinical improvement in patients with involuntary bladder contractions, in many cases only partial inhibition may result at clinically tolerated dosages. This may be partially attributed to low bioavailability, making it difficult to achieve sufficient drug concentration in the effector organ, to side-effects which limit the dose that can be given, or possibly to 'atropine resistance'.

In addition to its inability to suppress detrusor activity completely in clinical situations, atropine is unable to inhibit completely *in vitro* bladder contractility induced by both nerve and electrical stimulation in many animal smooth muscle models, although not in human bladder specimens. The resistance to atropine suggests that a portion of the neurotransmission in the final common pathway of bladder contraction may be non-cholinergic and non-adrenergic, secondary to release of a neurotransmitter other than acetylcholine or noradrenaline. Atropine resistance has not been demonstrated in human or porcine bladder muscle (Sibley 1984, Kinder & Mundy 1985, Wein et al 1987). Nevertheless, the concept is applied to explain the difficulty in abolishing involuntary bladder contractions with anticholinergic agents, and used also to support treatment of such types of persistent bladder activity with additional pharmacological agents which display different mechanisms of action.

Commonly prescribed agents with almost exclusively anticholinergic activity are propantheline bromide, L-hyoscyamine sulphate, methantheline bromide, and emepronium bromide. The use of these medications as first-line therapy, or in combination with other agents (musculotropics, tricyclic antidepressants, calcium channel antagonists) for the treatment of incontinence secondary to uninhibited contractions is widely accepted. However, patients who do not respond to or do not tolerate the side-effects of drugs which are purely anticholinergic will often benefit from other classes of medication.

The potential side-effects of anticholinergic therapy are due to the non-bladder-specific nature of antimuscarinic drugs. Muscarinic receptors in the bladder have not exhibited characteristics which clearly separate them from muscarinic receptors in other organs. In our experience, complaints of dry mouth, blurred vision, gastric reflux and constipation are most commonly elicited, but these side-effects are often willingly tolerated by patients who have experienced a good clinical response in terms of bladder control. Anticholinergics should be prescribed with extreme caution in patients with narrow-angle glaucoma, significant bladder outlet obstruction, obstructive, atonic or toxic gastrointestinal disease, cardiac arrhythmia and myasthenia gravis. Care should be taken in prescribing these agents to young children and the elderly, who may be more prone to the sequelae of dehydration and decreased perspiration. Many elderly patients, independent of their physicians' instructions or knowledge, may voluntarily restrict their fluid intake because of their incontinence and be more susceptible to these problems.

Variations in the dosage and route of administration during clinical evaluations of drug efficacy may affect the interpretation of the results. This problem can be illustrated by studies which utilized propantheline and emepronium. These agents have low biological availability when given orally, within the 5–10% range, and may vary markedly between individuals. The benefit of individual drug titration, which is rarely performed during clinical trials, was demonstrated in a study (Blaivas et al 1980) where the propantheline dose, usually 15 to 30 mg four times daily, was varied between 7.5 and 60 mg four times daily in order to obtain a complete response in 25 of 26 patients. Interestingly, the non-responder was unable to tolerate a dose of 15 mg four times daily.

The poor oral absorption of emepronium prompted several investigations of an intramuscular preparation to assess the drug's efficacy (Ekeland & Sander 1976, Cardozo et al 1980, Perera et al 1982). It was notable that in contrast to the efficacy demonstrated with the oral form, an absence of bladder response to 0.3 mg/kg given intramuscularly was found in one study (Perera et al 1982).

The necessity for double-blind controlled studies when establishing the clinical efficacy of medications used to treat urinary incontinence cannot be questioned. The placebo response during the evaluation of drugs for voiding dysfunction has been estimated to be approximately 30%. In one study (Hansen et al 1982) no difference between oral emepronium (200 mg, three times daily) and placebo was noted, with the overall subjective cure or improvement rate in the drug and the placebo groups being 79%!

Direct smooth muscle relaxants. Smooth muscle cells depend on the cytoplasmic concentration of calcium ions for activation of their contractile proteins. During smooth muscle stimulation, an increase in intracellular calcium levels occurs as a result of an increased permeability of the membrane and influx of extracellular calcium, and from a secondary release of calcium from intracellular stores. The rise in cytosolic calcium concentration initiates smooth muscle contraction by serving as a cofactor with calmodulin for the activation of myosin light-chain kinase.

Calcium antagonists have proved effective in a variety of cardiovascular disorders. They have been used to treat bladder dysfunction on the basis of their presumed ability to provide an additional action to suppress bladder smooth muscle contractility at a site metabolically distal to the cholinergic receptor. Differences in the degree and site of action may be used to explain the selective effects of various calcium antagonists on the inhibitory response to cholinergic and electrical field stimulation during *in vitro* studies on human detrusor muscle (Fovaeus et al 1987). Unfortunately, the information available from clinical trials does not suggest that systemic therapy with pure calcium antagonists is an effective way to treat bladder hyperactivity.

The mechanism of flavoxate has not been established, although it has been found to have moderate calcium antagonistic activity and an ability to inhibit phosphodiesterase, but no anticholinergic activity. The clinical effects of flavoxate have been studied and have demonstrated varying rates of success, as with the pure calcium channel antagonists.

Drugs with mixed actions (anticholinergic and smooth muscle relaxants). Some medications used in the treatment of the over-active bladder have been shown to have more than one mechanism of action *in vitro*, but all have a more or less pronounced anticholinergic effect which is usually associated with the dominant side-effects. The clinical efficacy of this group of agents may result predominantly from their atropine-like effect at clinically tolerated dosages, but their additional smooth muscle relaxant properties theoretically support their use both as primary therapy, as well as in combination with other agents.

Commonly prescribed agents include oxybutynin chloride (potent anticholinergic, papaverine-like direct smooth muscle relaxant, local anaesthetic), dicyclomine hydrochloride (anticholinergic, direct smooth muscle relaxant), terodiline (anticholinergic and calcium antagonist), and imipramine (weak central and peripheral anticholinergic, blocks the active transport system in the presynaptic nerve ending responsible for amine reuptake, antihistaminic and calcium antagonistic).

Clinical studies have shown that oxybutynin is effective in controlling the over-active bladder and that the dose-limiting side-effects, like those of other agents in this group, are anticholinergic in nature. A randomized double-blind controlled study which was performed in 30 patients with detrusor instability and which compared oxybutynin (Ditropan) (5 mg orally, three times daily) to placebo (Moisey et al 1980) is useful for illustrating the difficulty in objectively documenting, by urodynamic testing, the subjective improvements noted during treatment. Of the 23 patients who received oxybutynin, 17 had symptomatic improvement and nine had evidence of urodynamic improvement, mainly an increase in bladder volume at first contraction and an increase in total bladder capacity. However, although the efficacy of the medication was demonstrated and urodynamic parameters in the group improved, the individual clinical responses to the medication did not correlate with the objective responses to bladder filling in the urodynamic laboratory. The difficulty in establishing a correlation between the level of clinical improvement and objective urodynamic findings is common not only to this class of agents but to most of the drugs used to treat voiding dysfunction.

The beneficial effects of terodiline in patients with over-active bladders has also been demonstrated in several controlled trials. In the rabbit bladder, terodiline caused a complete inhibition of the response to electrical field stimulation (Husted et al 1980). Terodiline has been proposed to possess both anticholinergic and calcium antagonistic properties within the same relative concentration range. However, at low concentrations, it seems to have a mainly antimuscarinic action, whereas at higher concentration the calcium antagonist effect becomes evident. These two effects seem at least additive *in vitro*, but whether the drug is *in vivo* actually more effective than standard antimuscarinic agents alone remains to be established. The anticholinergic properties seem to dominate at clinically tolerated doses. The difficulty in extrapolating the dose-related pharmacological efficacy of vesical smooth muscle in an animal laboratory model to the clinical situation is obvious.

The clinical efficacy of terodiline has been established in a well-constructed and well-supervised multicentre study which used a randomized, double-blind, two-period cross-over protocol (Peters 1984). The results revealed a patient preference for terodiline over placebo of 63%. There was no significant difference in side-effects; however, 35% of the patients demonstrated side-effects on placebo. The frequency of voluntary micturition decreased from 9.6 to 8.9 per 24 hours on placebo, and from 9.9 to 7.3 on terodiline. Involuntary micturitions decreased from 2.3 to 1.7 on placebo and from 2.5 to 1.5 on terodiline. Volume at first desire to void increased on placebo from 159 to 162 and on terodiline from 151 to 198 ml. Bladder capacity increased from 312 to 318 ml on placebo and from 320 to 374 ml on terodiline. All these changes were shown to be statistically significant.

The results of this well-monitored study which demonstrated the efficacy of terodiline can be used to illustrate several points. The patient preference for the 73 of 89 patients who completed the trial showed that 31 of 46 patients favoured the drug over placebo. Although this difference is statistically significant, the number of patients preferring placebo and having side-effects on the placebo is notable. The cystometric volume increase, which was recorded before the first desire to void, was increased negligibly in the placebo group, and would and should not be expected to explain the improvement in voiding frequency or involuntary voiding. The results also reinforce the difficulty in correlating the improvement in voiding frequency with cystometric findings. The total volume voided per day is rarely recorded, even in studies which are testing agents that affect bladder function. The total urine output, which is dependent on fluid intake, is useful in eliminating the effects of increased fluid intake and output which are often associated with improved continence.

The difference between statistical significance and clinical significance should also be considered when one reviews any clinical efficacy trial. The improvements in voiding frequency (8.9 on placebo vs. 7.3 on terodiline) and in involuntary micturition (1.7 on placebo to 1.5 on terodiline) were statistically significant, but the clinical improvement of voiding every two hours and 41 minutes (placebo) or every three hours and 16 minutes (terodiline), or having 17 incontinence episodes (placebo) vs 15 incontinence episodes (terodiline) over ten days, may or may not cause notable improvement in the patients' lifestyles.

Prostaglandin inhibitors.   Prostaglandins have been proposed to have a role in excitatory neurotransmission and contractile activity, and perhaps as a cofactor in the response to ATP in the lower urinary tract. Although prostaglandins are not felt to be directly involved in bladder emptying, they may contribute to the tone or spontaneous activity of bladder muscle, act as modulators of transmission, or affect the sensory afferent nerves by increasing the activity at a given bladder volume. An effect on bladder epithelium by prostaglandins which mimics bladder irritation has been implicated (Downie & Karmazyn 1984). Studies have been performed with flurbiprofen and indomethacin, which provide some symptomatic effect but were not shown to completely abolish detrusor hyperactivity (Cardozo et al 1980).

Polysynaptic inhibitors.   Baclofen has been suggested to be effective both for patients with detrusor hyperreflexia secondary to spinal cord lesions (Roussan et al 1975) and for idiopathic detrusor instability (Taylor & Bates 1979). The high incidence of side-effects with this class of drugs limits their usefulness in the treatment of bladder over-activity.

β-Adrenergic agonists and α-adrenergic antagonists.   The presence of β-adrenergic receptors in human bladder muscle, which are responsible for smooth muscle relaxation during sympathetic stimulation, has prompted clinical attempts to increase bladder capacity by stimulating these receptors. The proposed mechanism of action of α-adrenergic blocking agents is that parasympathetic denervation of the bladder results in a marked increase in its adrenergic innervation, with a resulting conversion of the usual β (relaxant) response of the bladder body in response to sympathetic stimulation to an α (contractile) effect (Sundin et al 1977). Although these alterations in innervation have been disputed (Nordling et al 1980), the alteration in receptor function has not. Patients with myelodysplasia, or sacral spinal cord or infrasacral neural injury, and those with voiding dysfunction after radical pelvic surgery, often demonstrate decreased bladder compliance. There is also evidence that bladder outlet obstruction may result in an alteration of the β-receptor to an α-receptor response (Perlberg & Caine 1982). The supporting evidence for the use of α-adrenolytic therapy in these patients has been summarized (Norlén 1982). The use of these agents has not gained wide clinical acceptance. The use of α-adrenergic antagonists to decrease outlet resistance is discussed below in the section on the over-active bladder outlet.

Selection of patients for treatment of detrusor over-activity

Patients with uninhibited bladder contractions who demonstrate unobstructed emptying of the bladder are the main group of patients who will benefit from treatment for detrusor over-activity. The bladder is rarely inhibited completely, but the functional capacity will increase, the force of detrusor contractions will decrease, and voluntary control will be expected to improve. The findings of a normal flow rate, a low post-void residual and uninhibited bladder contractions on a cystometrogram make up the ideal urodynamic presentation. Although urodynamic equipment of varying sophistication is not always available, the post-void urinary residual may be followed by catheterization or ultrasound before and after instituting therapy.

Patients with uninhibited bladder contractions but with poor bladder emptying present a more complex therapeutic challenge. Many elderly patients with uninhibited bladder contractions demonstrate detrusor hyperactivity with impaired contractile function, resulting in increased residual urine (Resnick & Yalla 1987). The balance between the benefit of inhibiting bladder contractility and the problems associated with increasing the post-voiding residual volume is not yet clear. However, if the continence status of the patients is improved, the residual urine can be followed if it does not predispose to urinary tract infections or impaired renal function. If the residual urine compromises continence by decreasing the functional capacity of the bladder, then an intermittent catheterization schedule can be instituted or therapy may be discontinued.

Inhibition of detrusor contractility in the presence of outlet obstruction is not advocated, especially when therapy for outlet obstruction is relatively safe and quite effective. The use of anticholinergic agents in the presence of outlet obstruction may be associated with total urinary retention.

Cognitive impairment and decreased ability to perform toileting functions, which may be associated with the primary neurological disease that is responsible for loss of bladder inhibition, may also affect continence. Pharmacological therapy should be used in these patients with specific goals in mind. Decreasing the number of incontinence episodes, increasng the 'warning period', or increasing the functional capacity of the bladder may be helpful, in combination with a toileting or behavioural intervention programme.

Drugs which increase outlet resistance

α-Adrenergic agonists. The bladder neck and proximal urethra contain a preponderance of α-adrenergic receptor sites, which produce smooth muscle contraction. The maximal pressure and maximal closure pressure of the urethra are increased by stimulating these receptors (Ek et al 1978). Outlet resistance is increased to a variable degree by such an action. The α-adrenergic agonists phenypropanolamine and pseudoephedrine are available as non-prescription medications in the form of decongestants or appetite suppressants. α-Adrenergic stimulants should be used with caution in patients with hypertension, diabetes mellitus, heart disease, peripheral vascular disease, increased intraocular pressure, hyperthyroidism or prostatic hypertrophy.

The role of α-adrenoreceptors in the chronic treatment of stress urinary incontinence has not been established. Satisfactory results have been reported with short-term use, but the improvements in urethral closure pressure demonstrated in the urodynamics laboratory have not been translated to long-term clinical success.

Imipramine has been used to increase outflow resistance because of its ability to block noradrenaline uptake in peripheral nerves. This increase in adrenergic tone would be expected to enhance the closure pressure of the bladder neck and proximal urethra. Although beneficial effects have been reported, there are no controlled clinical trials demonstrating the efficacy of imipramine, and the profile of side-effects may limit its usefulness in stress urinary incontinence.

Oestrogen therapy.   This facilitates urinary storage in some women, especially those who are postmenopausal, by increasing urethral outlet resistance. Whether this effect is related to changes in the autonomic innervation or receptor content of the urethral smooth muscle, which results in improved function, or to changes in the non-muscular elements of the urethral wall (urethral mucosa, submucosal vasculature and connective tissue), has not been clearly established. Clinical experience also supports an augmented or additive effect when oestrogens are combined with α-adrenergic therapy.

The urethra and trigone are embryologically related to the female genital tract and signficant work has been done on the effects of oestrogenic hormones on the lower urinary tract. The sensitivity of α-adrenergic stimulation (Hodgson et al 1978), the α-adrenergic receptor content and autonomic innervation (Levin et al 1981), and the sensitivity of the urethral smooth muscle to noradrenaline stimulation, have all been shown to be oestrogen dependent. Oestrogen replacement increases the function of the urethral sphincter mechanism in castrated female baboons by a mechanism unrelated to the skeletal muscle component of the sphincter (Bump & Friedman 1986).

In addition to the broad range of side-effects associated with oestrogen therapy, known or suspected breast carcinoma, a history of thrombophlebitis or thrombotic disorders, and abnormal genital bleeding are specific contraindications to therapy. The risk of increased endometrial carcinoma is time and dose dependent, and an increased risk of breast carcinoma in postmenopausal women has been suggested.

Therapy designed to facilitate bladder emptying

Absolute or relative failure to empty the bladder results from decreased bladder contractility, increased outlet resistance, or both. Decreased bladder contractility may result from temporary or permanent alteration in the neurological or muscular mechanisms necessary for initiating and maintaining a normal detrusor contraction. Increased outlet resistance is generally secondary to anatomical obstruction, but may be secondary to a failure of coordinated relaxation of the smooth or striated muscle sphincters during bladder contraction usually observed in patients with spinal cord injury. An alteration in the normal dynamic interaction of the bladder and bladder outlet, characterized by an increase in outlet resistance, may result in poor bladder emptying despite normal or over-active bladder function.

Poor bladder emptying may precipitate a spectrum of urinary storage abnormalities, ranging from mild frequency and urgency to severe incontinence. The underlying pathophysiology may be poor detrusor function or increased outlet resistance, resulting in moderately elevated urinary residuals which decrease the functional capacity of the bladder. Significant retention may result in overflow incontinence. The pathophysiological relationship between bladder outlet obstruction and uninhibited bladder contractions is generally accepted, although not completely understood. The general improvement in both clinical symptoms and cystometric parameters, which has been measured after relief of the obstruction, supports the causal relationship with bladder outlet obstruction as an aetiology for uninhibited bladder contractions.

Treatment for failure to empty the bladder generally consists of attempts to increase intravesical pressure or to facilitate the micturition reflex, to decrease outlet resistance, or both. When increased outlet resistance is accompanied by increased bladder activity, relief of the obstruction may be necessary before treatment of the overactive detrusor in order to avoid urinary retention.

Drugs which increase bladder contractility

Parasympathomimetric agents. Because at least a major portion of the final common pathway in physiological bladder contraction is stimulation of the muscarinic cholinergic receptor sites at the postganglionic parasympathetic neuromuscular junction, agents that imitate the actions of acetylcholine might be expected to be useful in the management of patients who cannot empty because of inadequate bladder contractility. Many acetylcholine-like drugs are available, but only bethanechol chloride has a relatively selective action on the urinary bladder and gut with little or no effect at therapeutic dosages on autonomic ganglia or on the cardiovascular system (Taylor 1985). Bethanechol chloride is cholinesterase resistant and *in vitro* stimulates a contraction of smooth muscle from all areas of the bladder (Raezer et al 1973). Adverse reactions rarely occur after oral administration and many of the side-effects which are described for these agents are limited to the subcutaneous route of administration. The medications should be used cautiously in patients with bronchial asthma, coronary artery disease, hyperthyroidism, peptic ulcer, Parkinsonism, or obstructive gastrointestinal disease. Use of these agents in patients with anatomical or neurogenic bladder outlet obstruction may precipitate high pressure urinary retention and increase the risk of upper tract deterioration.

The use of bethanechol chloride given by a subcutaneous or oral route for the treatment of decreased bladder emptying or urinary retention is common, but the clinical data to support such use are rare. Several reports (Diokno & Koppenhoeffer 1976, Diokno & Lapides 1977) have claimed a beneficial effect of bethanecol in 'rehabilitating' atonic or hypotonic bladders. Bethanechol (50–100 mg/day) has also been given in combination with phenoxybenzamine (20–30 mg/day) to patients with atonic bladders and functional outlet obstruction (Khanna 1976). A subcutaneous dose of 5 mg of bethanecol does increase the intravesical pressure at all points along the accommodation curve of the cystometrogram and does decrease the bladder capacity threshold (Lapides 1964, Yalla et al 1977b). This response of detrusor muscle to bethanecol is also noted *in vitro*. However, a relatively constant increase in tension in all areas of the bladder smooth muscle should not be confused with the ability to stimulate a physiological bladder contraction in a patient who cannot normally initiate one. The evidence that repeated doses of bethanecol could conceivably affect the bladder smooth muscle or facilitate the micturition reflex arc in a manner which would help to stimulate a bladder contraction has also not been presented. The reported effects of the medication must be carefully distinguished from other simultaneous manoeuvres which are often performed for patients in urinary retention.

The results of various studies (Gibbon 1965, Merrill & Rota 1974, Yalla et al 1977a, Light & Scott 1982) have not supported the use of bethanecol to improve bladder emptying in patients with neurogenic bladder dysfunction. Non-neurogenic female patients with increased residual urine as well as 'normal' controls did not demonstrate significant changes in flow parameters or residual urine during treatment with bethanecol (Wein et al 1980). In a double-blind study in men, no significant dose-related or cystometric response was noted when the patients were treated with 100 mg orally (Wein et al 1978).

Prostaglandins. The use of prostaglandins to facilitate emptying is based upon the hypothesis that (along with other excitatory neurotransmitters) these substances are necessary for the maintenance of bladder tone and for bladder contractile activity (Bultitude et al 1976, Pavlakis et al 1983). Prostaglandins are produced in the bladder in response to mechanical and nerve stimulation, and E_2 and $F_{2\alpha}$ stimulate *in vitro* and *in vivo* bladder contractile responses. Instillation of 0.5–1.5 mg of prostaglandin (PGE_2) within the bladders of female patients was reported to improve emptying in approximately two-thirds of patients in studies by two different investigators (Bultitude et al 1976, Desmond et al 1980), but these results were not reproduced by others, who found no benefit (Delaere et al 1981). The clinical value of prostaglandins is at best controversial. The fact that some patients with chronic retention of urine may benefit cannot be discounted, although the mechanism of the effect is unclear.

Blockers of inhibition. A sympathetic reflex pathway has been demonstrated during bladder filling in the cat which promotes urine storage by exerting an inhibitory effect on pelvic parasympathetic ganglionic transmission. This effect is α-adrenergic in nature (de Groat & Booth 1984, de Groat & Kawatani 1985). The use of α-adrenergic antagonists or ganglionic blocking agents (Hartviksen 1966) to achieve clinical facilitation of bladder contractility has been proposed but has not been clinically substantiated. The proposed use of sympathetic blockade, although substantiated by the results of research, illustrates the difficulty in extrapolating from an animal model to the clinical situation.

Neuropeptide physiology and pharmacology research directed at understanding the role of endogenous opioids on lower urinary tract function has identified a tonic inhibitory role of these substances on the micturition reflex at various levels. The intrathecal application of narcotic antagonists for stimulating bladder activity in spinal injury patients is a promising area requiring further investigation.

Drugs which decrease outlet resistance

α-Adrenergic blocking agents. The smooth muscle of the bladder base and proximal urethra contains predominantly α-adrenergic receptors, though β-adrenoceptors are present. The bladder body contains both varieties of receptors, with the β-adrenoceptor being more common. Opinions on the role in voiding function and dysfunction of the postganglionic sympathetic nerve fibres which innervate the bladder base and proximal urethral area differ. Evidence has been presented for a physiological internal sphincter located at the bladder neck or within the proximal urethra which responds to α-adrenergic blockade with an increase in flow rate, decrease in residual urine, and improvement in upper tract appearance in patients with neurogenic lesions (Krane & Olsson 1973a,b). Dyssynergia of the bladder neck is seen with spinal cord lesions above the sympathetic outflow. The use of α-adrenergic blockade to treat increased outlet resistance in spinal cord injury patients has gained widespread acceptance. The ability of certain α-adrenergic blockers to decrease external (skeletal) sphincter activity is controversial, but several studies support the view that α-adrenergic agents which decrease electromyographic activity at the external sphincter probably have their effect at the central rather than the peripheral level. The successful use of α-adrenergic therapy to treat the increase in urethral tone which is presumed to result from denervation secondary to radical hysterectomy has also been reported (Norlén 1982).

Benign prostatic hyperplasia represents hyperplasia of both the stromal and glandular elements of the prostate. Although not invariably associated with outlet obstruction and voiding symptomatology, prostatic enlargement is commonly associated with both the symptoms and the objective urodynamic findings of an abnormality of bladder emptying secondary to outlet obstruction, and an abnormality of urinary storage secondary to the development of detrusor over-activity.

The increased outlet resistance has been proposed to be secondary to both an increase in prostatic size as well as an increase in the tone of the prostatic smooth muscle (Caine 1986). Therefore, α-adrenergic antagonists which relax the smooth muscle of the prostate and prostatic urethra have been proposed to be effective for the treatment of symptomatic benign prostatic hyperplasia. Specific characterization of the response of the prostatic smooth muscle has demonstrated a primary α_1-adrenoreceptor.

Ten clinical trials involving the use of α-adrenergic blockade in the treatment of benign prostatic enlargement have been cited in a recent review (Lepor 1989). Five studies used a non-specific α-blocker, phenoxybenzamine; three studies used prazosin, a specific α_1-blocker; and one study used terazosin, a long-acting α_1-blocker. One of the studies which utilized prazosin in a double-blind cross-over design involving 20 patients and lasting four weeks reported a statistically significant increase in maximal urinary flow rate (4.9 ml/s to 6.9 ml/s, with no increase in the placebo group) and reduced residual volume (Hedlund et al 1983). However, the majority of patients receiving the placebo or the active medication experienced an improvement in obstructive symptoms. A single-blind study utilizing terazosin was performed with 15 patients over 27 weeks. This study demonstrated a statistically significant improvement in peak and maximum flow rates, residual urine, and obstructive symptoms (Dunzendorfer 1988).

To support the laboratory evidence that this class of agents actively relaxes prostatic smooth muscle *in vitro*, further objective data from placebo-controlled double-blind studies which evaluate urinary flow rate, residual urine volume and patient symptomatology are necessary. 'Symptom scores' which provide an objective method of evaluating the obstructive and, more importantly, the irritative symptoms associated with prostatic obstruction should be used in all these studies. Irritative voiding symptoms (frequency, urgency and nocturia) have been demonstrated to improve with prostatic resection and are often the symptoms which motivate patients to seek treatment. Therefore, during any discussion on drug efficacy for the treatment of prostatic enlargement which draws its conclusions from symptom score analysis, an improvement in these symptoms may in fact be a more important variable than a statistically significant improvement in urinary flow rate. Currently, multicentre double-blind placebo-controlled studies are under way in the United States to further evaluate the efficacy of terazosin for the treatment of symptomatic benign prostatic hyperplasia.

The specific role of testosterone and its metabolites in the development of benign prostatic hyperplasia has not been clearly defined, but androgens are clearly required for both the development and maintenance of prostatic size. Testosterone suppression with oestrogens, luteinizing hormone-releasing agonists and antagonists, anti-androgens, and progestational agents has been investigated.

These forms of hormonal manipulation are limited by side-effects (gynaecomastia, hot flushes, decreased libidio, impotency). Laboratory studies in a canine model of benign prostatic hyperplasia have demonstrated that selective blockade of the enzyme 5α-reductase is associated with a decrease in prostatic size. The proposed mechanism of action is the inhibition of the production of dihydrotestosterone without producing a decrease in serum testosterone levels. This form of therapy appears promising because many of the side-effects of androgen deprivation can be avoided. Further clinical studies involving this type of therapy are required.

Centrally acting muscle relaxants. Obstruction at the level of the striated sphincter may result from lesions of the spinal cord above the sacral outflow. Currently, there is no pharmacological agent specific for the urethral striated sphincter, and drug therapy remains limited for this condition. The benzodiazepines have not been demonstrated to have a specific relaxant effect on skeletal muscle (Byck 1975) but patients without neurological disease may benefit primarily from the anti-anxiety effects of the medication. Dantrolene sodium is believed to directly affect excitation–contraction coupling (Bianchine 1980) but results in generalized muscle weakness. Transient euphoria, diarrhoea and hepatotoxicity have been observed. The use of this medication has been reported to have positive (Murdock et al 1976) and limited (Teague & Merrill 1978) effects in patients with detrusor–sphincter dyssynergia secondary to spinal cord injury. Baclofen, a derivative of γ-aminobutyric acid, inhibits the transmission of monosynaptic and polysynaptic spinal cord reflexes and has been found to be useful in the treatment of skeletal spasticity (Bianchine 1980). Baclofen appears to be the most efficacious medication for relaxation of the external sphincter associated with detrusor–sphincter dyssynergia, but is not selective for the sphincter and can rarely be used in the high dosages necessary to relieve the anatomical obstruction without prominent effects on other skeletal musculature.

Conclusions

Pharmacological therapy can have an impact on voiding dysfunction involving both the filling and emptying phases of the bladder and bladder outlet. The successful institution of pharmacological therapy requires both an understanding of the effects of the micturition disorder on the bladder and bladder outlet, and a knowledge of the clinical pharmacology of the medications that are available. Current and continuing advances in the understanding of the neurophysiology and pharmacology of the lower urinary tract, combined with controlled clinical studies which clarify the indications for and efficacy of existing and newly developed agents, will provide an increased ability for successful medical intervention for this disabling condition.

References

Bianchine J 1980 Drugs for Parkinson's disease: centrally acting muscle relaxants. In: Gilman AG et al (eds) The pharmacological basis of therapeutics, 6th edn. Macmillan, New York, p 475–493

Blaivas JG, Labib KB, Michalik SJ, Zayed AA 1980 Cystometric response to propantheline in detrusor hyperreflexia: therapeutic implications. J Urol 124:259–262

Bultitude MI, Hills NH, Shuttleworth KED 1976 Clinical and experimental studies on the action of prostaglandins and their synthesis inhibitors on detrusor muscle in vitro and in vivo. Br J Urol 48:631–637

Bump RC, Friedman CI 1986 Intraluminal urethral pressure measurements in the female baboon: effects of normal manipulation. J Urol 136:508–511

Byck R 1975 Drugs and the treatment of psychiatric disorders. In: Goodman LS, Gilman A (eds) The pharmacologic basis of therapeutics, 5th edn. Macmillan, New York, p 152–200

Caine M 1986 The present role of alpha-adrenergic blockers in the treatment of benign prostatic hypertrophy. J Urol 136:1–4

Cardozo L, Stanton S, Robinson H, Hole D 1980 Evaluation of flurbiprofen in detrusor instability. Br Med J 280:281–283

de Groat WC, Booth AM 1984 Autonomic systems to the urinary bladder and sexual organs. In: Dyck PJ et al (eds) Peripheral neuropathy. WB Saunders, Philadelphia, p 285–299

de Groat WC, Kawatani M 1985 Neural control of the urinary bladder: possible relationship between peptidergic inhibitory mechanisms and detrusor instability. Neurourol Urodyn 4:285–300

Delaere K, Thomas C, Moonen T, Debruyne F 1981 The value of prostaglandin E2 and F2α in women with abnormalities of bladder emptying. Br J Urol 53:306–309

Desmond AO, Bultitude M, Hills N, Shuttleworth K 1980 Clinical experience with intravesical prostaglandin E2. A prospective study of 36 patients. Br J Urol 52:357–366

Diokno AC, Koppenhoeffer R 1976 Bethanechol chloride in neurogenic bladder dysfunction. Urology 8:455–458

Diokno AC, Lapides J 1977 Action of oral and parenteral bethanechol on decompensated bladder. Urology 10:23–24

Downie JW, Karmazyn M 1984 Mechanical trauma to bladder epithelium liberates prostanoids which modulate neurotransmission in rabbit detrusor muscle. J Pharmacol Exp Ther 230:445–449

Dunzendorfer U 1988 Clinical experience with symptomatic management of BPH with Terazosin. Urology 32(Suppl 6):27–31

Ek A, Andersson K-E, Gullberg B et al 1978 The effects of long-term treatment with norephedrine on stress incontinence and urethral closure pressure profile. Scand J Urol Nephrol 12:105–110

Ekeland A, Sander S 1976 A urodynamic study of emepronium bromide in bladder dysfunction. Scand J Urol Nephrol 10:195–199

Fovaeus M, Andersson K-E, Batra S et al 1987 Effects of calcium channel blockers and Bay K 8644 on contractions induced by muscarinic receptor stimulation of isolated bladder muscle from rabbit and man. J Urol 137:798–803

Gibbon NOK 1965 Urinary incontinence in disorders of the nervous system. Br J Urol 37:624–629

Hansen W, Hansen L, Maegaard E, Mayhoff H, Nordling J 1982 Urinary incontinence in old age. A controlled clinical trial of emepronium bromide. Br J Urol 54:249–253

Hartviksen K 1966 Discussion. Acta Neurol Scand Suppl 42:180–181

Hedlund H, Andersson K-E, Ek A 1983 Effects of prazosin in patients with benign prostatic obstruction. J Urol 130:275–278

Hodgson BJ, Dumas S, Bolling BR, Heesch CM 1978 Effect of estrogen on sensitivity of rabbit bladder and urethra to phenylephrine. Invest Urol 16:67–69

Husted S, Andersson K-E, Sommer L, Østergaard JR 1980 Anticholinergic and calcium antagonistic effects of terodiline in rabbit urinary bladder. Acta Pharmacol Toxicol 46:20–30

Khanna OP 1976 Disorders of micturition: neuropharmacological basis and results of drug therapy. Urology 8:316–328

Kinder RB, Mundy AR 1985 Atropine blockade of nerve mediated stimulation of the human detrusor. Br J Urol 57:418–421

Krane RJ, Olsson C 1973a Phenoxybenzamine in neurogenic bladder dysfunction. I. A theory of micturition. J Urol 110:650–652

Krane RJ, Olsson C 1973b Phenoxybenzamine in neurogenic bladder dysfunction. II. Clinical considerations. J Urol 110:653–656

Lapides J 1964 Urecholine regimen for rehabilitating the atonic bladder. J Urol 91:658–659

Lepor H 1989 Nonoperative management of benign prostatic hyperplasia. J Urol 141:1283–1289

Levin RM, Jacobowitz D, Wein AJ 1981 Autonomic innervation of rabbit urinary bladder following estrogen administration. Urology 17:449–453

Light J, Scott F 1982 Bethanechol chloride and the traumatic cord bladder. J Urol 128:85–89

Merrill DC, Rotta J 1974 A clinical evaluation of detrusor denervation supersensitivity using air cystometry. J Urol 111:27–30

Moisey CU, Stephenson T, Brendler C 1980 The urodynamic and subjective results of treatment of detrusor instability with oxybutynin chloride. Br J Urol 52:472–475

Murdock MM, Sax D, Krane R 1976 Use of dantrolene sodium in external sphincter spasm. Urology 8:133–137

Nordling J, Christensen B, Gosling J 1980 Noradrenergic innervation of the human bladder in neurogenic dysfunction. Urol Int 35:188

Norlén L 1982 Influence of the sympathetic nervous system on the lower urinary tract and its clinical implications. Neurourol Urodyn 1:129

Pavlakis AJ, Siroky M, Leslie CA et al 1983 Prostaglandins in lower urinary tract. Neurourol Urodyn 2:105

Perera GLS, Ritch AES, Hall MRP 1982 The lack of effect on intramuscular emepronium bromide for urinary incontinence. Br J Urol 54:259–260

Perlberg S, Caine M 1982 Adrenergic response of bladder muscle in prostatic obstruction. Urology 20:524–527

Peters D 1984 Terodiline in the treatment of urinary frequency and motor urge incontinence. A controlled multicentre trial. Scand J Urol Nephrol Suppl 87:21–33

Raezer DM, Wein AJ, Jacobowitz D et al 1973 Autonomic innervation of canine urinary bladder. Cholinergic and adrenergic contributions and interaction of sympathetic and parasympathetic nervous systems in bladder function. Urology 2:211–221

Resnick NM, Yalla SV 1987 Detrusor hyperactivity with impaired contractile function. J Am Med Assoc 257:3076–3081

Roussan MS, Abramson A, Levine S, Feibel A 1975 Bladder training: its role in evaluating the effect of an antispasticity drug on voiding in patients with neurogenic bladder. Arch Phys Med Rehabil 56:463–468

Sibley GNA 1984 A comparison of spontaneous and nerve-mediated activity in bladder muscle from man, pig and rabbit. J Physiol (Lond) 354:431–443

Sundin T, Dahlstrom A, Norlén L et al 1977 The sympathetic innervation and adrenoreceptor function of the human lower urinary tract in the normal state and after parasympathetic denervation. Invest Urol 14:322–328

Taylor P 1985 Cholinergic agonists. In: Gilman AG et al (eds) Goodman and Gilman's
    The pharmacological basis of therapeutics, 7th edn. Macmillan, New York, p 100–109
Taylor MC, Bates CP 1979 A double-blind crossover trial of baclofen: a new treatment
    for the unstable bladder syndrome. Br J Urol 51:504–505
Teague CT, Merrill DC 1978 Effect of baclofen and dantrolene on bladder stimulator
    induced detrusor sphincter dyssynergia in dogs. Urology 11:531–535
Wein AJ 1981 Classification of neurogenic voiding dysfunction. J Urol 125:605–609
Wein AJ, Hanno PM, Dixon DO, Raezer DM, Benson GS 1978 The effect of oral
    bethanechol chloride on the cystometrogram of the normal adult male. J Urol
    120:330–331
Wein AJ, Malloy T, Shofer F, Raezer D 1980 The effects of bethanechol chloride on
    urinary parameters in normal women and in women with significant residual urine
    volumes. J Urol 124:397–405
Wein AJ, Levin RM, Barrett DM 1987 Voiding function: relevant anatomy, physiology
    and pharmacology. In: Gillenwater JY et al (eds) Adult and pediatric urology.
    Yearbook Medical Publishers, Chicago, p 800–862
Yalla SV, Blunt KJ, Fam BA, Constantinople NL, Gittes RF 1977a Detrusor sphincter
    dyssynergia. J Urol 118:1026–1029
Yalla SV, Rossier AB, Fam BA, Gabilondo FB, Di Benedetto M, Gittes RF 1977b
    Functional contribution of autonomic innervation to urethral striated sphincter: studies
    with parasympathetic, parasympatholytic and alpha adrenergic blocking agents in spinal
    cord injury and control male subjects. J Urol 117:494–499

DISCUSSION

Burnstock: There are many fine, non-myelinated fibres running in the bladder and I sometimes wonder whether they are vulnerable to drugs which have local anaesthetic action, or whether stretching of the urethra, for problems of urine retention, can damage these fibres, especially since the beneficial effects of stretching can apparently last for up to three months.

Staskin: The localized anaesthetic effect of oxybutynin is well known. Some people have tried to use it directly instilled into the bladder to inhibit bladder contractions. It also has a profound relaxing effect on the bowel. But the actual anaesthetic effect has not been really shown.

Andersson: When terodiline and oxybutynin are used systemically, it is difficult to attribute their clinical effects to other than their anticholinergic action (Andersson 1988). Even if we can show that *in vitro* they have other modes of action, and terodiline is certainly a calcium antagonist, there may be anticholinergic side-effects long before the calcium-antagonistic action becomes useful.

I think that oxybutynin's local anaesthetic effects and several of the non-specific effects of this drug might be useful when it is instilled intravesically. The intravesical administration of some of these 'spasmolytic' drugs to patients undergoing clean intermittent catheterization is an improved way of using such drugs, but we are unlikely to realize their potential in urinary incontinence by giving them systemically, because they are so non-selective that side-effects occur long before an optimum effect on the bladder is achieved.

Marsden: In the translation from *in vitro* to *in vivo* work in human beings, we know that millimolar, micromolar and nanomolar concentrations may have effects *in vitro*, but the crucial question is what concentrations of those drugs are obtained *in vivo*. What sort of concentrations at the effector organ would you expect from conventional clinical doses of these drugs given by mouth?

Andersson: Mostly they are in the nanomolar range.

Marsden: What sort of receptor concentrations would you expect from intravesical delivery?

Andersson: We used 10–100 µM concentrations. But we don't know much about penetration through the bladder epithelium; some of the drugs used might penetrate well, and others do not. We have to consider basic properties like pH and lipid solubility when we give drugs intravesically.

Marsden: But in rough terms, by systemic administration you may be producing no more than nanomolar concentrations at the effector site. With a drug that penetrates the uroepithelium, you could reach millimolar concentrations, theoretically.

Andersson: Yes.

Stanton: Most anticholinergic drugs are badly absorbed; Ritch pointed out that only 6% of emepronium bromide is absorbed, and at that level systemic side-effects were starting. We tend to give drugs individually, to titrate the dose, to determine their clinical benefit and side-effects. The exception is that with the elderly, we give small doses first and gradually build up. But we generally exceed the recommended doses for the drugs discussed here.

One should distinguish between centrally (neurogenically) induced instability and that due to psychosomatic causes. We haven't talked much about those at this meeting. There is a large group of women with psychosomatically induced bladder instability in whom drug treatment is probably not very helpful. It might be useful initially as a support, if one plans to give bladder retraining. Whereas for neurogenic instability, drug treatment is more effective.

Finally, a plea that we avoid the use of the term 'stress incontinence' as a diagnostic label. The International Continence Society has tried to define standards for terminology. We felt that stress incontinence is a symptom and a sign as much as urge incontinence is, but not a diagnostic label, because of the problems of interpreting results where these are used as diagnostic labels without urodynamic diagnosis.

Staskin: I agree totally. I would also agree with Dr Andersson's points and add an example of the difference between systemic and local effects. Taken orally, α-adrenergic blockers decrease blood pressure and cause impotence; injected directly into the penis they cause smooth muscle relaxation and produce an erection.

Toson: Oxybutynin is a lipophilic drug and therefore it could cross the blood–brain barrier. Are there reports of central side-effects with oxybutynin?

Stanton: Yes, mostly in the American literature, because it is one of the paradoxes that we can't yet use oxybutinin in the UK, because we still await a product licence for it; but it is available in the USA. There were central side-effects in a small number of patients.

Staskin: The problem is sometimes in differentiating a patient who complains of dizziness from someone who has difficulty in visual accommodation.

Marsden: On the relative lipid solubility and penetration into brain of different anticholinergic agents, Geoff Burnstock spoke about the role of the neurovascular barrier in access of drugs to autonomic ganglia via that barrier. Is this established as a functional entity, other than a physically visible structure?

Burnstock: Not really. Mike Gershon has promoted this idea. I think such a blood–ganglion barrier may exist in the gut, but it is unlikely to exist in the bladder, because the internal organization of ganglia in the bladder is little like that of the gut or the central nervous system.

Marsden: Could we define the cholinergic receptor subtypes concerned with bladder control, compared with neural control?

Andersson: So far as we know, in the human bladder the muscarinic receptors are M_2 receptors, using the M_1/M_2 nomenclature (Andersson et al 1988a). By pharmacological means of further subclassifying muscarinic receptors the rat bladder receptors have been classified as 'M_3' receptors (Monferini et al 1988). But there is no correlation between the pharmacological classification and the cloned acetylcholine receptors whose structure has been determined; there are five or more of these already.

There have been attempts to relate the type of muscarinic receptor to the second messenger system mediating the effects. This is not clarified for the human bladder yet, but probably there is an inositol trisphosphate (IP_3) mechanism linked to muscarinic receptor stimulation in the human bladder.

Marsden: So M_3 is linked to IP_3 in the human bladder, as against central nervous system neural muscarinic receptors, most of which are considered to be M_1 receptors. Do the anticholinergic drugs that are used for bladder symptoms have any specificity for $M_{1,2,3}$?

Andersson: No.

Burnstock: There are also muscarinic receptors on ganglion cells in the guinea pig bladder, occupation of which might lead to widespread effects on the smooth muscle.

Toson: Unfortunately, as far as we know from the available literature, the muscarinic receptor subtype mediating bladder contraction (Nilvebrant et al 1985, Monferini et al 1988) is widely distributed in the body, and also in the central nervous system (e.g. in the brainstem); consequently there is no opportunity to design an antimuscarinic drug that is selective for the bladder.

Kirby: In relation to the use of combinations of drugs for the treatment of instability, we used probanthine with quinidine to treat this condition, stimulated by Geoff Burnstock's ATP story. We compared this combination with probanthine and placebo. We didn't complete the study because there was not much difference between the two, but I think we should look more at the use of combinations of drugs, because single agents have been so disappointing.

Burnstock: Quinidine is not the right choice for a purinergic receptor antagonist, because it is non-specific. However, the calcium antagonist, nifedipine, turns out to be more effective in blocking the ATP contractile component in the bladder than the cholinergic contractile component. There is a clear parallel with the differential effects of ATP and noradrenaline released from sympathetic nerves supplying blood vessels.

Brading: Quinidine contracts bladder muscle, so it might have a detrimental effect.

Kirby: Nifedipine is rather fast acting; one needs a slow-release preparation.

Andersson: There is a slow-release preparation. But in general, if you combine an anticholinergic drug with nifedipine you get better inhibitory effects than if you combine it with verapamil and certain other calcium antagonists (Andersson et al 1986). And with the NANC (non-adrenergic, non-cholinergic) contraction in human bladder which is also resistant to tetrodotoxin, calcium antagonists are effective for relaxing that kind of contractile activation. We don't know what that means.

de Groat: The drug cocktail approach could be taken to the extreme. One could use β-adrenergic receptor agonists, in combination with potassium channel openers, anticholinergic agents, and direct muscle relaxants. Have drug combinations been tested in Dr Brading's model of the unstable bladder in the pig?

Brading: I have never tried mixing them; we have enough to do finding out what they do individually! But you may be right. We have only looked at the individual classes as potential detrusor muscle relaxants for unstable contractions.

Toson: This kind of experiment is difficult to do in an appropriate way. In fact, different drugs (e.g. β_2-agonists, calcium antagonists, potassium channel openers, etc.) could have different time courses, making it complicated to pick up additive effects.

de Groat: This drug combination approach is used in the treatment of hypertension. Some patients with severe hypertension may take four different drugs. Even if there are different time courses of drug action the drugs could be made to act simultaneously in an acute experimental animal by administering some early and some late, so that a combination of effects could be observed. In other words, if you knew the time course of each drug action, you could give them in a certain sequence and presumably have all present at the time of their peak action.

Andersson: Some combination experiments have been done *in vitro*. For example, in rabbit urinary bladder atropine causes 40% inhibition of electrically induced contractions, and a calcium antagonist about 70% inhibition. A combination of atropine and a calcium antagonist will completely inhibit bladder contractions (Husted et al 1980). That is also an interesting combination *in vivo* but, so far as I know, little systematic work has been done on drug combinations for effective treatment of unstable bladder contractions.

de Groat: I recognize the problems of extrapolating to the human situation from drug effects *in vitro*. This is why experiments like this should be done in the pig model, where you have identified unstable bladder contractions. You have determined the effects of these agents *in vitro* on single muscle cells and you can now look at their effects in the whole animal, to see if they reduce unstable bladder activity.

Brading: This is an area that drug companies may well get into. We should like to find out the basic mechanisms first, and then the drug companies with their greater resources should come in; we can advise them what types of drug, and which combinations, to look at.

de Groat: Unfortunately, drug companies may not be so interested in testing other companies' compounds. University investigators will have to do those studies, rather than drug companies.

Marsden: There also is the problem of persuading one drug company to use another company's products in a combined preparation.

Stanton: And nobody dies from bladder problems, whereas people die from cardiac problems, or suffer a great deal of unhappiness until they get the right pill formulation for contraception. Until drug manufacturers see bladder problems at a higher level, we shall not have much joy from them.

Toson: Dr Staskin, were you suggesting in your paper that the rationale for the use of drugs currently available for the treatment of urinary incontinence is wrong, or are the drugs themselves unsuitable?

Staskin: The point I was trying to make is that these combinations have not been used in a controlled way. It is very easy to add another drug if a patient is already on one. Many of us have patients on oxybutynin and imipramine together who don't respond to either drug alone; but although we think this is a good combination for these patients with bladder instability, we have not done a controlled study with urodynamic evaluation, to show that this combination works; nor would we imply that there was a theoretical advantage to it, other than the fact that we presume there is some difference in the mechanism of action of the medications, rather than the anticholinergic effect.

Toson: It is possible that some clinical trials were unsuccessful because they used non-selective drugs and consequently adequate doses could not be used, because of the risk of side-effects.

Staskin: I agree. All the clinical studies are flawed by such problems.

Andersson: It is always easy to criticize clinical trials but it is difficult to do good studies, particularly when testing drugs for bladder instability. A major problem is to pick out the right patients, because detrusor instability is a symptom and a clinical diagnosis that can have very different backgrounds. It is therefore wrong to expect that the same drug will benefit all patients. If you collect a patient material and are uncertain about the background to their detrusor instability, you will have a few responders, some who are in between, and some non-responders. And then you will end up with the kind of results in which, say, 62% do well on a drug and 42% do well on placebo. This high degree of placebo response is something we have to accept in experiments on this kind of patient. It is nothing new; in migraine treatment there is a very high degree of placebo response. For as long as we cannot pick out patients who for some reason are the ones who should be the target for a particular kind of therapy, we can't expect to get 100% responses.

Staskin: That reinforces what Mr Stanton said, and if you are going to divide a population into two, in order to do a controlled pharmacological study, you need to define the population. In the study on terodiline, the patients were identified as women with non-neurogenic bladder instability who on a cystometrogram demonstrated a wave-like set of uninhibited bladder contractions. A considerable attempt was made to evaluate these patients objectively, although this may not necessarily be the group that best represents an over-active bladder.

Maggi: Imipramine is used a lot to control enuresis in children (Kunin et al 1970, Wein 1984). Has it been tested in controlled double-blind clinical studies in relation to detrusor hyperreflexia and detrusor instability? Is there a differential ability of this drug to influence these two conditions? And do other tricyclic antidepressants, in addition to imipramine, act on enuresis or on these other conditions? Finally, what is known about the site of action of imipramine in enuresis and other conditions? Is it acting peripherally or centrally?

Staskin: Drs Levin and Wein looked at the anticholinergic and smooth muscle-relaxing effects of imipramine. Earlier, we looked at all the phenothiazines and tricyclic antidepressants in the muscle bath. They all had a calcium channel blocking effect and anticholinergic effect, to different degrees, and a smooth muscle relaxant effect.

I hesitate to comment on the use of imipramine in enuresis; I have not seen people respond to it.

Earlier Mr Stanton said that those with uninhibited bladder contractions (detrusor hyperreflexia) tend to do much better than patients with detrusor instability during any medication study. The reason may be that the hyperreflexic population is fairly well defined, whereas the aetiology of detrusor instability is not so obvious. But patients with severe hyperreflexia when selected for a study often need very large doses of medications. There have been reports in which imipramine overdosage in children caused several deaths. As a result, its use at least in England was severely curtailed.

Maggi: So is imipramine effective in detrusor hyperreflexia or in instability?

Staskin: Imipramine's anticholinergic effect suppresses bladder contractility; the smooth muscle effects may not be present with prescribed doses.

Marsden: Has anyone done a trial of tetracyclic antidepressants, for example drugs like mianserine with relatively little anticholinergic activity, as treatment for detrusor hyperreflexia or instability?

Staskin: Trazidone, an atypical antidepressant, has a very low anticholinergic effect but still has much of the calcium channel blocking effects of the tricyclics. It is reported that it doesn't cause significant bladder side-effects such as urinary retention, which seems to be an anticholinergic effect. The reason for using imipramine in enuresis was the idea that an additional central effect may be obtained.

Brindley: In a young paraplegic woman with a sacral anterior root stimulator who was well deafferented we completely cured the reflex incontinence, but revealed unsuspected pure stress incontinence. I put her on desipramine (50 mg per day) and she became drier; at 75 mg she was totally dry. She remained for three years on 75 mg/day, sometimes trying to reduce to 50 mg a day, but whenever she did that she became wet. After a couple of years I offered her an operation that would enable her to stop taking this drug. Linda Cardozo did a Stamey suspension and this patient is now dry without desipramine. When she was on the drug the stimulator worked exactly as well as it had worked before and now works after; she always voided with zero residual, and the bladder pressures were the same with as without the drug. So her continence under desipramine had nothing to do with anticholinergic effects; it was a reinforcement of urethral or bladder neck smooth muscle.

Andersson: There are studies on stress incontinence showing that you can improve both symptomatology and urethral pressures by giving imipramine to these patients. I don't know any controlled studies on the effects of imipramine in this condition, however.

Stanton: What is known about the use of desmopressin in nocturnal enuresis? What is its mechanism?

Andersson: Several well-controlled studies show a beneficial effect of this vasopressin analogue (Andersson et al 1988b) in enuresis. It has been accepted for the treatment of this condition in several countries. It is believed to work only by reducing urinary volume. This agent has also been used in patients with nocturia after prostatectomy, and here too it reduces the symptom just by reducing the volume.

de Groat: Jerry Blaivas said earlier that in many cases of unstable bladder the uninhibited contractions are essentially mini-micturition reflexes that use the same central neural mechanisms that are used to void normally. When we are using drugs which block the normal neural pathways, this creates a problem, because we are expecting the drug to block unwanted micturition reflexes and at the same time to permit normal voiding. That seems to be an impossible requirement. What is needed is a drug that works on the pathological process rather than on the normal physiological mechanism. You can't expect to block involuntary micturition and have the voluntary micturition unaffected.

We have drugs that are 'effective'; if you give a large dose of atropine or a ganglionic blocking agent to most patients, they will not be able to urinate. Developing new agents that block the normal control mechanism may not be very useful because we already have drugs that are effective, and we can't use them because of side-effects or because they produce such strong effects that a patient who is incontinent becomes a patient who can't urinate. We need new approaches or new combinations of drugs.

Staskin: Although the subtypes of muscarinic receptors have not been found to be organ specific, if there were organ-related structural conformation differences near the receptor, this might enable us to develop drugs that are more specific for the bladder because they have better access to the appropriate receptors.

Marsden: It strikes me as curious that here we have a collection of surgeons talking about drugs. That must mean that they are not happy about their operations! But also, the discussion is all between urologists; I haven't heard the bowel surgeons speak. Is that because they are happier in their operations, or because they don't think that drugs have useful effects on the bowel?

Stanton: With respect, we are talking about drugs for non-surgical conditions here!

Swash: We also don't have any evidence that the drugs actually work very well.

Marsden: I was being provocative.

Brading: As basic scientists, we agree with Dr de Groat that antimuscarinic drugs are not ideal for treating detrusor instability. We feel it would be better to use drugs that do not interfere with the normal micturition reflex, especially as this may be somewhat damaged in some instances. The class of drugs that is looking promising at the moment is the potassium channel openers (such as cromakalim and pinacidil). These drugs work directly on the smooth muscles to reduce their excitability. The drug cromakalim, for example, when applied to detrusor strips at low concentrations, reduces the frequency of the spontaneous electrical activity, and, as you increase the dose, so the activity is abolished; and as an increasing number of potassium channels are opened in the membrane, it hyperpolarizes towards the potassium equilibrium potential, which thus reduces the membrane excitability (Foster et al 1989a).

We have examined the effects of cromakalim on the mechanical activity of strips of detrusor smooth muscle dissected from unstable bladders. We have used mini-pigs, in which a silver ring has been placed to fit snugly round the urethra in the piglet. These animals get progressive obstruction as they grow, and develop detrusor instability. We have also examined material obtained from humans with unstable bladders, at open prostatectomy. In these unstable bladders, the spontaneous activity shows a different pattern from that of normal bladders. In normal bladders there is seldom any degree of maintained tone, each contraction relaxing to the baseline, whereas in the unstable bladders the contractions fuse to give a degree of tone. Cromakalim very effectively abolishes the spontaneous activity in both normal and unstable bladder strips.

Dr Andersson has looked at the hypertrophied rat bladder and shown that the spontaneous activity is also diminished very effectively by pinacidil and cromakalim (Malmgren et al 1989).

Since any drug used to treat detrusor instability ideally should not interfere with the normal micturition reflex, we have tested the effects of cromakalim on the excitatory innervation using transmural stimulation of the intrinsic nerves in the muscle strips. In our experiments (Foster et al 1989b), in both human and mini-pig strips the size of the response in the presence of cromakalim at a concentration sufficient to abolish spontaneous activity was not significantly different from the control response. The tissues also responded well to the application of muscarinic agonists, although the dose–response curves were shifted to the right in the presence of the cromakalim. Similar results were seen in the rat (Malmgren et al 1989).

The effect of these potassium channel openers has also been examined *in vivo* using cystometric techniques. In normal rats, pinacidil had very little effect on detrusor pressure, and bladder emptying was normal. In the unstable rat model, pinacidil given orally at 1 mg/kg resulted in the disappearance of the unstable contractions, and there was a reduction in the maximum detrusor pressure, although the rats could still empty their bladders completely. This decrease in micturition pressure was not found with cromakalim, although this drug too inhibited the spontaneous bladder contractions. There was no effect on bladder capacity.

In the obstructed unstable mini-pig, cromakalim infused intravenously at 0.3 mg/kg caused the disappearance of the unstable contractions, but the animal was still able to urinate apparently normally (Foster et al 1989b). At this concentration, however, the blood pressure falls, and the pigs do not look as happy as normal.

Andersson: There is some clinical experience with these drugs. We have recently finished a study on 10 patients with bladder instability secondary to outflow obstruction and all the symptoms that can be attributed to an unstable bladder contraction. We treated them with pinacidil at the maximum dose used to treat hypertension, for two weeks, which should be enough to produce a steady state. But we didn't find any effect on symptomatology or on urodynamic variables. This doesn't mean that the *principle* might not be useful, because the blood pressure-reducing effects of the drugs will limit the dosage that can be used for effects on the bladder. It would be interesting to see if these drugs work on bladder hyperactivity other than that associated with outflow obstruction. But, so far, we are a little frustrated by the clinical effects that we have seen.

Marsden: What is the theoretical mechanism whereby these drugs that affect potassium channels decrease spontaneous bladder hyperactivity but not normal micturition?

Brading: The spike potential frequency is dependent on membrane potential; if you hyperpolarize the membrane you slow the spikes down. The spikes trigger contraction and produce a lot of the spontaneous tone. Excitatory transmitters will cause contraction in two ways, by depolarizing the membrane and increasing spike activity in the tissues and, probably indirectly, by releasing calcium from internal stores. The idea is that if the general excitability of the smooth muscle is partially suppressed, you may lose a lot of the undesirable spontaneous activity, whereas if the normal nerve activity were still coming in and releasing transmitter synchronously onto the majority of the smooth muscle cells, you could still generate a good contractile response.

Marsden: That comes back to the old question of bladder excitability being abolished by deafferentation, or not, as the case may be.

Burnstock: Presumably the potassium channel openers produce hyperpolarization, which reduces the noise activity level, which is what you want. But if you are releasing a transmitter which produces substantial depolarization, you get up into the firing zone, which would lead to contraction. Interestingly, ATP produces depolarization of bladder smooth muscle, but acetylcholine doesn't.

Brading: This is certainly true in guinea pigs (Fujii 1988). We don't really know in the human how acetylcholine does work; in the guinea pig, it doesn't depolarize much, and probably works through releasing internal calcium stores (Mostwin 1985). This pathway may not be affected by potassium channel openers.

de Groat: I am encouraged by this work; it's exciting to see such a selective effect of a drug, even *in vitro.* Maybe pinacidil will be limited in its use by its side-effects on the vascular system. In addition, as Geoff was saying, the nervous system may be able to overcome the effect of pinacidil. Thus it would probably have to be administered in combination with some other agent that would suppress the neural input to the bladder.

Maggi: It has been shown that the exposure of smooth muscle of the canine trachea to potassium channel blockers increases the number of gap junctions (Kannan & Daniel 1978). Have you considered the possibility that the potassium channel openers have a morphological effect and for example might reduce the number of gap junctions?

Brading: Yes, we have. There is still argument about how these drugs work. We have been looking for other changes. I wouldn't be surprised if they had effects at the level of the interaction between cells.

Andersson: How do muscarinic receptors activate human smooth muscle? We don't know if there is an initial depolarization which opens up L-type calcium channels, leading to calcium inflow which in turn releases calcium from internal stores; or whether the muscarinic receptors generate IP_3 which causes intracellular calcium release. There is evidence favouring a calcium influx, because if extracellular calcium is removed by EGTA, there is almost no effect produced by carbachol, or any other muscarinic agonist, in human detrusor muscle.

Brading: The contractile response to carbachol takes some time to go, however.

Andersson: Yes, about 30 minutes. But in for example the guinea pig, there is a good correlation between the contraction induced by carbachol and the generation of phosphoinositides (Noronha-Blob et al 1989). Perhaps there is a difference in excitation–contraction coupling between man and smaller mammals, and this could explain some of the differences in experimental results.

References

Andersson K-E 1988 Current concepts in the treatment of disorders of micturition. Drugs 35:477–494

Andersson K-E, Fovaeus M, Morgan E, McLorie G 1986 Comparative effects of five different calcium channel blockers on the atropine-resistant contraction in electrically stimulated rabbit urinary bladder. Neurourol Urodyn 5:579–586

Andersson K-E, Fovaeus M, Hodlund H 1988a Urogenital muscarinic receptors and drug effects. Ann Clin Res 20:356–366

Andersson K-E, Bengtsson B, Paulsen O 1988b Desamino-8-D-arginine vasopressin (DDAVP): pharmacology and clinical use. Drugs Today 24(7):509–528

Foster CD, Fujii K, Kingdon J, Brading AF 1989a The effect of cromakalim on the smooth muscle of the guinea-pig urinary bladder. Br J Pharmacol 97:281–291

Foster CD, Speakman MJ, Fujii K, Brading AF 1989b The effects of cromakalim on the detrusor muscle of human and pig urinary bladder. Br J Urol 63:284–294

Fujii K 1988 Evidence for adenosine triphosphate as an excitatory transmitter in guinea-pig, rabbit and pig urinary bladder. J Physiol (Lond) 404:39–52

Husted S, Andersson K-E, Sommer L, Østergaard JR 1980 Anticholinergic and calcium antagonistic effects of terodiline in rabbit urinary bladder. Acta Pharmacol Toxicol 46 (Suppl I):20–30

Kannan MS, Daniel EE 1978 Formation of gap junctions by treatment in vitro with potassium conductance blockers. J Cell Biol 78:338–348

Kunin SA, Limbert DJ, Platzker AG, McGinley J 1970 The efficacy of imipramine in the management of enuresis. J Urol 109:385–387

Malmgren A, Andersson K-E, Sjögren C, Andersson PO 1989 Effects of pinacidil and cromakalim (BRL 34915) on bladder function in rats with detrusor instability. J Urol 142:1134–1138

Monferini E, Giraldo E, Ladinsky H 1988 Characterization of the muscarinic receptor subtypes in the rat urinary bladder. Eur J Pharmacol 147:453–458

Mostwin JL 1985 Receptor operated intracellular Ca stores in the smooth muscle of the guinea-pig bladder. J Urol 133:900–905

Nilvebrant L, Andersson K-E, Mattiasson A 1985 Characterization of the muscarinic cholinoceptors in the human detrusor. J Urol 134:418–423

Noronha-Blob L, Lowe V, Patton A, Canning B, Costello D, Kinnier WJ 1989 Muscarinic receptors: relationships among phosphoinositide breakdown, adenylate cyclase inhibition, in vitro detrusor muscle contractions and in vivo cystometrogram studies in guinea pig bladder. J Pharmacol Exp Ther 249:843–851
Wein A 1984 Applied pharmacology. In: Stanton SL (ed) Clinical gynecologic urology. CV Mosby, St Louis, Missouri, p 441–461

Final general discussion

Bourcier: I would like to present some of our findings on physiotherapy for incontinence. Let me comment on the new popularity of sport in many countries. Anatomical observations made according to Dr DeLancey's work have allowed us to understand better the functional aspects of urethral structure. The pelvic diaphragm, with slow- and fast-twich fibres, could be responsible for the supportive attachment of the vagina and for the voluntary control of the proximal urethra. In the vertical position, during sports, the urethra leaves the bladder at a point of combined intra-abdominal pressure and maximum gravity force. This situation probably accounts for the occurrence of symptoms of genuine stress incontinence in the standing position and while exercising. To avoid this problem a strong pelvic floor musculature is necessary, with a normal reflex pelvic floor contraction.

We already know that the incidence of incontinence is related to age, but we are less aware of the prevalence of stress incontinence in association with sports. Each time there is an increase in intra-abdominal pressure the pelvic floor musculature must respond: thus stress incontinence can present during vigorous activities, such as sports. During strenuous sporting activity the intra-abdominal pressure in the erect position may be two or three times greater than in the normal situation. This downward pressure from the abdominal viscera has to be offset by the tone and power of the levator ani. This suggests that strong abdominal contractions during sports constitute a factor in the onset of pelvic floor disorders in young nulliparous women.

Since 1987 we have been classifying sports according to the risk they present for the pelvic floor. Three main categories can be suggested:

High risk factors: for example, hurdling, triple jump, trampolining, and body-building.

Moderate risk factors: for example, tennis and jogging.

No risk factors: for example, swimming and rowing.

Comparing the three different criteria of strength/endurance of the levator ani (pelvic floor activity), reflex pelvic floor contraction (reflex activity), and urethral closure during stress (volitional control), we have three groups of sportswomen, as shown in Table 1.

In Group I, the patient needs to have information concerning peri-urethral muscular contraction during stress by means of biofeedback. In Group II, the first stage of treatment is to relearn reflex pelvic floor contraction, using cones and standard biofeedback. Patients in Group III are in a different situation because they have either pelvic floor damage or a congenital weakness. They

TABLE 1   (Bourcier) Classification of sportswomen with pelvic floor disorders

Disordered function	Group I	Group II	Group III
Levator ani activity	+	+	−
Reflex pelvic activity	+	−	−
Urethral closure during stress	−	−	−

need electrostimulation and other techniques available to strengthen the perineal and pelvic floor muscles, including physiotherapy and pelvic floor exercises.

Special equipment, with a large video screen connected to a computerized unit, is used to monitor two EMG channels from an intravaginal probe and surface abdominal electrodes. This machine provides continuous monitoring and gives information to the patient during the treatment programmes. A mobile base with a remote unit allows the patient to move freely.

During the fitness programme each woman undergoes a standard exercise regimen for 20 minutes. With applied biofeedback, levator ani muscles must be contracted before any intra-abdominal pressure rise, particularly in strenuous activities such as skipping, jogging or weight-lifting. This learning process provides information on responses to varied conditions and focuses the patient's efforts on control of the pelvic floor during sports. Applied biofeedback is probably the most efficient modality of the treatment and prevention of pelvic floor problems in sportswomen.

In France, emphasis is now placed on the conservative treatment of pelvic floor disorders. New therapies have been developed which have proved very successful. New methods of rehabilitation are based on advances in computerized instruments which enable these exercises to be carried out more objectively. The popularity of these new methods is due to their ease of use, to the patient's comfort, to the absence of side-effects and to the low cost compared to surgery. Physiotherapy should improve the state of the pelvic floor, and improve disordered urinary and faecal continence. It therefore leads to an improvement in the woman's quality of life.

A final but very important point is the French postpartum classification based upon obstetric risk factors (including birth weight, skull circumference and length of the second stage of labour). Although it is difficult to isolate individual risk factors, it is possible to classify deliveries into two groups in order to better understand the possible immediate incidence and long-term consequences.

First group. No problem is apparent; after practising Kegel's exercises and the use of cones, these women can carry out minimum physical activity.

Second group. Anomalies are found on obstetrical examination of the perineum; there may be obvious prolapse or postpartum urinary incontinence. Physical activities may be restarted, but cautiously. Above all the patient must be advised not to undertake abdominal straining, for example during gymnastics, too early. Depending on the results obtained, the correct time for carrying out toning-up exercises of the abdominal wall can be determined, usually after several weeks. In this group, biofeedback and electrostimulation could be used to promote recovery.

Marsden: I think you are not alone in France in beginning to see this group of nulliparous incontinent young women appearing with increasing frequency.

Stanton: Your clinical approach is essential as a complement to drug therapy and surgery. It has always struck me that where we have gone slightly awry in the UK is that for many years we have allowed physiotherapists to give postnatal exercises to all women who come to delivery in our hospitals, with no accountability as to whether it has been effective. Are you 'controlling' what you are doing, for example in a group without treatment, or with an alternative procedure, as well as carefully assessing patients in your treatment programme? I think it's essential to have some objectivity.

Bourcier: Different methods are suggested for women referred to physiotherapy. The patient has the choice between attending sessions in a physiotherapy department for six weeks or using equipment at home. For the latter method to work, the patient has to be highly motivated to train herself every day, with electrical stimulation and/or cones. The major problem is to be sure that the pelvic muscles are properly trained; the most common misunderstanding is to exercise the gluteal muscles or adductors. A second problem is the daily use of the stimulator. These two points could explain much of the failure of home care compared to the supervised programme.

Fowler: Female athletes are not best known for their extreme femininity. One wonders to what extent there may be some hormonal imbalance. I would also be interested to know what proportion of such incontinent women have polycystic ovaries. Could it be that either hormonal changes induced by heavy exercise, or the pre-existing hormonal profiles of these women, predispose them to neuromuscular disorders of the pelvic floor? If sex hormones play an important part as co-transmitters in female pelvic floor muscles, a hormonal imbalance might result in abnormal weakness.

Bourcier: Hormonal imbalance could be one of the problems in these sportswomen.

Stanton: We recognize that women who take exercise to excess become amenorrhoeic, and therefore there is a decrease in the secretion of gonadotropins by the pituitary. What effect this has on their habitus is not really known, but obviously there is an imbalance there, of oestrogen and even progesterone output. As regards hormonal effects on bladder control, not much is known, because there is little objective analysis of the clinically obvious fact that women who take energetic sport very seriously are more likely to have episodes of urinary incontinence. These women will also have modified their hormone output, and this may affect the end-organs and the transmitters and the receptors.

Burnstock: Young women who go in for heavy training often get severely osteoporotic bones, due to changes in hormone levels. My guess is that Dr Fowler is right and that such hormone changes might also alter the expression of neurotransmitters and receptors in the bladder. We need to look at this possibility.

Kirby: I suppose that if you can build up your biceps or deltoid muscles, there is no reason why you shouldn't body-build your pelvic floor! What is the mechanism by which striated muscle hypertrophy occurs? Is it an increase in innervation, or in muscle cell number or cell size?

Fowler: It is due to an increase in cell size.

Kirby: And is it possible to achieve that in the pelvic floor? Can you for example double the size of your pelvic floor musculature?

Bourcier: Not at all. Sometimes, as I said earlier in this meeting, we can try to strengthen the perineal muscles, through our physiotherapy programme, but the results are poor in this special group.

Stanton: I think the answer is in the end-point. The description I use for patients who want a conservative approach based on pelvic floor exercises, as opposed to surgery, is to say that if they wanted to go in for a 100 or 200 yards race at international or national level, they would have to train for at least three months, for a couple of hours a day—rigorous athletic training. You have to translate that training image into pelvic floor exercises. That kind of intensity has probably never been achieved. It is very difficult to persuade a patient to do Kegel exercises, or use your biofeedback apparatus, Dr Bourcier, or even use the Plevnik metal cones and practise for 2–3 hours each day. Nothing less than that will suffice to build up the pelvic floor muscles.

Swash: There is a problem about using physiotherapy and attempting to make a muscle hypertrophy when that muscle is damaged. I would be more enthusiastic about the possibility of your treatment working, Dr Bourcier, if it was started *before* there was any injury to the pelvic floor. If you wait until six weeks after delivery, or until a woman has presented with some symptom, there must be some damage to the pelvic floor already. It is then less likely that an attempt to cause hypertrophy will be effective.

Bourcier: Yes; we have been talking about sportswomen, but with women suffering from stress incontinence in their daily activities, physiotherapy also seems to be an effective treatment. Three months of treatment with 12 sessions of stimulation and biofeedback are necessary to cure female patients complaining of urinary incontinence. In the case of sportswomen, as the pelvic floor is weaker, the results are poor, because the intra-abdominal pressure is too high for the pelvic floor support.

Marsden: Have obstetricians and gynaecologists recognized that women actively engaged in sports have a greater risk of developing urinary incontinence after parturition and obstetric procedures?

Stanton: That's not known, to the best of my knowledge.

Staskin: Perhaps the problem is not as complex as we are supposing. The proper urodynamic studies needed to identify the aetiology of urinary loss during these types of strenuous physical activity may be more practically performed as the technology for ambulatory urodynamic studies becomes available.

The aetiology of the urinary loss may be uninhibited bladder contractions or inadequate sphincter resistance during excessive activity. If it is uninhibited contractions, anticholinergic therapy would not be possible because of the side-effects of dry mouth and decreased perspiration.

The pathophysiological mechanism of urinary loss where decreased sphincter resistance is found is more interesting, because sphincter resistance is multifactorial. At rest there is a positive closure pressure. During exercise, if the intra-abdominal pressure transmission is slightly greater to the bladder than to the continence mechanism and voluntary sphincter closure pressure, the latter may give way during exercise.

Voluntary sphincter relaxation (urethral instability) is easy to explain, but unequal pressure transmission is more difficult to conceptualize. Where the pressure transmission is unequal, at higher pressures the net effect to bladder and bladder outlet is greater and may overcome other compensatory mechanisms which are sufficient at lower levels of activity to produce continence. It may be 'normal' for females to lose a small amount of urine with unusually high increases in intra-abdominal pressure.

Stanton: I think that is absolutely right. I don't think it's urethral instability; rather, as you say, the level of intra-abdominal pressure is much higher than normal, and may exceed the normal (although not very high) urethral pressure. Certainly, the two anecdotal examples that I recall were both women who had stable bladders. One said that every time she played squash (and it only happened when she played squash) she was incontinent on using a powerful forehand stroke. The other woman said that every time she screamed at her husband, she leaked!

Index of contributors

Non-participating co-authors are indicated by asterisks. Entries in bold type indicate papers; other entries refer to discussion contributions.

Indexes compiled by John Rivers

323

Subject index

325